Clinical Manual
for the
Treatment of Autism

Clinical Manual for the Treatment of Autism

Edited by

Eric Hollander, M.D.
Esther and Joseph Klingenstein Professor and
Chair, Department of Psychiatry;
Director, Seaver and New York Autism Center of Excellence
Mount Sinai School of Medicine
New York, New York

Evdokia Anagnostou, M.D.
Child Neurologist and Assistant Professor,
Department of Psychiatry;
Clinical Director, Seaver and New York Autism Center of Excellence
Mount Sinai School of Medicine
New York, New York

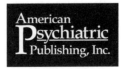

American
Psychiatric
Publishing, Inc.

Washington, DC
London, England

If you would like to buy between 25 and 99 copies of this or any other APPI title, you are eligible for a 20% discount; please contact APPI Customer Service at appi@psych.org or 800-368-5777. If you wish to buy 100 or more copies of the same title, please e-mail us at bulksales@psych.org for a price quote.

Manufactured in Canada on acid-free paper
11   10   09   08   07   5   4   3   2   1
First Edition

Typeset in Adobe's Formata and AGaramond.

American Psychiatric Publishing, Inc.
1000 Wilson Boulevard, Arlington, VA 22209-3901
www.appi.org

Library of Congress Cataloging-in-Publication Data
Clinical manual for the treatment of autism / edited by Eric Hollander, Evdokia Anagnostou. — 1st ed.
       p. ; cm.
    Includes bibliographical references and index.
    ISBN 978-1-58562-222-1 (pbk. : alk. paper)
    1. Autism in children—Treatment. 2. Autism—Treatment. I. Hollander, Eric, 1957–
II. Anagnostou, Evdokia, 1971– [DNLM: 1. Autistic Disorder—drug therapy.
2. Autistic Disorder—psychology. WM 203.5 C64 2008]
    RJ506.A9C546 2008
    618.92′85882—dc22

                                                                                    2007018818

British Library Cataloguing in Publication Data
A CIP record is available from the British Library.

Contents

1 **Clinical Diagnosis of Autism. 1**
   Fred R. Volkmar, M.D., and
   Marc Woodbury-Smith, M.D., Ph.D.

2 **Evaluation and Testing for Autism. 27**
   Audrey Thurm, Ph.D., Latha Soorya, Ph.D., and
   Ann Wagner, Ph.D.

List of Tables and Figures

Contributors

Evdokia Anagnostou, M.D.
Child Neurologist and Assistant Professor, Department of Psychiatry; Clinical Director, Seaver and New York Autism Center of Excellence, Mount Sinai School of Medicine, New York, New York

Michael G. Chez, M.D.
Director, Pediatric Neurology, Sutter Neuroscience Institute, Sacramento, California

Geoffrey Collins, B.A.
Department of Psychiatry, Mount Sinai School of Medicine, New York, New York

Carolyn Coughlin
Rosalind Franklin University/The Chicago Medical School, North Chicago, Illinois

Craig A. Erickson, M.D.
Resident, Department of Psychiatry, Indiana University School of Medicine, Indianapolis, Indiana

Aaron Jason Fisher, B.A.
Doctoral Candidate, Penn State University, State College, Pennsylvania

Stanley I. Greenspan, M.D.
Clinical Professor, George Washington University Medical School, Washington, D.C.; Chair, Interdisciplinary Council on Developmental and Learning Disorders, Silver Spring, Maryland

Eric Hollander, M.D.
Esther and Joseph Klingenstein Professor and Chair of Psychiatry; Director, Seaver and New York Autism Center of Excellence, Mount Sinai School of Medicine, New York, New York

Connie Kasari, Ph.D.
Professor, Department of Education, University of California, Los Angeles, California

Matthew Kominsky
Rosalind Franklin University/The Chicago Medical School, North Chicago, Illinois

Lee Marcus, Ph.D.
Clinical Director and Professor, Chapel Hill TEACCH Center, Department of Psychiatry, University of North Carolina at Chapel Hill

Christopher J. McDougle, M.D.
Albert E. Sterne Professor and Chairman, Department of Psychiatry, Indiana University School of Medicine, Indianapolis, Indiana

Cynthia A. Molloy, M.D., M.S.
Assistant Professor, Center for Epidemiology and Biostatistics, Cincinnati Children's Hospital Medical Center; Department of Pediatrics, University of Cincinnati College of Medicine, Cincinnati, Ohio

Dennis Mozingo, Ph.D.
Assistant Professor, Department of Pediatrics, University of Rochester Medical Center, Rochester, New York

Daniel W. Mruzek, Ph.D.
Assistant Professor, Department of Pediatrics, University of Rochester Medical Center, Rochester, New York

Yann Poncin, M.D.
Assistant Professor of Child Psychiatry, Yale University Child Study Center, New Haven, Connecticut

David J. Posey, M.D.
Associate Professor of Psychiatry, Indiana University School of Medicine and Chief of the Christian Sarkine Autism Treatment Center, James Whitcomb Riley Hospital for Children, Indianapolis, Indiana

Erin Rotheram-Fuller, Ph.D.
Assistant Research Psychologist, Department of Family Medicine, David Geffen School of Medicine at UCLA, Los Angeles, California

Lawrence Scahill, M.S.N., Ph.D.
Professor of Nursing and Child Psychiatry, Yale University Child Study Center and School of Nursing, New Haven, Connecticut

Melissa L. Schapiro, B.A.S.
Department of Psychiatry, Seaver and New York Autism Center of Excellence, The Mount Sinai School of Medicine, New York, New York

Eric Schopler, Ph.D.
Professor Emeritus, TEACCH Division, Department of Psychiatry, University of North Carolina at Chapel Hill

Tristram Smith, Ph.D.
Assistant Professor, Department of Pediatrics, University of Rochester Medical Center, Rochester, New York

Latha Soorya, Ph.D.
Assistant Professor, Mount Sinai School of Medicine, New York, New York

Kimberly A. Stigler, M.D.
Assistant Professor of Psychiatry and Daniel X. Freedman Psychiatric Research Fellow, Indiana University School of Medicine, Indianapolis, Indiana

Audrey Thurm, Ph.D.
Staff Scientist, Pediatric and Developmental Neuropsychiatry Branch, National Institute of Mental Health, Bethesda, Maryland

Fred R. Volkmar, M.D.
Irving B. Harris Professor and Director, Yale Child Study Center, Departments of Child Psychiatry, Pediatrics, and Psychology, Yale University School of Medicine, New Haven, Connecticut

Ann Wagner, Ph.D.
Chief, Neurodevelopmental Disorders Branch, Division of Pediatric Translational Research and Treatment Development, National Institute of Mental Health, Bethesda, Maryland

Stacey Wasserman, M.D.
Research Fellow, Department of Psychiatry, Seaver and New York Autism Center of Excellence, The Mount Sinai School of Medicine, New York, New York

Serena Wieder, Ph.D.
Associate Chair, Interdisciplinary Council on Developmental and Learning Disorders, Silver Spring, Maryland

Marc Woodbury-Smith, M.D., Ph.D.
Consultant Psychiatrist, Section of Developmental Psychiatry, Cambridge University, Cambridge, United Kingdom

Jennifer R. Zarcone, Ph.D.
Associate Professor, Department of Pediatrics, University of Rochester Medical Center, Rochester, New York

Michelle Zimmer, M.D.
Assistant Professor of Clinical Pediatrics, Cincinnati Children's Hospital Medical Center, The Kelly O'Leary Center for Autism Spectrum Disorders, Division of Developmental Disabilities, Cincinnati, Ohio

Disclosure of Competing Interests

The following authors have competing interests to declare:

Evdokia Anagnostou, M.D.—Receives consultation fees from IntegraGen.

Craig A. Erickson, M.D.—*Grant support:* Bristol-Myers Squibb.

Eric Hollander, M.D.—*Grant support:* Abbott, Bristol-Myers Squibb, National Institute of Mental Health, National Institute of Neurological Disorders and Stroke, CAN, National Institute on Drug Abuse; *Consultant:* Neuropharm, Nastech, Forest; *Intellectual property:* oxytocin, memantine.

Christopher J. McDougle, M.D.—*Grant support:* Janssen, Bristol-Myers Squibb; *Consultant:* Janssen, Eli Lilly, Forest Research Institute, Bristol-Myers Squibb; *Speaker's bureau:* Janssen, Bristol-Myers Squibb.

David J. Posey, M.D.—*Grant support:* Eli Lilly, Forest, Janssen; *Stock:* Shire; *Speaker honoraria:* Pfizer, Janssen; *Consultant:* Eli Lilly, Forest.

Lawrence Scahill, M.S.N., Ph.D.—*Consultant:* Janssen, Bristol-Myers Squibb, Supernus. Provided training to Janssen and Bristol-Myers Squibb.

Kimberly A. Stigler, M.D.—Receives support from Bristol-Myers Squibb, Janssen and Eli Lilly (Pilot Research Award).

The following authors have no competing interests to report:

Michael G. Chez, M.D.
Geoffrey Collins, B.A.
Carolyn Coughlan
Aaron Jason Fisher
Stanley I. Greenspan, M.D.
Connie Kasari, Ph.D.
Matthew Kominsky
Lee Marcus, Ph.D.
Cynthia A. Molloy, M.D., M.S.
Dennis Mozingo, Ph.D.
Daniel W. Mruzek, Ph.D.
Yann Poncin, M.D.
Erin Rotheram-Fuller, Ph.D.

Melissa L. Schapiro, B.A.S.
Tristram Smith, Ph.D.
Latha Soorya, Ph.D.
Audrey Thurm, Ph.D.
Fred R. Volkmar, M.D.
Ann Wagner, Ph.D.
Stacey Wasserman, M.D.
Serena Wieder, Ph.D.
Marc Woodbury-Smith, M.D., Ph.D.
Jennifer R. Zarcone, Ph.D.
Michelle Zimmer, M.D.

Foreword

Autism has exploded into public awareness in recent years amid frequent reports in the popular media of a dramatic rise in the number of patients with autism seeking treatment services. In fact, careful systematic reviews of the available data suggest that the true incidence of autism spectrum disorders may be in the range of 30–60 per 10,000 as opposed to the original estimate of 4 per 10,000. The question is whether this increase is a result of an ascertainment bias, a broadening of the boundaries of the autism spectrum, or diagnostic substitution. Systematic literature review suggests that to a large extent this is a result of all of the above. However, a true rise in the incidence of autism spectrum disorders cannot be ruled out. It is possible that there are as yet undetermined environmental factors that may have an epigenetic effect in turning on various genes of minor effect; this, in turn, may have an interactive effect in coding for the various core and associated symptom domains that make up this complex and heterogeneous syndrome of autism.

Whatever the cause for this increase in the demand for services of people with autism of all ages and at all levels of ability and severity, it is clear that there is a real need for clear, up-to-date, and evidence-based treatments. These treatments may address the target symptoms that cause distress and interfere with functioning, or alternatively may aim to improve the developmental trajectory of the illness. It is also clear that no one treatment fits all such individuals, because patients with autism greatly vary in intelligence, language abilities, age at first presentation, disruptive behaviors, and presence of comorbid neurological disorders such as epilepsy, and comorbid psychiatric disorders such as obsessive-compulsive disorder, bipolar disorder, and attention-deficit/hyperactivity disorder.

There have been substantial efforts in recent years to study a range of treatments and services in a systematic, rigorous fashion in order to determine whether such approaches are efficacious and safe and to clarify which target symptoms and which individuals are likely to benefit. It is clear that early intervention with a broad range of services is critical to improving outcome. These services may include psychosocial approaches such as behavioral and social skills interventions; specialized educational programs; occupational, speech and language, and physical therapies; and, in some cases, medications to address specific target symptoms that cause distress and interfere with functioning.

In the following chapters, the contributors describe, in a clear and straightforward fashion, how to diagnose autism and which testing and evaluation instruments to use with which patients. The authors highlight the appropriate role of various medications for specific target symptoms and individuals, including selective serotonin reuptake inhibitors and antidepressants; anticonvulsants and mood stabilizers; antipsychotics; cholinesterase inhibitors; and stimulants and nonstimulants for attention and hyperactivity. Psychosocial treatments—including applied behavior analysis; developmental individual-difference, relationship-based (DIR)/floortime treatment; and peer relationship interventions—are then discussed. Educational approaches are described, as are complementary and alternative treatments. Of course, we were not able to discuss all available treatments in the context of this book. We focused on well-accepted psychoeducational models that have some evidence for their use. As such, new models that have no empirical data for their use or are not widely available, as well as focused treatment approaches such as occupational, physical, and speech and language therapy, have not been included in this book. Finally, promising new avenues and future treatment directions are explored.

The contributors to this book are internationally known experts who have actually developed these treatments, or who have conducted pivotal studies to determine the safety and efficacy of such treatments. In addition, they are also experienced clinicians who actually treat patients with autism and are widely recognized for their clinical skills.

We believe that this book will be an essential resource for a broad range of clinicians and investigators, including pediatricians; psychiatrists; neurologists; psychologists; behavioral, speech, and occupational therapists; educators; and even highly informed family members who are actively involved in treatment planning. The field has made tremendous gains over the past decade in its understanding of the causes of autism, and our hope is that this state-of-the-art compendium of treatments for autism will help advance the care that people with autism receive.

Acknowledgments

We acknowledge the contributions of Rachel Rafferty, Stephanie Hemmert, and Dr. Ilana Slaff at the Seaver and New York Autism Center of Excellence, Department of Psychiatry, Mount Sinai School of Medicine, in the preparation of this manuscript.

Eric Hollander, M.D.
Evdokia Anagnostou, M.D.

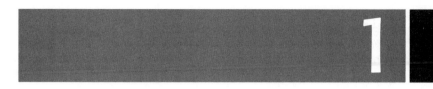

Clinical Diagnosis of Autism

Fred R. Volkmar, M.D.

Marc Woodbury-Smith, M.D., Ph.D.

Historical Background

Development of Diagnostic Concepts

Although our current conceptualization of autism and Asperger's disorder is based on the clinical accounts of Kanner (1943) and Asperger (1944), respectively, children presenting in a similar way were probably described much earlier as "wild" or "feral" (Wing 1997a). Similarly, other diagnostic concepts have arisen for children with social interaction impairments whose difficulties shade off into either personality disorder or psychosis. For example, Wolff (2000)

The support of National Institute of Child Health and Human Development Program Project Grants 1PO1HD35482 and 5-P01-HD03008 and of STAART (Studies to Advance Autism Research and Treatment) Autism Center Grant U54 MH66494, as well as the Simons Foundation, is gratefully acknowledged.

coined the term *schizoid disorder of childhood* to describe a group of children who were socially loners and exhibited ritualistic and repetitive patterns of behavior. Nonetheless, it was Kanner's description of 11 socially impaired boys and Asperger's study of 4 boys with difficulty relating to their peers that have been the most influential.

Kanner (1943) described 11 children with "autistic disturbances of affective contact," astutely observing that this group shared a common impairment relating to others, particular communicative abnormalities, and a pattern of unusual behaviors. He noted that the children did not display the usual motivation toward social and affective interaction with others and borrowed the term *autism* from Bleuler (1911/1951) to suggest that such children live in their own world. In addition, he noted that communication was marked by either its complete absence (with two of the series being mute) or its qualitatively odd nature (e.g., literalness, echolalic quality, or lack of use of the first person). Regarding odd behaviors, he noted that the children were sensitive to certain environmental stimuli such as particular sounds and resisted change in their routine and in their environment. This triad of impairments has endured in both clinical descriptions and subsequent nosology. Kanner also suggested that autism was an inborn, constitutional disorder in which children were born lacking the typical motivation for social interaction and affective contact.

In contrast, however, some of the other observations Kanner noted have since been shown to be incorrect. For example, he suggested that parents of such children are more likely to be middle class and that relationship problems exist between the parents and their children. Epidemiological research has failed to observe any class bias (Fombonne 2005), and studies of attachment have suggested that children with autism do form attachment to their parents (Sigman et al. 1995). Importantly, there is also no evidence for abnormal parenting (Wing 1997a). Kanner also suggested that there was no association with mental retardation, but it is now recognized that profiles on assessments of intellectual functioning are remarkable in their scatter, with relative strengths offset by areas of vulnerability (Klin et al. 2005c) and with overall scores often in the intellectually impaired range (Fombonne 2005). Overall, however, the outcome gradually appears to be improving with earlier detection and intervention (Howlin 2005).

One year after Kanner's publication, Asperger (1944), unaware of Kanner's paper, described four boys ages 6–11 years who had difficulty relating to others despite adequate cognitive and verbal skills. Recognizing the core difficulties with social interaction, and conceptualizing the disorder as fundamentally one of personality, Asperger coined the term *autistic psychopathy,* with *psychopathy* better translating as *personality disorder* rather than its more contemporary usage. He also described a number of other features: First, despite the apparently normal verbal skills, conversations were marked by idiosyncrasies, such as circumlocution, overinclusive and long-winded accounts, and one-sidedness. Moreover, a marked impairment in the use of nonverbal communicative strategies such as eye contact and gesture were noted. Asperger also remarked on the subjects' egocentric preoccupations with interests that were unusual in either focus or intensity. Other observations included their motor clumsiness and conduct problems.

While clearly there are similarities in the cases described by Asperger and Kanner, there are also differences in the original descriptions of these conditions. For example, Asperger believed the condition did not manifest until later in childhood, and a normal pattern of early development has been retained in current nosology. He also noted that all the initial cases occurred exclusively in boys. The two groups of children were also different in terms of their verbal and cognitive skills, with Asperger's having apparently fluent verbal skills, whereas Kanner's were mute or exhibited severe language difficulties. As will become apparent later in this chapter, the relationship between Asperger's disorder and autism has been the focus of much research (see Klin et al. 2005a for a discussion), which has been plagued by tautological and changing definitions. Currently, and based on clinical similarities, the two disorders, along with pervasive developmental disorder not otherwise specified (PDDNOS), are conceptualized as forming a spectrum, termed *autism spectrum disorders* (ASDs). Strikingly, however, there is evidence both in favor of and refuting such a conceptualization.

Besides autism and Asperger's disorder, a number of other disorders of social interaction have also been described. In the absence of strong evidence to the contrary, some of these are currently conceptualized as synonymous with, or closely related to, autism and Asperger's disorder, such as schizoid disorder of childhood (Wolff 2000), right-hemisphere learning disability (Weintraub and Mesulam 1983), and nonverbal learning disability (Rourke 1994; Rourke and Tsatsanis 2000), whereas others are almost definitely distinct. Most notable are Rett's disorder (Van Acker et al. 2005) and childhood disintegrative disorder (Volkmar et al. 2005), both included within the pervasive developmental disorders (PDDs) category of DSM-IV-TR (American Psychiatric Association 2000). Rett's disorder was first described in 1966 by Rett, who observed similar hand-wringing movements in two girls and subsequently described 22 subjects with a syndrome consisting of stereotypic hand movements, dementia, autistic traits, and ataxia (Rett 1966). What is perhaps most striking about the presentation is that these developmental insults follow a period of relatively normal development. Although now classified along with autism, Asperger's disorder, and other disorders of social interaction, Rett's disorder in the majority of cases is known to be associated with mutations in a single gene, namely, the gene for methyl-CpG-binding protein 2 (*MeCP2*) (Amir et al. 1999). Childhood disintegrative disorder was first described a century ago by Heller (1908), who described six children between the ages of 3 and 4 years who had severe developmental regression following a period of apparently normal development. This condition appears to be extremely rare and remains poorly understood.

From Clinical Description to Nosology

Clinical descriptions such as those of Kanner and Asperger are useful in bringing to light symptom clusters that may represent clinical syndromes with etiological and treatment implications. However, because these descriptions are generally based on small numbers of cases, their nosological validity is limited initially (i.e., until others can repeat and refine the initial clinical observations). Thus, Kanner's and Asperger's case studies were complemented by further descriptions by the authors themselves and by other clinicians who reported similar symptom clusters. Given the early confusion about the relationship of these conditions to other conditions, particularly schizophrenia, it was not until much later that these descriptions were formally recognized within the diagnostic nomenclature of the ICD and DSM (Volkmar and Klin 2005). Their inclusion represented an important step, because formally classifying disorders in this way and setting out diagnostic criteria ensures that researchers who are interested in etiology and in underlying neurobiology are indeed investigating the same group of people. Moreover, "official recognition" means that authorities may identify those with the diagnosis as being entitled to special provisions or services, and educators will be able to offer special education services.

Classifying disorders for which the etiology is by and large unknown, as is the case for autism, relies on the grouping together of specific behaviors that "capture" the disorder and that differentiate it from disorders with similar features. Such an approach must provide sufficient detail to allow diagnoses to be made consistently and reliably by clinicians and researchers alike. This approach originates prima facie from observation rather then solid empirical data, with core defining criteria being modified subsequently in light of emerging evidence for the reliability and validity of the criteria being used. Notably, this method of phenomenological classification is atheoretical (i.e., based not on what is known of pathogenesis but, rather, on observable behaviors). From the outset this approach presents particular difficulties with regard to autistic disorder, because the disorder lacks pathognomonic behaviors or other defining characteristics, and there is a wide variation in expression over both age and level of development.

Importantly, it must be borne in mind that diagnostic systems lose value if they are overly broad or overly narrow. This issue has been particularly apparent during the development of DSM criteria. In DSM-III-R (American Psychiatric Association 1987), the work group adopted purposefully broad criteria and made some significant changes—most strikingly the removal of the age at onset criteria that had characterized previous nosological and clinical definitions (Volkmar et al. 1992). However, although this approach led to increased sensitivity, it also had the effect of reducing the specificity of the diagnosis, with a high rate of false positives, especially among individuals with retardation, in whom the rate of false positives reached 60% (Volkmar and Klin 2005).

Similarly, certain factors need to be considered in the choice of which diagnostic behaviors will be included in the nosological definition. For example, social disability has always been a central defining feature of ASDs, and consequently all diagnostic systems have added extra weight to this category, with both ICD-10 (World Health Organization 1992) and DSM-IV-TR requiring the presence of two items from this category. This emphasis is based on work suggesting that the social difficulties (the "autism," as it were) carry much of the weight diagnostically (Siegel et al. 1989; Volkmar et al. 1994). In contrast, motor mannerisms do not clearly separate people with autism from those with intellectual disability (mental retardation) who do not have autism.

Most notably, over the years consensus has emerged that the social impairment is, consistent with Kanner's original description of the syndrome of early infantile autism, the sine qua non of ASDs. Without some form of social impairment, therefore, a positive diagnosis would be doubtful. Nonetheless, the research literature has described as many as 20% of children "growing out" of autism as they reach adulthood (Seltzer et al. 2003), and other adults with autism, particularly the intellectually more able ones, can develop strategies to mask their impairment. Such individuals will not necessarily be picked up at assessment if the diagnostician is not alert to such issues. Importantly, although a social impairment is crucial, it is not pathognomonic of autism, because it is found in a number of other developmental disorders, such as schizoid personality disorder, schizotypal personality disorder, and schizophrenia. Thus, the current DSM-IV-TR and ICD-10 criteria emphasize the presence of social features more than others in formal diagnostic criteria. These two systems also require some significant difficulties in the areas of communication/play and in the domain of restricted interests and repetitive behaviors. The data from the DSM-IV (American Psychiatric Association 1994) field trial (Volkmar et al. 1994), discussed later in this chapter, show that relative to the diagnosis of experienced clinicians (which remains the gold standard), these guidelines yield a relatively good balance of sensitivity and specificity across the range of chronological age and developmental level. These criteria have proved reasonably robust and useful in various contexts and countries (Volkmar and Klin 2005). There are also data that show that the use of these criteria by less experienced clinicians significantly increases diagnostic reliability (Klin et al. 2000).

In contrast to the social impairments, other behaviors that are perhaps more pathognomonic, such as an attachment to objects, are not seen universally or are, in the case of unusual attachments, more frequent in certain age groups. Even when they are not essential diagnostic features, aspects of autism symptomatology may be important foci for intervention (e.g., behavioral strategies and/or medication). Although the restricted interests and behaviors are seen almost universally among individuals with autism and may be important targets of treatment, they are as a single diagnostic feature less diagnostically specific than the social deficits. Repetitive mannerisms, albeit usually in rather mild forms, can be seen among typically developing children up to age 5 years.

Other core autism impairments are also seen among typically developing children. Most notable is echolalia, which occurs when children are first learning to talk. However, echolalia among children with autism is noted for its nonfunctionality and its failure to develop into meaningful communicative language. Moreover, it can persist into later childhood, adolescence, and adulthood.

Autism as a diagnosis first appeared in DSM-III (American Psychiatric Association 1980). Before 1980, the category "childhood schizophrenia" broadly encompassed the whole range of psychiatric experiences of childhood. However, this was deemed problematic as it became clear that disorders such as autism differed significantly from schizophrenia, with its essential features being identified as deviant social development, deviant communicative development, and a group of behaviors characterized by resistance to change, with onset in the first years of life (Rutter 1978). Infantile autism was subsequently included for the first time in DSM-III, which recognized the core impairments of social interaction and communication, and the restricted and repetitive patterns of behavior, and explicitly differentiated the disorder from schizophrenia by making the two mutually exclusive. Moreover, autism was placed in the PDD category, which included, in addition to infantile autism, childhood-onset pervasive developmental disorder (COPDD), residual autism, and atypical PDD. The term *pervasive developmental disorders* was introduced to convey that individuals with disorders in this category were impaired in multiple domains of development. COPDD was included for individuals with no early developmental impairments, and residual autism was included for individuals who at some point had met the criteria for infantile autism but who no longer did. Finally, atypical PDD was used for individuals who did not meet the full set of criteria for infantile autism or another explicit PDD. The syndromes described by Rett and Heller were not included within this category.

Although inclusion of autism in DSM allowed clinicians an objective set of criteria by which to judge autism as an entity distinct from other childhood psychiatric disorders, there were some problems. First, the criteria applied to younger children and did not take into consideration the impact of age on modifying the presentation. Second, the criteria more appropriately applied to more intellectually and functionally impaired individuals. Third, diagnoses of autism and schizophrenia were represented as orthogonal constructs, precluding the possibility of comorbidity and reflecting the hierarchical and parsimonious approach of this version of DSM.

Recognizing some of the limitations of DSM-III, the work group for DSM-III-R modified the diagnostic criteria in several ways. Most notably, the criteria were broadened to allow for the changes that result from age, level of functioning, and intellectual ability. The work group also excluded the onset criterion and the schizophrenia exclusion criterion and renamed the diagnostic subthreshold category pervasive developmental disorder not otherwise specified (PPDNOS). The COPDD category was excluded. Again, the syndromes of Rett and Heller were not included in the PDDs category. There were several problems with the DSM-III-R criteria. Most strikingly, exclusion of the age at onset criterion was inconsistent with Kanner's report and with those of other clinicians (e.g., Rutter 1978). The criteria were also complex and detailed, making them difficult to use in everyday clinical practice, and the drastic changes from the DSM-III, such as the exclusion of the COPDD category, complicated research. Nonetheless, the applicability of diagnostic criteria across age and developmental level categories was a major advance (Volkmar et al. 1992).

The DSM-IV Field Trial

In 1994, a DSM-IV field trial was conducted involving nearly 1,000 patients seen by 125 raters in 21 international sites (Volkmar et al. 1994). Diagnoses for all patients were clinician assigned and made independently of the various diagnostic systems being evaluated. These diagnoses served as a first approximation of a diagnostic gold standard. Patients were included only if they exhibited difficulties that would reasonably include autism in the differential diagnosis. The field trial provided data to allow 1) the pattern of agreement among several diagnostic systems, including DSM-III, DSM-III-R, and ICD-10, in terms of their sensitivity and specificity, and positive and negative predictive values, and 2) aspects of the reliability of criteria and of diagnoses made by the various diagnostic systems. The results indicated that DSM-III had a good balance of sensitivity and specificity but, as discussed previously, was limited by not being applicable beyond the developmental period. In contrast, DSM-III-R, although having a high sensitivity, had a low specificity. This finding was expected in light of DSM-III-R's broad criteria and the lack of an age at onset criterion. The ICD-10 performed the best overall, and overall agreement between clinicians was greatest for this system. Ultimately, given the superior performance of the ICD-10 criteria, the development of the DSM-IV criteria was based on these criteria with certain modifications. Moreover, given the problems associated with having two divergent sets of diagnostic criteria, convergence between DSM-IV and ICD-10 was considered desirable (see Table 1–1).

Although the focus of the field trial was autism, it also commented on the diagnosis of Asperger's disorder. Only 48 cases of Asperger's disorder were included. Compared with their intellectually able counterparts with autism, those who had received a clinical diagnosis of Asperger's disorder were 1) less likely to exhibit language and communication deviance, 2) more likely to have motor delays, and 3) more likely to have abnormal preoccupations. Although the validity of Asperger's disorder vis-à-vis high-functioning autism was not clear, it was deemed appropriate to include this diagnostic category for research purposes, and, aware that such individuals experience difficulties as a result of their impairments, to facilitate these subjects' access to educational and other services (see Table 1–2).

In addition to autism and Asperger's disorder, DSM-IV included Rett's disorder and childhood disintegrative disorder. Moreover, the residual category PDDNOS was retained for subthreshold cases (see Table 1–3).

Alternative Approaches to Classification

The Zero to Three/National Center for Clinical Infant Programs (NCCIP) (National Center for Clinical Infant Programs 1994) has developed an alternative diagnostic taxonomy for emotional, behavioral, attachment, and developmental disorders of childhood, which, as in DSM-IV, is multiaxial but, in contrast, places less emphasis on diagnostic labels in an attempt to avoid the problem of multiple diagnostic labels in any one individual. This diagnostic system addresses the manifestation of such disorders observed in infants and very young children up to age 4 years. It is not intended to replace existing taxonomies as described in the nosology of ICD-10 and DSM-IV-TR, but to supplement and, by providing alternative conceptualizations, encourage an evolving heuristic of childhood mental disorders.

This system is designed around five axes: Axis I reflects the most prominent features of the disorder, and diagnostic labels are replaced by seven diagnostic categories; Axis II describes relationship problems between the infant and his or her primary caregiver; Axis III includes medical conditions not nec-

Table 1–1.   DSM-IV diagnostic criteria for autistic disorder

A.   A total of six (or more) items from (1), (2), and (3), with at least two from (1), and one each from (2) and (3):

(1)   qualitative impairment in social interaction, as manifested by at least two of the following:

(a)   marked impairment in the use of multiple nonverbal behaviors such as eye-to-eye gaze, facial expression, body postures, and gestures to regulate social interaction

(b)   failure to develop peer relationships appropriate to developmental level

(c)   a lack of spontaneous seeking to share enjoyment, interests, or achievements with other people (e.g., by a lack of showing, bringing, or pointing out objects of interest)

(d)   lack of social or emotional reciprocity

(2)   qualitative impairments in communication as manifested by at least one of the following:

(a)   delay in, or total lack of, the development of spoken language (not accompanied by an attempt to compensate through alternative modes of communication such as gesture or mime)

(b)   in individuals with adequate speech, marked impairment in the ability to initiate or sustain a conversation with others

(c)   stereotyped and repetitive use of language or idiosyncratic language

(d)   lack of varied, spontaneous make-believe play or social imitative play appropriate to developmental level

(3)   restricted repetitive and stereotyped patterns of behavior, interests, and activities, as manifested by at least one of the following:

(a)   encompassing preoccupation with one or more stereotyped and restricted patterns of interest that is abnormal either in intensity or focus

(b)   apparently inflexible adherence to specific, nonfunctional routines or rituals

(c)   stereotyped and repetitive motor mannerisms (e.g., hand or finger flapping or twisting, or complex whole-body movements)

(d)   persistent preoccupation with parts of objects

B.   Delays or abnormal functioning in at least one of the following areas, with onset prior to age 3 years: (1) social interaction, (2) language as used in social communication, or (3) symbolic or imaginative play.

C.   The disturbance is not better accounted for by Rett's disorder or childhood disintegrative disorder.

Source.   Reprinted with permission from American Psychiatric Association: *Diagnostic and Statistical Manual of Mental Disorders,* 4th Edition, Text Revision. Washington, DC, American Psychiatric Association, 2000. Copyright 2000, American Psychiatric Association. Used with permission.

Table 1–2.   DSM-IV diagnostic criteria for Asperger's disorder

A.   Qualitative impairment in social interaction, as manifested by at least two of the following:

   (1)   marked impairment in the use of multiple nonverbal behaviors such as eye-to-eye gaze, facial expression, body postures, and gestures to regulate social interaction

   (2)   failure to develop peer relationships appropriate to developmental level

   (3)   a lack of spontaneous seeking to share enjoyment, interests, or achievements with other people (e.g., by a lack of showing, bringing, or pointing out objects of interest to other people)

   (4)   lack of social or emotional reciprocity

B.   Restricted repetitive and stereotyped patterns of behavior, interests, and activities, as manifested by at least one of the following:

   (1)   encompassing preoccupation with one or more stereotyped and restricted patterns of interest that is abnormal either in intensity or focus

   (2)   apparently inflexible adherence to specific, nonfunctional routines or rituals

   (3)   stereotyped and repetitive motor mannerisms (e.g., hand or finger flapping or twisting, or complex whole-body movements)

   (4)   persistent preoccupation with parts of objects

C.   The disturbance causes clinically significant impairment in social, occupational, or other important areas of functioning.

D.   There is no clinically significant general delay in language (e.g., single words used by age 2 years, communicative phrases used by age 3 years).

E.   There is no clinically significant delay in cognitive development or in the development of age-appropriate self-help skills, adaptive behavior (other than in social interaction), and curiosity about the environment in childhood.

F.   Criteria are not met for another specific pervasive developmental disorder or schizophrenia.

Source.   Reprinted with permission from American Psychiatric Association: *Diagnostic and Statistical Manual of Mental Disorders,* 4th Edition, Text Revision. Washington, DC, American Psychiatric Association, 2000. Copyright 2000, American Psychiatric Association. Used with permission.

essarily related to the Axis I presentation and disorders included in other diagnostic systems; Axis IV includes psychosocial stressors; and Axis V includes the infant's functional and emotional developmental level according to specified criteria.

In the absence of strong empirical or scientific support for contemporary conceptualizations of childhood emotional and behavioral disorders, these

Table 1–3.   DSM-IV diagnostic criteria for pervasive developmental disorder not otherwise specified (including atypical autism)

This category should be used when there is a severe and pervasive impairment in the development of reciprocal social interaction associated with impairment in either verbal or nonverbal communication skills or with the presence of stereotyped behavior, interests, and activities, but the criteria are not met for a specific pervasive developmental disorder, schizophrenia, schizotypal personality disorder, or avoidant personality disorder. For example, this category includes "atypical autism"—presentations that do not meet the criteria for autistic disorder because of late age at onset, atypical symptomatology, or subthreshold symptomatology, or all of these.

Source.   Reprinted with permission from American Psychiatric Association: *Diagnostic and Statistical Manual of Mental Disorders,* 4th Edition, Text Revision. Washington, DC, American Psychiatric Association, 2000. Copyright 2000, American Psychiatric Association. Used with permission.

criteria are based on expert consensus and are in this respect similar to other nosological systems. In contrast, however, there are two major differences in the approach employed. First, the NCCIP system utilizes, at least in the case of autism, a very different set of diagnostic conceptualizations without a firm empirical basis. Second, unlike DSM-IV-TR and ICD-10, this system also focuses on the relevance of the interaction between an infant and his or her caregiver.

Although attractive in its novel approach, the NNCCIP system has a number of difficulties. First, stress is known to be an important etiological factor that precedes many emotional and behavioral disorders or, at least, precedes their onset or acute manifestation. Therefore, giving primacy to it may be an inappropriate simplification and may result in failure to identify important interindividual pathological differences. Second, dismissing preexisting syndromal constructs fails to recognize that, although they are born from heuristic and descriptive methods, their continuing usage over the years derives in part from the supporting empirical and scientific evidence, in particular the etiological significance of conceptualizing and classifying them in this way. Third, treatments have been designed and their usefulness empirically established around existing taxonomies; it would therefore be difficult to argue the case for dismissing any system unless the alternative had equal or better etiological and treatment implications.

Areas of Diagnostic Controversy

Asperger's Disorder

Asperger's disorder has perhaps been associated with the most controversy. People have used Asperger's disorder as a diagnostic concept in very different ways, such as a mild form of autism (Gillberg and Gillberg 1989), as a synonym for PDDNOS (Szatmari et al. 1989), or as a way to describe higher functioning people with autism (those with so-called high-functioning autism) (Wing 1997b). Moreover, several different diagnostic algorithms have also been suggested (Klin et al. 2005b). The diversity of approaches reflects confusion over the use of the term and inconsistency in its use.

Despite Asperger originally stating that he believed "autistic psychopathy" was different from autism, its definition in both DSM-IV-TR and ICD-10 closely aligns the two diagnoses by using almost identical criteria. Asperger's disorder differs from autism only in its apparent later onset, with no abnormalities being present during the first few years of life (the onset rule); its association with a normal level of intellectual functioning; and its absence of the communicative impairments of autism. Moreover, the precedence rule dictates that a diagnosis of autism takes precedence if a person meets those criteria. Much research has focused on the relationship between autism and Asperger's disorder, but the results have been conflicting. The main problem has been one of tautology: as the two syndromes are defined by almost the same set of criteria, there is no reason to expect that any external validity for differentiating between them will be demonstrated.

One other problem has been that because of the onset and precedence rules, some researchers have argued that assigning a diagnosis of Asperger's disorder is almost impossible. Subjects with Asperger's disorder almost certainly have a communication impairment, and they are likely to have been developmentally impaired from a young age. Indeed, Asperger highlighted a number of communicative impairments as core features of the disorder, pragmatic in nature, and also later noted that early abnormalities appear to be common.

DSM and the ICD have overlooked a number of core factors described by Asperger. These include pragmatic language impairments, motor clumsiness, and sensory preoccupations. Indeed, when these factors are included in the diagnosis, some evidence for differentiation from autism is demonstrated (Klin et al. 2005b). DSM-IV-TR has taken this into consideration, but, sadly, these recommendations have not as yet been incorporated into the diagnostic criteria. These limitations notwithstanding, including Asperger's disorder is beneficial in terms of service and educational provision, a growing body of research activity, and a better informed debate about the best approaches to diagnosis of more verbal and able individuals with severe social impairments (Klin et al. 2005a).

Subtypes of Autism

Although the relationship between autism and Asperger's disorder has been the focus of research, another area of nosological consideration has been whether autism is clinically and etiologically heterogeneous and can be broken down into distinct subgroups. Several previous studies have used factor and cluster analytic approaches to examine patterns of symptoms in people with autism. Spiker et al. (2002) examined 171 autism multiplex sibships, using cluster analysis to investigate patterns of symptom clustering on the Autism Diagnostic Interview—Revised (ADI-R). They demonstrated a continuous severity gradient with three clusters describing mild, moderate, and severe impairments. This clustering along a severity gradient is consistent with the idea of a spectrum of disorders. Similarly, Constantino et al. (2004) examined autistic symptoms in 226 singletons as measured by the Social Responsiveness Scale. They found symptoms loaded onto a single factor. In contrast, Silverman et al. (2002) examined 212 sibships and looked at the degree to which the core impairments, as measured on the ADI-R, clustered within families. They found that certain aspects of communication and repetitive patterns of behavior all showed significant familiality.

Although the evidence is conflicting, the clinical heterogeneity supports the idea that there may be distinct subtypes of autism. Indeed, Wing and colleagues suggested the existence of at least three clinical subtypes: "active but odd," "passive," and "aloof" (Wing and Gould 1979). The suggestion is that distinct clinical subtypes reflect the differential effect of different etiological factors. Interestingly, recent genetic linkage studies have begun to support this idea, with improved linkage signals at previously identified loci when subgroups are examined, notably a phrase speech delay subgroup and a repetitive patterns of behavior subgroup (see Rutter 2005).

Comorbidity

Autism has been reported to co-occur with various other developmental and behavioral conditions. Some of these associations seem relatively frequent, others much less so. The critical issues are whether such associations occur at levels greater than would be expected by chance alone, and whether the symptoms and behavioral manifestations observed are best viewed as part of autism or as the manifestation of some other condition (Tsai 1996).

Focusing on symptoms rather than disorder makes it clear that individuals with PDDs exhibit many behavioral difficulties, including hyperactivity, attentional problems, obsessive-compulsive–like phenomena, self-injury, stereotypy, tics, and affective symptoms. Although such behaviors can be very appropriate targets for intervention, there is currently some disagreement about whether such symptoms justify an additional diagnosis (Volkmar and Klin 2005). Nonetheless, a number of conclusions may be drawn regarding prevalence of major mental disorders among people with ASDs.

Schizophrenia

The investigation of comorbidity for schizophrenia among clinic samples of both adults and children with ASDs has indicated that the rates are probably low across the spectrum of intellectual ability (Ghaziuddin et al. 1992, 1998; Volkmar and Cohen 1991). It therefore seems reasonable to conclude that the prevalence of schizophrenia is not elevated in this population. Nonetheless, a small number of these individuals may develop schizophrenia, and this can be associated with diagnostic challenges. Moreover, one study (Wing and Shah 2000) has suggested that catatonia may be associated with ASDs, although it is not clear whether this condition is most appropriately conceptualized as psychotic, related to a mood disorder, or a manifestation of the autism phenotype.

Mood Disorders

A number of studies have indicated a risk of mood disorders, particularly depressive disorder, among people with ASDs. Mood disorders can occur during childhood and adolescence as well as adulthood, and across the spectrum of intellectual ability (Ghaziuddin et al. 2002, 2005). In fact, these studies strongly suggest that depression is perhaps the most common psychiatric diagnosis among people with ASDs (see also Klin et al. 2005a, 2005c). Importantly, although mood disorders can be diagnosed at any level of intellectual ability, cognitive ability and the autism phenotype itself will both have a modifying effect on presentation. For example, a depressive disorder may present as an increase in social withdrawal or stereotypic movements, or manifest as catatonia (see above) or anxiety. Although the risk factors are likely to be the same as in the general population, it has been suggested that a subgroup of people with ASDs are at risk for major mood disorders (DeLong 2004), reflecting a common genetic mechanism. Moreover, people with ASDs may experience a disproportionate number of negative life events such as bullying and social exclusion at school, particularly during the adolescent years.

Obsessive-Compulsive Disorder

Features suggesting obsessive-compulsive disorder (OCD) are frequently observed in adults with autism and Asperger's disorder. However, even though certain behavioral features are suggestive, the question of whether an additional diagnosis of OCD is justified in autism remains controversial (Baron-Cohen 1989). While, as suggested earlier, differentiating between comorbidity and behaviors that are manifestations of the disorder should be possible, it is important to recognize that treatment may be indicated irrespective of the underlying phenomenology if such symptoms are having a negative impact.

Attention-Deficit/Hyperactivity Disorder

Similarly, symptoms of inattention and hyperactivity are frequently noted among individuals with PDDs, with some reports suggesting that attention-deficit/hyperactivity disorder (ADHD) should be considered an additional diagnosis and target of treatment in persons with autism, but solid empirical data on this question are lacking. Moreover, whether it is appropriate to assign an additional diagnosis of ADHD among people with autism remains controversial (Verte et al. 2005). The additional comorbid diagnosis of ADHD may be made more easily in individuals with Asperger's disorder or PDDNOS (Barkley 1990). Once again, however, treatment may be indicated if such symptoms are having a negative impact on well-being.

Tic Disorders

Unusual motor mannerisms and stereotypies are common in autism. These behaviors change in intensity, type, and frequency over time, and as a function of variables such as adequacy of educational programming. Verbal stereotypies and perseveration may also be observed. As noted previously, the stereotyped movements of autism do not justify an additional diagnosis of stereotypic movement disorder. On the other hand, several case reports and a few series have suggested possible associations between autism and Asperger's disorder with Tourette's disorder (Nelson and Pribor 1993; Realmuto and Main 1982). One large-scale survey of 447 children with ASDs (Baron-Cohen et al. 1999) found that 19 (4.3%) met the diagnostic criteria for Tourette's disorder. This notwithstanding, the differentiation of tics versus stereotyped movements and other motor problems can be difficult.

Clinical Diagnostic Assessment and Differential Diagnosis

The diagnosis of autism and other PDDs is made following a clinical evaluation that includes 1) a thorough developmental history, which includes interviews with a key person who knew the patient during his or her formative years; 2) direct observation/interview with the patient; 3) review of clinical and educational records; 4) physical examination when indicated (e.g., to identify specific patterns of medical abnormality and dysmorphology associated with known genetic syndromes); 5) blood tests when indicated (principally for genetic evaluation); and 6) cognitive, neuropsychological assessments when indicated, such as measures of IQ and executive capacities (Volkmar et al. 1999).

A number of clinical interviews, notably the ADI-R (Lord et al. 1994), have been developed to facilitate and standardize the history. A companion instrument to the ADI-R, the Autism Diagnostic Observation Schedule (ADOS), has been developed as a procedure that places the patient in naturalistic social situations demanding specific social reactions (Lord et al. 2000). Although the protocol follows standard administration, the situations themselves are very unstructured, providing no guidelines to the child as to how to conduct him- or herself. In this way, a sample of naturalistic interaction is approximated. Assessment procedures are discussed in more detail in Chapter 2 ("Evaluation and Testing for Autism"). When assessing a child or adolescent with symptoms suggestive of a PDD, a detailed diagnostic evaluation is required to rule out disorders that have a similar presentation.

Autism and General Medical Conditions

All children with developmental impairments in the domains of social inter-action and communication should receive a thorough evaluation to rule out the possibility of an organic cause for their presentation. The list of potential organic etiologies of significant developmental delay that are associated with features of autism is relatively large, but the etiologies fall into the categories of infective (e.g., encephalitis or meningitis), endocrinopathic (e.g., hypothy-roidism), metabolic (e.g., homocystinuria), traumatic (e.g., head injury), or toxic (e.g., fetal alcohol syndrome). As a practical matter, for more strictly de-fined autism the list of associated medical conditions is somewhat shorter and includes fragile X syndrome and tuberous sclerosis as well as epilepsy (Filipek 2005; Fombonne et al. 1997). In addition, certain other disorders need to be ruled out. For example, Landau-Kleffner syndrome is characterized by acquired aphasia with epilepsy. The communication disorder and manifestation of the seizures may be mistaken for a PDD. In this condition a highly distinctive electroencephalographic abnormality is present and associated with devel-opment of a marked aphasia (Deonna 1991), rather than with a primary social disability.

Differentiation From Other Psychiatric Disorders

Autism and related disorders must also be differentiated from other psychiat-ric and developmental conditions. Several issues complicate this task. As may be inferred from the previous discussion of psychiatric comorbidity, there is no reason to expect that having autism or a related condition would protect against developing other disorders. On the other hand, sometimes complex issues of syndrome boundaries can arise, and the somewhat different ap-proaches taken in DSM and the ICD to the problem of comorbidity further complicate the task of differential diagnosis (see Volkmar and Klin 2005 for a discussion). Interest has centered on differentiation of autism from a range of other conditions, including OCD, anxiety disorders, schizophrenia, specific developmental disorders (particularly specific language disorders), and intel-lectual deficiency (mental retardation),

When children with social or communicative difficulties display habits or other repetitive patterns of behavior, it can sometimes be difficult to distin-guish between OCD and a PDD. However, a diagnosis of autism is supported in the context of 1) severe social and communicative impairments that have an early onset and that form the prominent presenting picture, 2) an early onset of the repetitive patterns of behavior, and 3) nonfunctional patterns of repetitive behavior (such as lining up or ordering objects) or those that are egosyntonic. Indeed, among higher functioning individuals with autism, the repetitive patterns of behavior are often associated with pleasure and mastery rather than distress (Grelotti et al. 2005). It is important to note that these behaviors in autism often interfere with everyday functioning and may require treatment to overcome the deleterious effect they may have on more general learning and development (Gabriels et al. 2005). Asperger (1944) made this point relative to the circumscribed interests so frequently seen in the condition that he described.

This notwithstanding, comorbid OCD can occur among individuals with autism, although recognizing this is often difficult in the context of preexisting repetitive patterns of behavior. Importantly, however, even if the exact phenomenological morphology has not been ascertained, if the behaviors are interfering with development, then some form of treatment may be warranted.

Although comorbidity for anxiety is not uncommon among people with autism, some of the symptoms that characterize these disorders such as excessive concern, the need for reassurance, the inability to relax, and feelings of self-consciousness are also seen in autism, particularly among higher functioning individuals. In some cases an additional diagnosis of an anxiety disorder may be warranted. Differentiating between the two disorders is generally not difficult because of the early onset of symptoms in autism, the characteristic early developmental delays seen in autism, the prominent and characteristic social and communicative impairments seen in autism but not anxiety disorders, and the developed social insight of children with anxiety disorders, whose anxiety is sometimes caused by a heightened awareness of other people. It is important to recognize that whether the symptoms are an integral part of the autism or represent a comorbid anxiety disorder, treatment may be required if they are affecting development.

Differentiating childhood schizophrenia from a diagnosis of autism can be difficult because both are characterized by social impairments and odd patterns of thinking. Nonetheless, florid delusions and hallucinations are not seen in autism and if present should alert to the alternative diagnosis or the possibility of comorbidity. Regarding the latter, it is important to bear in mind that comorbidity is relatively rare (Volkmar and Cohen 1991). In addition, the hierarchical nature of the DSM nosology means that a diagnosis of schizophrenia supplants that of Asperger's disorder or PDDNOS, whereas comorbidity in autism requires the presence of delusions and hallucinations for 1 month or more before both diagnoses are warranted. In assessing cases in which uncertainty of diagnosis exists, certain developmental factors may point toward one diagnosis over the other. In particular, autism is associated with an earlier age at onset of abnormalities, more severe social and communicative impairments, and the existence of associated developmental impairments.

Developmental language disorders such as expressive and/or receptive language impairments often affect socialization and may be mistaken for PDDs. The distinction is particularly difficult in preschool children, in whom formal evaluation may indeed highlight the impact developmental language delay has on other aspects of functioning (Paul and Sutherland 2005). However, there is evidence that two items on the ADI-R consistently differentiated an autism group from their language-impaired peers at 20 and 42 months, namely, point for interest and the use of conventional gestures (Chawarska and Volkmar 2005). Importantly, although other behaviors at 42 months, such as seeking to share enjoyment and imaginative play, appeared to differentiate between groups, repetitive and stereotypic patterns of behavior did not.

Differentiating between more global developmental delay and a PDD is often difficult, particularly when evaluating the younger infant (see Chawaska and Volkmar 2005 for a detailed discussion). One study (Paul and Sutherland 2005), however, identified a number of items on the ADI-R that differentiated between these two groups. Namely, at 24 months the following items differentiated between groups: seeking to share own enjoyment, directing attention, using the other's body as a tool, showing interest in other children, greeting, exhibiting social reciprocity, paying attention to voice, pointing, and understanding gestures. Two of these behaviors, directing attention (showing) and attention to voice, particularly differentiated between groups. At 36 months, four items correctly classified all subjects: use of other's body, attention to voice, pointing, and finger mannerisms. Similarly, when the ADOS was used, children with autism of ages between 38 and 61 months were more likely to show impaired nonverbal behaviors (such as eye contact) to regulate social interaction. Standardized assessments such as the ADI-R and ADOS may therefore be particularly useful in this context.

Conclusions

The descriptions of Kanner, Asperger, and other early clinician-investigators have proved remarkably enduring. Over the past decades considerable progress has been made in clarifying early sources of diagnostic confusion, issues of essential diagnostic features, and aspects of clinical phenomenology so that, for example, there is now rather general (and reasonably good) agreement on the diagnosis of autism relatively strictly defined (Lord and Volkmar 2002). In some ways, having achieved relatively good agreement on essential features, it is not surprising that much effort is now focused on better understanding the relationship of autism to other conditions within the PDD category as well as to the much larger broader spectrum of social difficulties.

For example, for Rett's disorder the discovery of a genetic basis, at least in some cases, has opened an important new area of work, and indeed the recent focus on the genetic basis of autism has confirmed the strong contribution of genetic factors to these conditions (Rutter 2005). The similarly dramatic regression (but of later onset) observed in childhood disintegrative disorder may be a fruitful area for study in the coming decade.

Areas of syndrome boundaries and syndrome relationships remain to be resolved. Considerable debate still exists around the differentiation of autism and Asperger's disorder relative to each other and other disorders not presently included in the PDDs class (Klin et al. 2005a). The relationship of these conditions to the most common (and also most poorly defined) condition in the PDDs category—PDDNOS—remains an area of active work and controversy (Rutter 2005; Volkmar and Klin 2005).

Although DSM-IV-TR and ICD-10 have provided a useful and well evaluated diagnostic framework for clinical diagnosis, they are undoubtedly not the last word on diagnosis. Although generally similar (at least for autism and related conditions) these two overarching approaches do have some practical differences (e.g., ICD-10 adopts explicit research criteria as well as more general clinical guidelines). The merits of each approach for autism remain to be clearly established, although it is clear that the trend toward more operational definitions (e.g., as exemplified in the ADOS and ADI-R) has tended to obviate this potential problem. Tensions between clinical and research diagnosis and the use (particularly in the United States) of labels for eligibility for services continue to exist.

References

American Psychiatric Association: Diagnostic and Statistical Manual of Mental Disorders, 3rd Edition. Washington, DC, American Psychiatric Association, 1980

American Psychiatric Association: Diagnostic and Statistical Manual of Mental Disorders, 3rd Edition, Revised. Washington, DC, American Psychiatric Association, 1987

American Psychiatric Association: Diagnostic and Statistical Manual of Mental Disorders, 4th Edition. Washington, DC, American Psychiatric Association, 1994

American Psychiatric Association: Diagnostic and Statistical Manual of Mental Disorders, 4th Edition, Text Revision. Washington, DC, American Psychiatric Association, 2000

Amir R, Van den Veyver I, Wan M, et al: Rett syndrome is caused by mutations in X-linked MECP2, encoding methyl-CpG-binding protein 2. Nat Genet 23:185–188, 1999

Asperger H: Die autistichen Psychopathen im Kindersalter. Arch Psychiatry Nervenkrank 117:76–136, 1944

Barkley R: Attention-Deficit Hyperactivity Disorder: A Handbook for Diagnosis and Treatment. New York, Guilford, 1990

Baron-Cohen S: Do autistic children have obsessions and compulsions? Br J Clin Psychol 28 (part 3):193–200, 1989

Baron-Cohen S, Scahill VL, Izaquirre J, et al: The prevalence of Gilles de la Tourette's syndrome in children and adolescents with autism: a large scale study. Psychol Med 29(5):1151–1159, 1999

Bleuler E: [Dementia Praecox or the Group of Schizophrenias] (1911). Translated by Zinkin J. New York, International Universities Press, 1951

Chawarska K, Volkmar F: Autism in infancy and early childhood, in Handbook of Autism and Pervasive Developmental Disorders, Volume 1: Diagnosis, Development, Neurobiology, and Behavior, 3rd Edition. Edited by Volkmar F, Paul R, Klin A, et al. Hoboken, NJ, Wiley, 2005, pp 223–246

Constantino JN, Gruber CP, Davis S, et al: The factor structure of autistic traits. J Child Psychol Psychiatry 45:719–726, 2004

DeLong R: Autism and familial major mood disorder: are they related? J Neuropsychiatry Clin Neurosci 16:199–213, 2004

Deonna TW: Acquired epileptiform aphasia in children (Landau-Kleffner syndrome). J Clin Neurophysiol 8:288–298, 1991

Filipek PA: Medical aspects of autism, in Handbook of Autism and Pervasive Developmental Disorders, Volume 1: Diagnosis, Development, Neurobiology, and Behavior, 3rd Edition. Edited by Volkmar F, Paul R, Klin A, et al. Hoboken, NJ, Wiley, 2005, pp 534–582

Fombonne E: Epidemiological studies of pervasive developmental disorders, in Handbook of Autism and Pervasive Developmental Disorders, Volume 1: Diagnosis, Development, Neurobiology, and Behavior, 3rd Edition. Edited by Volkmar F, Paul R, Klin A, et al. Hoboken, NJ, Wiley, 2005, pp 42–69

Fombonne E, Du Mazaubrun C, Cans C, et al: Autism and associated medical disorders in a French epidemiological survey. J Am Acad Child Adolesc Psychiatry 36:1561–1569, 1997

Gabriels RL, Cuccaro ML, Hill DE, et al: Repetitive behaviors in autism: relationships with associated clinical features. Res Dev Disabil 26:169–181, 2005

Ghaziuddin M, Tsai L, Ghaziuddin N: Comorbidity of autistic disorder in children and adolescents. Eur Child Adolesc Psychiatry 1:209–213, 1992

Ghaziuddin M, Weidmer-Mikhail E, Ghaziuddin N: Comorbidity of Asperger syndrome: a preliminary report. J Intellect Disabil Res 42 (part 4):279–283, 1998

Ghaziuddin M, Ghaziuddin N, Greden J: Depression in persons with autism: implications for research and clinical care. J Autism Dev Disord 32:299–306, 2002

Ghaziuddin M, Leininger L, Tsai L: Brief report: Thought disorder in Asperger syndrome: comparison with high-functioning autism. J Autism Dev Disord 25:311–317, 2005

Gillberg IC, Gillberg C: Asperger syndrome—some epidemiological considerations: a research note. J Child Psychol Psychiatry 30:631–638, 1989

Grelotti DJ, Klin A, Gauthier I, et al: fMRI activation of the fusiform gyrus and amygdala to cartoon characters but not to faces in a boy with autism. Neuropsychologia 43:373–385, 2005

Heller T: Dementia infantilis. Zeitschrift fur die Erforschung und Behandlung des Jugenlichen Schwachsinns 2:141–165, 1908

Howlin P: Outcomes in autism spectrum disorders, in Handbook of Autism and Pervasive Developmental Disorders, Volume 1: Diagnosis, Development, Neurobiology, and Behavior, 3rd Edition. Edited by Volkmar FR, Klin A, Paul R, et al. Hoboken, NJ, Wiley, 2005, pp 201–222

Kanner L: Autistic disturbances of affective contact. Nerv Child 2:217–250, 1943

Klin A, Lang J, Cicchetti DV, et al: Brief report: Interrater reliability of clinical diagnosis and DSM-IV criteria for autistic disorder: results of the DSM-IV autism field trial. J Autism Dev Disord 30:163–167, 2000

Klin A, McPartland J, Volkmar FR, et al: Asperger syndrome, in Handbook of Autism and Pervasive Developmental Disorders, Volume 2: Assessment, Interventions, and Policy, 3rd Edition. Edited by Volkmar F, Paul R, Klin A, et al. Hoboken, NJ, Wiley, 2005a, pp 88–125

Klin A, Pauls D, Schultz R, et al: Three diagnostic approaches to Asperger syndrome: implications for research. J Autism Dev Disord 35:221–234, 2005b

Klin A, Saulnier C, Tsatsanis K, et al: Clinical evaluation in autism spectrum disorders: psychological assessment within a transdisciplinary framework, in Handbook of Autism and Pervasive Developmental Disorders, Volume 2: Assessment, Interventions, and Policy, 3rd Edition. Edited by Volkmar F, Paul R, Klin A, et al. Hoboken, NJ, Wiley, 2005c, pp 772–798

Lord C, Volkmar F: Genetics of childhood disorders: XLII. Autism, part 1: diagnosis and assessment in autistic spectrum disorders. J Am Acad Child Adolesc Psychiatry 41:1134–1136, 2002

Lord C, Rutter M, Le Couteur A: Autism Diagnostic Interview—Revised: a revised version of a diagnostic interview for caregivers of individuals with possible pervasive developmental disorders. J Autism Dev Disord 24:659–685, 1994

Lord C, Risi S, Lambrecht L, et al: The Autism Diagnostic Observation Schedule—Generic: a standard measure of social and communication deficits associated with the spectrum of autism. J Autism Dev Disord 30:205–223, 2000

National Center for Clinical Infant Programs: Diagnostic Classification of Mental Health and Developmental Disorders of Infancy and Early Childhood. Washington, DC, National Center for Clinical Infant Programs, 1994

Nelson EC, Pribor EF: A calendar savant with autism and Tourette syndrome: response to treatment and thoughts on the interrelationships of these conditions. Ann Clin Psychiatry 5:135–140, 1993

Paul R, Sutherland D: Enhancing early language in children with autism spectrum disorders, in Handbook of Autism and Pervasive Developmental Disorders, Volume 2: Assessment, Interventions, and Policy, 3rd Edition. Edited by Volkmar F, Paul R, Klin A, et al. Hoboken, NJ, Wiley, 2005, pp 946–976

Realmuto GM, Main B: Coincidence of Tourette's disorder and infantile autism. J Autism Dev Disord 12:367–372, 1982

Rett A: [On a unusual brain atrophy syndrome in hyperammonemia in childhood]. Wein Med Wochenschr 118:723–726, 1966

Rourke B: Syndrome of Nonverbal Learning Disabilities: Manifestations in Neurological Disease Disorder and Dysfunction. New York, Guilford, 1994

Rourke BP, Tsatsanis KD: Nonverbal learning disabilities and Asperger syndrome, in Asperger Syndrome. Edited by Klin A, Volkmar FR. New York, Guilford, 2000, pp 231–253

Rutter M: Diagnosis and definition of childhood autism. J Autism Child Schizophrenia 8:139–161, 1978

Rutter M: Genetic influences and autism, in Handbook of Autism and Pervasive Developmental Disorders, Volume 1: Diagnosis, Development, Neurobiology, and Behavior, 3rd Edition. Edited by Volkmar F, Paul R, Klin A, et al. Hoboken, NJ, Wiley, 2005, pp 425–452

Seltzer MM, Krauss MW, Shattuck PT, et al: The symptoms of autism spectrum disorders in adolescence and adulthood. J Autism Dev Disord 33:565–581, 2003

Siegel B, Vukicevic J, Elliott GR, et al: The use of signal detection theory to assess DSM-III-R criteria for. J Am Acad Child Adolesc Psychiatry 28:542–548, 1989

Sigman M, Arbelle S, Dissanayake C: Current research findings on childhood autism. Can J Psychiatry 40:289–294, 1995

Silverman JM, Smith CJ, Schmeidler J, et al: Symptom domains in autism and related conditions: evidence for familiality. Am J Med Genet 114:64–73, 2002

Spiker D, Lotspeich LJ, Dimiceli S, et al: Behavioral phenotypic variation in autism multiplex families: evidence for a continuous severity gradient. Am J Med Genet 114:129–136, 2002

Szatmari P, Bremner R, Nagy J: Asperger's syndrome: a review of clinical features. Can J Psychiatry 34:554–560, 1989

Tsai LY: Brief report: comorbid psychiatric disorders of autistic disorder. J Autism Dev Disord 26:159–163, 1996

Van Acker R, Loncola JA, Van Acker EY: Rett's syndrome: a pervasive developmental disorder, in Handbook of Autism and Pervasive Developmental Disorders, Volume 1: Diagnosis, Development, Neurobiology, and Behavior, 3rd Edition. Edited by Volkmar F, Paul R, Klin A, et al. New York, Wiley, 2005, pp 126–184

Verte S, Geurts HM, Roeyers H, et al: Executive functioning in children with autism and Tourette syndrome. Dev Psychopathol 17:415–445, 2005

Volkmar FR, Cohen DJ: Comorbid association of autism and schizophrenia. Am J Psychiatry 148:1705–1707, 1991

Volkmar FR, Klin A: Issues in the classification of autism and related conditions, in Handbook of Autism and Pervasive Developmental Disorders, Volume 1: Diagnosis, Development, Neurobiology, and Behavior, 3rd Edition. Edited by Volkmar F, Paul R, Klin A, et al. Hoboken, NJ, Wiley, 2005, pp 5–41

Volkmar FR, Cicchetti DV, Bregman J, et al: Three diagnostic systems for autism: DSM-III, DSM-III-R, and ICD-10. J Autism Dev Disord 22:483–492, 1992

Volkmar FR, Klin A, Siegel B, et al: Field trial for autistic disorder in DSM-IV. Am J Psychiatry 151:1361–1367, 1994

Volkmar F, Cook EH Jr, Pomeroy J, et al: Practice parameters for the assessment and treatment of children, adolescents, and adults with autism and other pervasive developmental disorders. American Academy of Child and Adolescent Psychiatry Working Group on Quality Issues. J Am Acad Child Adolesc Psychiatry 38 (suppl 12):32S–54S, 1999 [erratum: J Am Acad Child Adolesc Psychiatry 39:938, 2000]

Volkmar FR, Koenig K, State M, et al: Childhood disintegrative disorder, in Handbook of Autism and Pervasive Developmental Disorders, Volume 1: Diagnosis, Development, Neurobiology, and Behavior, 3rd Edition. Edited by Volkmar F, Paul R, Klin A, et al. Hoboken, NJ, Wiley, 2005, pp 70–78

Weintraub S, Mesulam MM: Developmental learning disabilities of the right hemisphere: emotional, interpersonal, and cognitive components. Arch Neurol 11:463–468, 1983

Wing L: The history of ideas on autism. Autism 1:13–23, 1997a

Wing L: Syndromes of autism and atypical development, in Handbook of Autism and Pervasive Developmental Disorders, 2nd Edition. Edited by Cohen DJ, Volkmar FR. New York, Wiley, 1997b, pp 148–172

Wing L, Gould J: Severe impairments of social interaction and associated abnormalities. J Autism Dev Disord 9:11–29, 1979

Wing L, Shah A: Catatonia in autistic spectrum disorders. Brit J Psychiatry 176:357–362, 2000

Wolff S: Schizoid personality in childhood and Asperger syndrome, in Asperger Syndrome. Edited by Klin A, Volkmar FR. New York, Guilford, 2000, pp 278–305

World Health Organization: International Classification of Diseases, 10th Revision. Geneva, World Health Organization, 1992

Evaluation and Testing for Autism

Audrey Thurm, Ph.D.

Latha Soorya, Ph.D.

Ann Wagner, Ph.D.

As was illustrated in the previous chapter, individuals with autism spectrum disorders (ASDs) fall within a broad range of severity and ability levels. The vast amount of heterogeneity found among individuals within this category poses challenges for the clinician. Obtaining a diagnosis is an important step, and the diagnosis conveys critical information about the core difficulties the individual is likely to encounter. However, a diagnosis in itself does not give a complete picture of the individual's strengths and weaknesses, nor does it convey

The views expressed in this chapter are those of the authors and do not necessarily reflect the official position of the National Institute of Mental Health, the National Institutes of Health, or any other part of the U.S. Department of Health and Human Services. Mention of trade names, commercial products, or organizations does not imply endorsement by the U.S. Government.

complete information about overall adaptive functioning or prognosis. A comprehensive evaluation is needed. The evaluation becomes the basis for a treatment plan as well as a measurement of baseline functioning by which progress can be measured. In this chapter we discuss general principles and guidelines for the assessment of individuals with autism as well as some examples of tools and measures.

The nature of ASDs necessitates special consideration and challenges for evaluators. There is often a high degree of variability within individuals across domains of functioning, making it a challenge to find appropriate assessment tools. Social withdrawal or anxiety can make it difficult for the individual with an ASD to tolerate the directive and interactive nature of the testing situation. Difficulty with receptive or expressive verbal and nonverbal communication can make it difficult for the individual being tested to follow directions and for the clinician to interpret the responses. Individuals with ASDs often do not understand the social context of an evaluation and may not appreciate the importance of trying to do one's best and conforming to instructions. Repetitive behaviors, stereotypies, or rigidity may interfere with efficient administration and smooth transitions from one type of task to another. Learning difficulties such as stimulus overselectivity and poor generalization also often contribute to a variable presentation of skills. Thus, standardized testing may yield inconsistent or invalid data from children with ASDs because the standardized procedures may be compromised by these behavioral, attention, and motivational problems.

A developmental approach to assessment is critical (Klin et al. 2004; National Research Council 2001). A diagnosis of an ASD is based in large part on the discrepancy between an individual's social and communication skills and his or her other abilities, as well as departure from normal development. Therefore, multiple skills and areas of functioning must be assessed, and the assessment must be done within a context of the individual's age and overall developmental or intellectual level. Obtaining an assessment of intellectual ability and adaptive functioning is an essential step in a comprehensive evaluation. Assessment tools should allow separate assessment of cognitive skill areas rather than offering only a total score. At a minimum, cognitive assessment instruments should result in separate scores for verbal and nonverbal abilities. Further evaluation of scatter within subtest scores and development of a profile of strengths and weaknesses are useful when interpreted by an experienced clinician.

Use of standardized instruments is important for assessing an individual's functioning relative to normative expectations and for assessment at multiple time points. However, instruments standardized on the general population might result in standard scores that obscure intra-individual variability. Tests that allow conversion of raw scores to age equivalents as well as standard scores can be particularly helpful. The clinician must also be aware of floor effects when evaluating individuals with low functioning, in terms of both overall standard scores and subtest scores. Evaluating developmental progress poses challenges as well. Repeating tests too frequently can result in "practice effects," with scores artificially inflated because the individual is familiar with the items. Because choice of tests used depends on age and developmental level, as an individual grows it is sometimes necessary to switch to a new test or to a different version of the same test. Even within the same test, items used will be different at different ages and developmental levels.

Evaluation should not be limited to domains that reflect the core features of ASDs. The pervasive nature of the core features, as well as commonly occurring cognitive impairments, affects many other domains of functioning. It is important to understand the individual's strengths and challenges to develop a comprehensive intervention plan that capitalizes on abilities while addressing areas of weaknesses. The need for expert evaluation across a wide domain of behaviors and skills often necessitates a team approach to evaluation. Clinicians with different areas of expertise and parents or other primary caregivers work together to form a comprehensive profile and intervention plan.

Individuals with ASDs often function differently in different settings and under different task demands. The assessor can obtain important information by varying the context and demands of the evaluation. Observations of behaviors in structured versus unstructured situations, in response to verbal and nonverbal cues, and in novel versus familiar settings can yield information critical to determining intervention goals and strategies. Reports from parents, teachers, or other caregivers are often necessary for information about infrequent behaviors that might not be observed in a clinical setting as well as for information about functioning at home and in the community. If communication skills are adequate, the individual with an ASD can provide important information about his or her own thoughts and experience through self-report. The opportunity to ask about individuals' perceptions of their relationships, of their interests, and what they find difficult or challenging should not be overlooked.

Initial (or diagnostic) psychological and medical evaluations are critical for profiling an individual's unique strengths and weaknesses and providing baseline levels of functioning in pertinent domains. Periodic evaluations subsequent to the initial diagnosis assess treatment efficacy and an individual's developmental progression. It is recommended that the design of periodic evaluations be considered during the initial evaluation stage, because the initial evaluation will serve as a baseline comparison, and test selection for comparable assessments is critical (Martin et al. 2003). Factors to be considered in planning with periodic or follow-up evaluations in mind include using tests with a broad age range to facilitate comparisons at different developmental stages and selecting measures sensitive to treatment effects. For instance, IQ tests may not be the most useful for frequent reevaluations, because IQ scores have been shown to remain relatively stable over time in persons with ASDs (Venter et al. 1992).

In the following sections we describe domains and give examples of specific tests used for screening and subsequent comprehensive evaluation. Although the domains being evaluated may be the same across individuals, the choice of instrument depends on age and level of functioning. In this chapter we aim to provide examples and guidelines for evaluation and testing of individuals with autism of all ages and levels of functioning, but with a focus on initial diagnostic evaluation. Particular tests and considerations may be more applicable to children and adolescents than to older individuals. We do make some specific references to distinctions in tests and/or procedures for adults.

Diagnostic Evaluations

Although early diagnosis is critical to appropriate early intervention, the initial diagnosis of autism can occur at various ages. Although the mean age at diagnosis has decreased over time, it remains greater than 3 years (Chakrabarti and Fombonne 2005). According to several professional organizations, including the American Academy of Child and Adolescent Psychiatry (Volkmar et al. 1999), the American Academy of Neurology (Filipek et al. 2000), and the American Academy of Pediatrics (Committee on Children With Disabilities 2001), a comprehensive assessment is required for diagnosis of autism. In fact, a two-tiered diagnostic process, including developmental screening, is recommended, followed by a comprehensive diagnostic evaluation when indicated. In the following subsections we describe domains and provide examples of specific tests that may be considered for screening and comprehensive evaluation. Examples of specific tests are also provided in Table 2–1.

Screening

Developmental screening is recommended for all children. Appropriate development screeners include instruments such as the Ages and Stages Questionnaires (Bricker and Squires 1999), the Parents' Evaluation of Developmental Status (Glascoe 1997), and the Child Development Inventory (Ireton 1992; Ireton and Glascoe 1995). If the screener indicates that the child fails to meet developmental milestones, the American Academy of Neurology recommends an autism-specific screener before proceeding to a second-stage evaluation for autism (Filipek et al. 2000). Autism-specific screeners include the Social Communication Questionnaire (Rutter et al. 2003), the Checklist for Autism in Toddlers (CHAT) (Baron-Cohen et al. 2000), the Modified CHAT (Robins et al. 2001), and the Pervasive Developmental Disorder Screening Test (Siegel 2004). In addition, observation-based autism screeners include the Screening Tool for Autism in Two-Year-Olds (Stone et al. 2004).

When scores on an autism screener fall within the risk range, or concern is raised by parents or professionals, the second stage of the diagnostic process is recommended to rule in or rule out an ASD or other developmental problem. This comprehensive diagnostic evaluation is optimally performed by a multidisciplinary team that includes a psychologist, a neurologist, a psychiatrist, a speech therapist, or other professionals who are familiar with the diagnosis of ASDs. In conjunction with or before the multidisciplinary evaluation, an audiologic evaluation is indicated to rule out hearing difficulties. The second-stage comprehensive developmental approach (see Klin et al. 2004 for such an approach with young children) should utilize multiple settings, multiple observations, and parental and/or caregiver involvement to accurately capture the variability and profile scatter common in children with autism. As outlined in the next section, in addition to autism-specific diagnostic instruments, measures of cognition (or development), communication (including speech), and adaptive functioning are essential. In addition, particularly if follow-up evaluations for assessment of change are to be considered, assessments of behaviors within all core domains of autism, as well as comorbid and medically related conditions, are warranted.

Table 2–1.   Examples of measures used in comprehensive autism assessment

Scale/instrument	Format	Age(s)	Rater	Administration time
Screening				
Social Communication Questionnaire	Checklist	>4 years	Parent/caregiver	5–10 minutes
Modified Checklist for Autism in Toddlers	Checklist	18–36 months	Parent/caregiver	5–10 minutes
Checklist for Autism in Toddlers	Checklist (caregiver report and primary healthcare worker observation)	18–36 months	Parent/caregiver and clinician	5–10 minutes
Diagnosis				
Autism Diagnostic Interview—Revised	Semistructured interview	>18 months mental age	Clinician or paraprofessional	1.5–2.5 hours
Autism Diagnostic Observation Schedule	Observation-based assessment	>15 months mental age	Clinician or paraprofessional	35–40 minutes
Childhood Autism Rating Scale	Checklist	>2 years	Clinician or paraprofessional	20–30 minutes
Communication and language				
Communication and Symbolic Behavior Scales, Developmental Profile	Parent screening, parent questionnaire, direct observation	6–24 months	Parents/caregivers, clinicians, and/or paraprofessionals	Parent screening: 5–10 minutes Parentquestionnaire: 15–25 minutes Behavior sample: 30 minutes

Table 2–1. Examples of measures used in comprehensive autism assessment (*continued*)

Scale/instrument	Format	Age(s)	Rater	Administration time
Communication and language (*continued*)				
Children's Communication Checklist–2	Checklist	4–16 years	Clinician or paraprofessional	5–15 minutes
Sequenced Inventory of Communication Development	Standardized assessment	4 months to 4 years	Clinician or paraprofessional	60–90 minutes
Reynell Scales of Language Abilities	Standardized assessment	1–6 years	Clinician or paraprofessional	35–40 minutes
Social interaction				
Social Responsiveness Scale	Questionnaire	4–18 years	Teacher or parent/ caregiver	15–20 minutes
Social Skills Rating System	Questionnaire	3–18 years	Teacher or parent/ caregiver/self	15–25 minutes
Matson Evaluation of Social Skills With Youngsters	Questionnaire	4–18 years	Teacher/self	15 minutes
Repetitive and stereotyped behavior				
Repetitive Behavior Scale—Revised	Questionnaire	Preschool–adulthood	Parent/caregiver	15–25 minutes

Cognitive/Developmental Assessment

Cognitive assessment is critical in making a diagnosis of an ASD. A significant portion of individuals diagnosed with autism have cognitive impairments, often indicating a comorbid diagnosis of mental retardation. Even in individuals without severe cognitive deficits, a variable profile of cognitive skills is common. Cognitive assessment is necessary to make a differential diagnosis between autism and Asperger's disorder, because lack of clinically significant cognitive delay is a defining feature of Asperger's disorder as per DSM-IV-TR (American Psychiatric Association 2000). Cognitive assessment typically includes an IQ measure, or for young children, a measure of developmental quotient (DQ).

In assessing individuals with autism, there are several considerations in determining which IQ or DQ test may be optimal for use. First, because by definition individuals with autism have deficits in communication, verbal scores on cognitive tests are often lower, particularly in younger children (Joseph et al. 2002; Mayes and Calhoun 2003), and nonverbal (or performance) scores are considered to be more preserved. In Asperger's disorder, defined without cognitive impairments and language delay, a reverse pattern of verbal scores higher than nonverbal abilities has been reported (Klin et al. 1995). Thus, it is recommended that a cognitive test that separates out scores between these domains be administered. Second, both verbal and nonverbal IQ may be different in the same individual with autism when measured with different cognitive tests because some tests are more verbally loaded, even on the nonverbal components, than others. For instance, scores on the Wechsler scales may be affected by comparably higher verbal demands, compared with other tests (Klin et al. 2005). Because of these issues, along with other specific test demands (e.g., scoring based on timed performance), cognitive tests are often chosen that are outside the standardized age range for the particular test. For young children under the age of 6 years, the Mullen Scales of Early Learning (Mullen 1995) is often used in the ASD population because it provides both verbal and nonverbal scores (as well as a gross motor domain) and covers the entire infant, toddler, and preschool age range. Another commonly used measure, designed for individuals ages 2½ years through 17 years, is the Differential Ability Scales (Elliott 1990), which also includes verbal and nonverbal clusters and allows for comparability of scores over a long period of childhood and adolescence.

Functioning: Adaptive and Global

Alongside cognitive assessment, evaluation of day-to-day functioning or adaptive behavior is essential in diagnosing mental retardation that may be associated with autism. Studies in individuals with ASDs suggest that adaptive behavior scores are substantially below those predicted by overall IQ (Schatz and Hamdan-Allen 1995). Thus, even individuals with an ASD and a high IQ can score poorly in life skills. Use of adaptive behavior measures in all groups can provide information for therapeutic and legal purposes, especially for high-IQ individuals with poor integration and limited independence in the community.

The most commonly used instrument for measurement of adaptive behavior is the Vineland Adaptive Behavior Scales (Sparrow et al. 1984), which was recently revised (Sparrow et al. 2005). In fact, supplemental norms for individuals with autism were published on the 1984 edition (Carter et al. 1998). Adaptive behavior scales such as the Vineland are also particularly useful because of their separate domain scores in areas such as communication, socialization, daily living, and motor skills, facilitating profile analysis across domains, which can be reevaluated over time. In fact, scores on the communication domain at early ages are quite predictive of later language functioning in children with autism (Thurm et al. 2006). Another commonly used adaptive behavior measure is the Scales of Independent Behavior—Revised (Bruininks et al. 1996).

Adaptive functioning measures may also be used for outcome evaluation. The Vineland Adaptive Behavior Scales was recently found to show change (with respect to maladaptive behavior) in a psychopharmacological treatment study (McDougle et al. 2005). Use of the age-equivalent scores, but not standard scores, measured change in a longitudinal study of children from ages 2 through 7 years (Charman et al. 2004).

Global functioning scales are also commonly used, particularly to assess change during treatment. A commonly used clinician rating of global functioning is the Children's Global Assessment Scale (Shaffer et al. 1983), which has now been modified for use with the ASD population (Wagner et al. 2007). In adults, the Global Assessment Scale (Endicott et al. 1976) and Global Assessment of Functioning Scale (American Psychiatric Association 2000) are frequently used. Such measures take into account multiple sources of information and fulfill the Axis V requirement of assessing functioning for a DSM-IV-TR diagnosis (American Psychiatric Association 2000). These scales measure psychological, social, and vocational or school functioning on a 100-point scale and are both efficient and reliable for use by professionals in clinical settings. A Clinical Global Impression scale, which includes baseline and improvement components, has also been developed for research (e.g., clinical trial) purposes (Aman et al. 2004).

Diagnostic Measures

Diagnostic measures have become integral in making a DSM-IV-TR diagnosis of autism (for a review, see Lord and Corsello 2005). Such instruments were initially developed for research purposes but are now used quite widely in both clinical and research settings because they 1) maximize sensitivity and specificity of diagnosis over time and 2) create standardized methods for diagnosis that are consistent across assessors.

Gold-standard diagnostic measures include the Autism Diagnostic Interview—Revised (ADI-R) (Le Couteur et al. 2003) and the Autism Diagnostic Observation Schedule (ADOS) (Lord et al. 1999, 2000). Combined, these two measures assess the four domains required for the diagnosis of autism: 1) qualitative abnormalities in reciprocal social interaction, 2) qualitative abnormalities in communication, 3) restricted repetitive and stereotyped patterns of behavior, and 4) abnormality of development evident at or before 36 months. The ADOS includes an algorithm with cutoffs for autism or ASD, whereas the ADI-R algorithm includes only autism. The manuals for these instruments recommend that they both be used in the context of a comprehensive assessment to make a diagnosis. The ADOS alone does not include repetitive behavior/restricted interests in its algorithm, does not assess for peer relationships, and does not capture the diagnostic requirement of whether symptoms were present before the age of 3 years. The ADOS does allow for direct observation and/or interview, whereas the ADI-R relies on caregiver report. The ADI-R includes questions about lifetime history of symptoms (with comparison to earlier functioning).

Although the ADI-R and the ADOS are developed for use throughout the lifespan, consideration of their use in young children requires special attention because of the lowered specificity and sensitivity of these instruments in very young children, particularly those with mental ages under 18 months. This poses a serious dilemma, in that an increasing number of children under the age of 3 years, and even 2 years, are undergoing comprehensive diagnostic evaluation. Although research instruments focusing on early "markers" are currently under development (Wetherby et al. 2004; Zwaigenbaum et al. 2005), there is currently no standardized, psychometrically tested assessment tool designed specifically for use in diagnosis of ASDs in children under 2 years or under 18 months mental age. Part of the problem is that DSM-IV-TR criteria may not be particularly useful for young children (Zwaigenbaum et al. 2007), because early characteristics of autism include subtle deficits such as variable eye gaze, inconsistent joint-attention skills, and reduced vocal and/or motor imitation (Zwaigenbaum et al. 2005).

There are several other measures designed for the exclusive purpose of autism diagnosis. For instance, the Childhood Autism Rating Scale (Schopler et al. 1988) and the Autism Behavior Checklist (Krug et al. 1980) are behavioral rating scales developed for clinical settings that provide quantitative measurements and have cutoffs for a diagnosis of autism. Other interviews used in the diagnosis include the Diagnostic Interview for Social and Communication Disorders (Wing et al. 2002) and the Parent Interview for Autism (Stone et al. 2003). The Psychoeducational Profile, 3rd Edition (PEP-3) (Schopler et al. 2005), designed for children, and the adult version of the Adolescent and Adult Psychoeducational Profile (Mesibov et al. 1988) are instruments that may be used in the diagnostic process as well, particularly for obtaining severity ratings of specific domains for treatment planning.

In general, the instruments described previously provide measures for the diagnosis of autism according to categorical cutoffs (based on continuous measures of the core domains of autism). However, severity is not explicitly quantifiable on these measures (Lord and Volkmar 2002). That is, once over the cutoff for diagnosis, these measures have not been rigorously studied with respect to meaningful categories (or dimensions) that could translate into a mild to severe status for an individual.

Diagnostic Formulation

As outlined by Klin et al. (2004), both qualitative and quantitative data should be integrated to form a complete differential diagnosis that not only considers DSM-IV-TR criteria but encapsulates information about functioning level and recommendations for intervention. This is particularly important because of the heterogeneity inherent in the autism diagnosis. Underscoring the significance of language and communication impairments, as well as cognitive deficits, for instance, is often essential information for service planning and prognosis evaluation.

For higher functioning individuals (i.e., those with cognitive functioning in the normal range and relatively intact language abilities), differential diagnosis between autistic disorder (which may be labeled as high-functioning autism), Asperger's disorder, or pervasive developmental disorder not otherwise specified requires careful analysis of current quantitative data on cognitive and sociocommunicative skills, historical information on whether language delay existed (absent in the Asperger's disorder diagnosis), and qualitative judgment of the severity of core autism impairments.

Assessment of Core Autism Spectrum Disorder Domains

In addition to measuring overall levels of functioning, measures of core deficits (i.e., communication, socialization, stereotyped and repetitive behaviors/restricted interest patterns) are often needed both at initial intake and at follow-up evaluations to determine the specificity and efficacy of an individualized treatment program or overall program evaluation for children with ASDs.

Communication

Communication is assessed via cognitive ability tests, autism diagnostic measures, and adaptive behavior instruments. However, additional assessment of specific communication skills such as speech and language are typically part of a comprehensive diagnostic evaluation. Speech and language are typically impaired in children with autism. In addition, a subset of individuals with autism also have specific language impairments (De Fosse et al. 2004). Early speech abilities (but not necessarily other communication skills) are typically spared in children with Asperger's disorder. Thus, in-depth language measures are necessary for differential diagnosis of ASDs.

For young children, parent reports such as the MacArthur Communicative Development Inventories (Fenson 1989) are helpful. The Communication and Symbolic Behavior Scales (Wetherby and Prizant 2002) include both parent report and observation of social communication skills. These tools may also be used periodically to evaluate developmental progression and response to treatment. For preschool-age children and older children, language measures that include both receptive and expressive components are often used.

These include the Sequenced Inventory of Communication Development (Hedrick et al. 1975), the Preschool Language Scale, 4th Edition (Zimmerman et al. 2003), and the Clinical Evaluation of Language Fundamentals (Semel et al. 1995). Language tests that are standardized across a wide age range, such as the Peabody Picture Vocabulary Test (L.M. Dunn and Dunn 1997), the Expressive One-Word Picture Vocabulary Test (Brownell 2000), and the Expressive Vocabulary Test (Williams 1997), are commonly used for their ability to capture changes throughout a wide range of development. In addition, language samples such as mean length of utterance should be considered in language evaluations because they can provide a wealth of information on language production and content (Hewitt et al. 2005).

Social Interaction

Measures of social behaviors relevant to autism that cover a broad age span and are sensitive to change are relatively scarce. Commonly used measures for social behavior include the social subdomain of the Vineland Adaptive Behavior Scales, the social domain of the ADI-R, the social domain of the ADOS, the Social Responsiveness Scale (Constantino et al. 2000), the Matson Evaluation of Social Skills (Matson et al. 1983), and the Social Skills Rating System (Gresham and Elliott 1990). These measures have been used with mixed success in showing outcomes in behavioral and medication treatment research (e.g., Aldred et al. 2004; Bauminger 2002).

Repetitive Behaviors and Stereotyped, Restricted Interests

A few measures have been developed or modified to facilitate evaluation of repetitive behavior/circumscribed interests in ASDs. Assessments such as the Yale-Brown Obsessive Compulsive Scale (Y-BOCS) (Goodman et al. 1989a, 1989b), the Children's Y-BOCS (CY-BOCS) (Scahill et al. 1997), and the Repetitive Behavior Scale—Revised (Bodfish et al. 2000) have been used in clinical drug trials targeting reductions in repetitive behaviors associated with ASDs. The Y-BOCS and CY-BOCS are brief (10–15 minutes) clinician-administered structured interviews that have been shown to be sensitive to change during short intervals and are often used in clinical practice. The CY-BOCS has now been modified for use with children with pervasive developmental disorders (McDougle et al. 2005).

Other Critical Domains for Assessment

Neurological and Medical Testing

As part of a comprehensive, interdisciplinary evaluation, neurological and genetic assessments should complement behavioral measures. There are many conditions associated with autism that require such testing. The American Academy of Child and Adolescent Psychiatry (Volkmar et al. 1999) recommends medical history and physical examination in an autism assessment, including examination for macrocephaly/megalencephaly, motor apraxia, and epilepsy or seizures (including potential testing for abnormal activity on the electroencephalogram). Given the high occurrence of medical problems involving both sleep and feeding habits in individuals with autism, these domains should be covered in an exam. Genetic and other laboratory testing that may be indicated include fragile X syndrome testing and screening for tuberous sclerosis (Volkmar et al. 1999), as well as karyotyping and other chromosomal analysis for inherited metabolic disorders or other abnormalities. In addition, formal audiologic hearing evaluation and lead screening tests are often recommended.

Assessment for Physical Therapy and Occupational Therapy

Motor apraxia, including hypotonia, is found in a significant minority of children with autism. If initial medical examination indicates, further evaluation for physical therapy may be warranted.

Occupational therapy is often utilized for individuals with autism to address impairments in activities of daily living, which often include lack of skills for play, dressing, and caretaking. In addition, sensory integration issues are found quite commonly in individuals with ASDs, which may also be addressed via occupational therapy. Although there are many checklists and direct observation tests of sensorimotor skills, the Sensory Profile (W. Dunn 1999) is a commonly used questionnaire that specifically measures sensory dysfunction.

Comorbid Psychiatric and Behavioral Problems

For a comprehensive evaluation, consideration of associated behavioral and psychiatric conditions is necessary because such comorbidity can cause considerable interference in social and family adjustment. For younger children, measures of self-regulation and temperament, including the Temperament and Atypical Behavior Scale (Neisworth et al. 1999) and the Children's Behavior Questionnaire (Rothbart et al. 2001) are available, as well as the recently developed Infant-Toddler Social and Emotional Assessment (Carter et al. 2003). For older individuals, psychiatric comorbidity such as anxiety, attention-deficit/hyperactivity disorder, and depression may be assessed via well-normed instruments such as the Child Behavior Checklist (Achenbach and Rescorla 2001) or the Behavior Assessment System for Children (Reynolds and Kamphaus 2004). The Aberrant Behavior Checklist (Aman et al. 1985), developed specifically for individuals with mental retardation, is often used for this purpose. It includes five subscales: 1) Irritability, Agitation, 2) Lethargy, Social Withdrawal, 3) Stereotypic Behavior, 4) Hyperactivity, Noncompliance, and 5) Inappropriate Speech. In addition, with the use of behavioral interventions to treat target negative or interfering behaviors in autism, functional analysis is often used as a baseline assessment of antecedents and consequences to targeted behaviors (Fisher et al. 2005). Finally, although individuals with autism may not be responsive to psychiatric interviews, parent reports of psychiatric instruments may be warranted if additional psychiatric diagnoses are apparent.

Neuropsychological and Learning Disability Assessment

Neuropsychological deficits associated with autism involve specific attentional abilities, executive functions, central coherence, and theory of mind (Volkmar et al. 2004). Although used to some degree in individuals of all ages and developmental levels, in-depth neuropsychological evaluation is most often administered to higher functioning individuals and older individuals with autism, and may be used for specific education and treatment planning (Ozonoff et al. 2005). Indications for this type of testing include the possibility of a specific learning disability (e.g., dyslexia), or when significant executive function impairment or comorbid attention-deficit/hyperactivity disorder is suspected. As with the other domains assessed, caution should be warranted when using standardized neuropsychological assessments in individuals with ASDs because issues such as cognitive and/or receptive communication impairments may interfere with meeting basic test demands.

Specific Outcome Measures

As specified, measures designed to capture change over time are critical to assessing intervention effectiveness. One type of outcome measure is a standardized questionnaire. The Pervasive Developmental Disorders Behavior Inventory (PDDBI) is a relatively new measure designed specifically to evaluate responsiveness to interventions for adaptive and maladaptive behaviors specific to individuals with ASDs (Cohen 2003; Cohen et al. 2003). The PDDBI has separate parent and teacher ratings forms. The four adaptive subscales are Social Approach Behaviors, Learning/Memory/Receptive Language, Phonological Skills, and Semantic/Pragmatic Ability. The maladaptive subscales evaluate self-stimulatory sensory behaviors, specific fears, arousal problems, aggression, social approach problems, and language problems (e.g., echolalia, odd intonation/pitch). The PDDBI has been shown to have good sensitivity and specificity, but it is a relatively new instrument and its sensitivity to change has not yet been demonstrated.

Another type of outcome measure is a criterion-referenced assessment. The Assessment of Basic Language and Learning Skills (ABLLS) is a comprehensive, criterion-based behavioral assessment tool originally designed for use in applied behavior analytic educational approaches, based on Skinner's analysis of verbal behavior (Sundberg and Partington 1998). The ABLLS provides an assessment of behavior in 26 domains, including language, self-help, academic, and autism-specific behaviors, and provides detailed assessments of skills. Data from the ABLLS can be directly translated for curriculum development and treatment evaluation. Furthermore, the ABLLS assesses many autism-specific learning problems such as poor generalization and motivation, providing valuable information for treatment planning.

Functional Behavioral Assessments

Functional behavioral assessments (FBAs) are assessment strategies (e.g., informant report, direct observation of behaviors, experimental manipulation of variables) that should be used in parallel with the standardized assessments described previously. FBAs yield information on factors (e.g., common antecedents and consequences) that are correlated with behavior problems. Results of FBAs include situations and conditions that predict the occurrence and non-occurrence of problem behavior (e.g., when, where, why) and hypotheses on the potential functions for a problem behavior (e.g., to escape from difficult tasks, to gain social attention). The utility of FBAs has been widely recognized, because information from FBAs has led to more efficient and effective treatment of problem behaviors for children with disabilities (O'Neill et al. 1997). As such, the Individuals with Disabilities Education Improvement Act of 2004 mandates the use of FBAs for students with disabilities and disruptive behavior problems. Although a full description of FBA procedures is beyond the scope of this text, manuals such as *Functional Assessment and Program Development for Problem Behavior: A Practical Handbook* (O'Neill et al. 1997) provide a useful discussion of the purpose and methods of FBAs for use in clinical settings.

Psychoeducational Testing

Children with ASDs are often enrolled in special education and have individualized education programs guiding initial pyschoeducational evaluations and progress evaluations at regular intervals, typically every 3 years. In most states, the triennial evaluation involves administration of standardized IQ, academic, and speech tests. Standardized tests allow global comparisons of an individual's skills to same-age peers. However, substantial changes are needed before improvement can be reflected on standardized test scores, such as IQ.

Traditional triennial evaluations using standardized cognitive and academic tests can be supplemented with measures to evaluate commonly impaired cognitive domains in ASDs, such as executive functions and motor planning. In addition, use of curriculum-based measurement (CBM) strategies is recommended to supplement traditional, standardized academic tests. CBM involves the ongoing, direct assessment of academic skills using frequent, brief (e.g., 5 minutes), regularly scheduled probes. These probes are linked to the individual student's classroom curriculum and are timed assessments of skills (e.g., brief reading passages, short spelling lists, samples of math items from the curriculum). Probes are used to establish periodic (e.g., weekly) goals and to measure progress toward short-term and long-term goals. CBM strategies have been shown to influence student progress and teacher instruction (Fuchs et al. 1984). CBM procedures can be valuable additions to progress evaluations in subjects with autism. First, CBM methods can help document small changes in academic skills that may not be captured in traditional standardized testing procedures. CBM procedures can also accommodate the unique attentional and motivational characteristics of children with ASDs. Research has shown that adjustments to motivational and attentional cues can change outcomes on traditional standardized tests (Koegel et al. 1997). Therefore, in some cases, CBM procedures may help capture a more accurate picture of an individual's skills.

Conclusions

In this chapter we have outlined some of the assessment issues and aspects of autism that are critical to consider when conducting diagnostic and follow-up psychological evaluation of individuals with ASDs. To give specific examples, we have focused on tests that are typically administered in outpatient settings with children and adolescents.

In summary, we again state the importance of using basic psychological assessment principles in evaluation and testing of individuals with ASDs. Included among these is the need to tailor assessment batteries to the specific needs of each individual with an ASD, paying particular attention to developmental/cognitive level, level of speech or alternative communication strategies, and other behavioral problems that might challenge the "testability" of that individual. Further, although quantitative scores from tests are invaluable for comparing individuals with autism with other individuals (and with themselves over time), they are not always feasible for individuals with autism who cannot cooperate with the testing situation. In addition, the norming samples for individual instruments should be considered carefully in making decisions about particular tests. Use of the "multi" method and informant assessment techniques (including testing over various sessions and in diverse settings) and use of multiple informants (including observation) are critical to the effective diagnostic and follow-up evaluation of individuals with autism.

References

Achenbach TM, Rescorla LA: Manual for the ASEBA School-Age Forms and Profiles. Burlington, University of Vermont, Research Center for Children, Youth, and Families, 2001

Aldred C, Green G, Adams C: A new social communication intervention for children with autism: pilot randomized controlled treatment study suggesting effectiveness. J Child Psychol Psychiatry 45:1420–1430, 2004

Aman MG, Singh NN, Stewart AW, et al: The Aberrant Behavior Checklist: a behavior rating scale for the assessment of treatment effects. Am J Ment Defic 89:485–491, 1985

Aman MG, Novotny S, Samango-Sprouse C: Outcome measures for clinical drug trials in autism. CNS Spectr 9:36–47, 2004

American Psychiatric Association: Diagnostic and Statistical Manual of Mental Disorders, 4th Edition, Text Revision. Washington, DC, American Psychiatric Association, 2000

Baron-Cohen S, Wheelwright S, Cox A, et al: The early identification of autism: the Checklist for Autism in Toddlers (CHAT). J R Soc Med 93:521–525, 2000

Bauminger N: The facilitation of social-emotional understanding and social interaction in high-functioning children with autism: intervention outcomes. J Autism Dev Disord 32:283–298, 2002

Bodfish JW, Symons FJ, Parker DE, et al: Varieties of repetitive behaviors in autism. J Autism Dev Disord 30:237–243, 2000

Bricker D, Squires J: The Ages and Stages Questionnaires, 2nd Edition. Baltimore, MD, Paul H Brookes Publishing, 1999

Brownell R: Expressive One-Word Picture Vocabulary Test, 2000 Edition. Minneapolis, MN, Pearson Assessments, 2000

Bruininks RH, Woodcock RW, Weatherman RE, et al: Scales of Independent Behavior, Revised. Itasca, IL, Riverside Publishing, 1996

Carter AS, Volkmar FR, Sparrow SS, et al: The Vineland Adaptive Behavior Scales: supplementary norms for individuals with autism. J Autism Dev Disord 28:287–302, 1998

Carter AS, Briggs-Gowan MJ, Jones SM, et al: The Infant-Toddler Social and Emotional Assessment (ITSEA): factor structure, reliability, and validity. J Abnorm Child Psychol 31:495–514, 2003

Chakrabarti S, Fombonne E: Pervasive developmental disorders in preschool children: confirmation of high prevalence. Am J Psychiatry 162:1133–1141, 2005

Charman T, Howlin P, Berry B, et al: Measuring developmental progress of children with autism spectrum disorders using parent report. Autism 8:89–100, 2004

Cohen I: Criterion related validity of the PDD Behavior Inventory. J Autism Dev Disord 33:47–53, 2003

Cohen IL, Schmidt-Lackner S, Romanczyk R, et al: The PDD Behavior Inventory: a rating scale for assessing response to intervention in children with pervasive developmental disorder. J Autism Dev Disord 33:31–45, 2003

Committee on Children With Disabilities: American Academy of Pediatrics: The pediatrician's role in the diagnosis and management of autistic spectrum disorder in children. Pediatrics 107:1221–1226, 2001

Constantino JN, Przybeck T, Friesen D, et al: Reciprocal social behavior in children with and without pervasive developmental disorders. J Dev Behav Pediatr 21:2–11, 2000

De Fosse L, Hodge SM, Markis N, et al: Language-association cortex asymmetry in autism and specific language impairment. Ann Neurol 56:757–766, 2004

Dunn LM, Dunn LM: The Peabody Picture Vocabulary Test, 3rd Edition. Circle Pines, MN, American Guidance Service, 1997

Dunn W: Sensory Profile. San Antonio, TX, Psychological Corporation, 1999

Elliott C: Manual for the Differential Abilities Scales. San Antonio, TX, Psychological Corporation, 1990

Endicott J, Spitzer R. Fleiss J, et al: The Global Assessment Scale: a procedure for measuring overall severity psychiatric disturbance. Arch Gen Psychiatry 33:766–771, 1976

Fenson L: The MacArthur Communicative Development Inventory: Infant and Toddler Versions. San Diego, CA, San Diego State University, 1989

Filipek PA, Accardo PJ, Ashwal S, et al: Practice parameter: screening and diagnosis of autism. Neurology 55:468–479, 2000

Fisher WW, Adelinis JD, Volkert VM, et al: Assessing preferences for positive and negative reinforcement during treatment of destructive behavior with functional communication training. Res Dev Disabil 26:153–168, 2005

Fuchs LS, Deno SL, Mirkin PK: Effects of frequent curriculum-based measurement of evaluation on pedagogy, student achievement, and student awareness of learning. Am Educ Res J 21:449–460, 1984

Glascoe FP: PEDS: Parents' Evaluation of Developmental Status. Nashville, TN, Ellsworth & Vandermeer Press, 1997

Goodman WK, Price L, Rasmussen S, et al: The Yale-Brown Obsessive Compulsive Scale. I. Development, use, and reliability. Arch Gen Psychiatry 46:1006–1011, 1989a

Goodman WK, Price L, Rasmussen S, et al: The Yale-Brown Obsessive Compulsive Scale. II. Validity. Arch Gen Psychiatry 46:1012–1016, 1989b

Gresham FM, Elliott SN: The Social Skills Rating System. Circle Pines, MN, American Guidance Service, 1990

Hedrick DL, Prather EM, Tobin AR: Sequenced Inventory of Communication Development. Seattle, WA, University of Washington Press, 1975

Hewitt L, Hammer C, Yont K, et al: Language sampling for kindergarten children with and without SLI: Mean Length of Utterance, IPSYN, and NDW. J Commun Disord 38:197–213, 2005

Ireton H: Child Development Inventories. Minneapolis, MN, Behavior Science Systems, 1992

Ireton H, Glascoe FP: Assessing children's development using parents' reports. The Child Development Inventory. Clin Pediatr 34:248–255, 1995

Joseph RM, Tager-Flusberg H, Lord C: Cognitive profiles and social-communicative functioning in children with autism spectrum disorder. J Child Psychol Psychiatry 43:807–821, 2002

Klin A, Volkmar FR, Sparrow SS, et al: Validity and neuropsychological characterization of Asperger syndrome: convergence with nonverbal learning disabilities syndrome. J Child Psychol Psychiatry 36:1127–1140, 1995

Klin A, Chawarska K, Rubin E, et al: Clinical assessment of young children at risk for autism, in Handbook of Infant, Toddler and Preschool Mental Health Assessment. Edited by DelCarmen-Wiggens R, Carter A. New York, Oxford University Press. 2004, pp 311–336

Klin A, Saulnier C, Tsatsanis K, et al: Clinical evaluation in autism spectrum disorders, in Handbook of Autism and Pervasive Developmental Disorders, Vol 2: Assessment, Interventions, Policy, 3rd Edition. Edited by Volkmar F, Paul R, Klin A, et al. Hoboken, NJ, Wiley, 2005, pp 772–798

Koegel L, Koegel R, Smith A: Variables related to differences in standardized test outcomes for children with autism. J Autism Dev Disord 27:233–243, 1997

Krug DA, Arick J, Almond P: Behavior checklist for identifying severely handicapped individuals with high levels of autistic behavior. J Child Psychol Psychiatry 21(3):221–229, 1980

Le Couteur A, Lord C, Rutter, M: The Autism Diagnostic Interview, Revised (ADI-R). Los Angeles, CA, Western Psychological Services, 2003

Lord C, Corsello C: Diagnostic instruments in autistic spectrum disorders, in Handbook of Autism and Pervasive Developmental Disorders, Volume 1: Diagnosis, Development, Neurobiology, and Behavior, 3rd Edition. Edited by Volkmar F, Paul R, Klin A, et al. Hoboken, NJ, Wiley, 2005, pp 730–771

Lord C, Volkmar F: Genetics of childhood disorders: XLII. Autism, part 1: diagnosis and assessment in autistic spectrum disorders. J Am Acad Child Adolesc Psychiatry 41:1134–1136, 2002

Lord C, Rutter M, DiLavore P, et al: Autism Diagnostic Observation Schedule. Los Angeles, CA, Western Psychological Services, 1999

Lord C, Risi S, Lambrecht L, et al: The Autism Diagnostic Observation Schedule–Generic: a standard measure of social and communication deficits associated with the spectrum of autism. J Autism Dev Disord 30:205–223, 2000

Martin NT, Bibby P, Mudford OC, et al: Toward the use of standardized assessment for young children with autism: current assessment practices in the UK. Autism 7:321–330, 2003

Matson JL, Rotatori AF, Helsel WJ: Development of a rating scale to measure social skills in children: the Matson Evaluation of Social Skills With Youngsters (MESSY). Behav Res Ther 21:335–340, 1983

Mayes SD, Calhoun SL: Analysis of WISC-III, Stanford-Binet IV, and academic achievement test scores in children with autism. J Autism Dev Disord 33:329–341, 2003

McDougle CJ, Scahill L, Aman MG, et al: Risperidone for the core symptom domains of autism: results from the study by the autism network of the Research Units on Pediatric Psychopharmacology. Am J Psychiatry 162:1142–1148, 2005

Mesibov GB, Schopler E, Schaffer B, et al: Adolescent and Adult Psychoeducational Profile (AAPEP), Volume 4. Austin, TX, Pro-Ed, 1988

Mullen EM: Mullen Scales of Early Learning: AGS Edition. Circle Pines, MN, American Guidance Service, 1995

National Research Council: Educating Children With Autism. Washington, DC, National Academy Press, 2001

Neisworth J, Bagnato S, Salvia J, et al: Temperament and Atypical Behavior Scale (TABS): Early Childhood Indicators of Developmental Dysfunction: TABS Assessment and Intervention Manual. Baltimore, MD, Paul H Brookes, 1999

O'Neill RE, Horner RH, Albin RW, et al: Functional Assessment and Program Development for Problem Behavior: A Practical Handbook, 2nd Edition. Pacific Grove, CA, Brooks/Cole, 1997

Ozonoff S, Goodlin-Jones BL, Solomon M: Evidence-based assessment of autism spectrum disorders in children and adolescents. J Clin Child Adolesc Psychol 34:523–540, 2005

Reynolds WM, Kamphaus RW: Behavior Assessment System for Children, II. Circle Pines, MN, American Guidance Service, 2004

Robins DL, Fein D, Barton et al: The Modified Checklist for Autism in Toddlers: an initial study investigating the early detection of autism and pervasive developmental disorders. J Autism Dev Disord 31:131–144, 2001

Rothbart MK, Ahadi SA, Hershey KL, et al: Investigations of temperament at three to seven years: the Children's Behavior Questionnaire. Child Dev 72:1394–1408, 2001

Rutter M, Bailey A, Berument SK, et al: Social Communication Questionnaire (SCQ) Manual. Los Angeles, CA, Western Psychological Services, 2003

Scahill L, Riddle MA, McSwiggin-Hardin M, et al: Children's Yale-Brown Obsessive Compulsive Scale: reliability and validity. J Am Acad Child Adolesc Psychiatry 36:844–852, 1997

Schatz J, Hamdan-Allen G: Effects of age and IQ on adaptive behavior domains for children with autism. J Autism Dev Disord 25:51–60, 1995

Schopler E, Reichler RJ, Renner BR: The Childhood Autism Rating Scale (CARS). Los Angeles, CA, Western Psychological Services, 1988

Schopler E, Lansing MD, Reichler RJ, et al: The Psychoeducational Profile, 3rd Edition. Austin, TX, Pro-Ed, 2005

Semel EM, Wiig, EH, Secord W: Clinical Evaluation of Language Fundamentals, 3rd Edition. San Antonio, TX, Psychological Corporation, 1995

Shaffer D, Gould MS, Brasic J, et al: Children's Global Assessment Scale (CGAS). Arch Gen Psychiatry 40:1225–1231, 1983

Siegel B: Pervasive Developmental Disorder Screening Test. San Antonio, TX, Harcourt Assessment, 2004

Sparrow S, Balla D, Cicchetti DV: Vineland Adaptive Behavior Scales. Circle Pines, MN, American Guidance Service, 1984

Sparrow S, Cicchetti DV, Balla D: Vineland Adaptive Behavior Scales, 2nd Edition. Circle Pines, MN, American Guidance Service, 2005

Stone WL, Coonrod EE, Pozdol SL, et al: The Parent Interview for Autism Clinical Version (PIA-CV): a measure of behavioral change for young children with autism. Autism 7:9–30, 2003

Stone WL, Coonrod EE, Turner LM, et al: Psychometric properties of the STAT for early autism screening. J Autism Dev Disord 34:691–701, 2004

Sundberg ML, Partington JW: The Assessment of Basic Language and Learning Skills (ABLLS). Pleasant Hill, CA, Behavioral Analysts, 1998

Thurm A, Lord C, Lee LC, et al: Predictors of language acquisition in preschool children with autism. J Autism Dev Disord 2006 Dec 19 [Epub ahead of print]

Venter A, Lord C, Schopler E: A follow-up study of high-functioning autistic children. J Child Psychol Psychiatry 33(3):489–507, 1992

Volkmar F, Cook EH Jr, Pomeroy J, et al: Practice parameters for the assessment and treatment of children, adolescents, and adults with autism and other pervasive developmental disorders. American Academy of Child and Adolescent Psychiatry Working Group on Quality Issues. J Am Acad Child Adolesc Psychiatry 38 (suppl 12):32S–54S, 1999 [erratum: J Am Acad Child Adolesc Psychiatry 39:938, 2000]

Volkmar FR, Lord C, Bailey A, et al: Autism and pervasive developmental disorders. J Child Psychol Psychiatry 45(1):135–170, 2004

Wagner A, Lecavalier L, Arnold LE, et al: Developmental disabilities modification of the Children's Global Assessment Scale. Biol Psychiatry 61(4):504–511, 2007

Wetherby A, Prizant B: Communication and Symbolic Behavior Scales Developmental Profile. Baltimore, MD, Paul H Brookes Publishing, 2002

Wetherby A, Woods J, Allen L, et al: Early indicators of autism spectrum disorders in the second year of life. J Autism Dev Disord 34:473–493, 2004

Williams KT: Expressive Vocabulary Test. Circle Pines, MN, American Guidance Service, 1997

Wing L, Leekam SR, Libby SJ, et al: The Diagnostic Interview for Social and Communication Disorders: background, inter-rater reliability, and clinical use. J Child Psychol Psychiatry 43:307–325, 2002

Zimmerman IL, Steiner VG, Pond RE: The Preschool Language Scale, 4th Edition. San Antonio, TX, Harcourt Assessment, 2003

Zwaigenbaum L, Bryson S, Rogers T, et al: Behavioral manifestations of autism in the first year of life. Int J Dev Neurosci 23:143–152, 2005

Zwaigenbaum L, Thurm A, Stone W, et al: Studying the emergence of autism spectrum disorders in high risk infants: methodological and practical issues. J Autism Dev Disord 2007 Aug 4 [Epub ahead of print]

Treatment of Autism With Selective Serotonin Reuptake Inhibitors and Other Antidepressants

Melissa L. Schapiro, B.A.S.

Stacey Wasserman, M.D.

Eric Hollander, M.D.

Antidepressant medications, particularly selective serotonin reuptake inhibitors (SSRIs), have been used for many years in the treatment of autism. These drugs can target core symptom domains by reducing repetitive preoccupations and perseverative behaviors, lessening social anxiety, and improving communication deficits, but they may cause adverse events such as increased motor

The work reported in this chapter is supported by funding from STAART Autism Center of Excellence Grant No. 5U54 MH06673–02, the Seaver Foundation, and U.S. Food and Drug Administration Grants FD-R-002026 and FD-R-001520.

activity, disinhibition, and mood disturbances. Also, certain SSRIs have not been shown to be effective in all populations. In this chapter we review antidepressant medications used to treat symptoms of autism, focusing particularly on the rationale for their use and clinical trials in autism.

Mechanism of Action

Selective Serotonin Reuptake Inhibitors

After the neurotransmitter serotonin (5-hydroxytryptamine [5-HT]) has been released by a presynaptic neuron, the serotonin transporter (SERT) is the primary mechanism for removing 5-HT from the synapse. The transporter terminates the synaptic activity of 5-HT and recycles it for later reuse (Stahl 1998). SSRIs work by blocking reuptake of 5-HT into the presynaptic nerve terminal, thus increasing the availability of 5-HT in the synapse. Because SSRIs all share the ability to block the SERT and alter 5-HT metabolism, the extent of reuptake blockade attained can be of critical importance and can affect the clinical response to SSRIs. However, it generally takes several weeks for many of the therapeutic effects of SSRIs to appear, which suggests that in addition to blocking the SERT, these medications also initiate neurobiological changes that result in delayed actions (Stahl 1998). For example, SSRIs appear to desensitize certain 5-HT receptors, which may mediate the effects of the receptor blockade (El Mansari and Blier 2006).

In addition, although the primary mechanism of action for all SSRIs relates to blockade of 5-HT reuptake, each has a characteristic profile that relates to effects outside the 5-HT system. Fluvoxamine has effects on σ_1 receptors (Narita et al. 1996), which are involved in dopamine regulation and modulation of N-methyl-D-aspartate receptors. Fluoxetine is a potent inhibitor of 5-HT$_{2C}$ receptors, which modulate noradrenergic and dopaminergic systems. Such actions may be associated with agitation and insomnia in anxious patients but may be of benefit in low-energy patients. Sertraline has significant dopamine uptake–blocking properties. Fluoxetine and sertraline have the highest dopamine D$_2$ receptor affinity among the SSRIs and have been reported in rare cases to induce extrapyramidal dysfunction. Citalopram is one of the most selective SSRIs. However, it has the highest affinity among SSRIs for the histamine H$_1$ receptor; this may make it more likely to cause weight gain. Escitalopram is the S-enantiomer of citalopram. Like citalopram, escitalopram has no affinity for norepinephrine or dopamine receptors but has some affinity for the H_1 receptor (Carrasco and Sandner 2005). In summary, SSRIs act by inhibiting the reuptake of 5-HT in the synaptic cleft and cause long-term changes in the 5-HT receptors, but each SSRI also has other characteristic pharmacological properties that may explain the variation in efficacy and side-effect profiles of this drug category.

Serotonin-Norepinephrine Reuptake Inhibitors

As the name implies, serotonin-norepinephrine reuptake inhibitors block the reuptake of both 5-HT and norepinephrine in the synaptic cleft. These drugs enhance norepinephrine and 5-HT neurotransmission but have little affinity for receptors mediating tricyclic-like side effects. However, venlafaxine, like tricyclic antidepressants, increases the responsiveness of α_1-adrenergic and dopaminergic (mainly D_3) systems and decreases the responsiveness of the 5-HT_2 system. Mirtazapine specifically enhances 5-HT_1 neurotransmission and blocks 5-HT_2 and 5-HT_3 receptors, but, in contrast to venlafaxine, lacks SSRI-like and adverse cardiovascular side effects (Gorman 1999).

Rationale for Use of Selective Serotonin Reuptake Inhibitors in the Treatment of Autism

Autistic individuals often demonstrate stereotyped motor behaviors, adherence to routines and rituals, and intense preoccupations with particular subjects or objects of interest. Repetitive behaviors and obsessive preoccupations can be so severe that they prevent the individual from participating in regular activities, interacting appropriately with others, and learning new skills. Coping with these behaviors is difficult not only for autistic individuals but also for their caregivers. Although researchers have little understanding of the causality and function of these behaviors, some have noted their similarity to the symptoms of obsessive-compulsive disorder (OCD).

OCD, which affects 2%–3% of people in the United States and in several other countries, is characterized by obsessions (persistent, intrusive thoughts) and/or compulsions (repetitive or ritualistic behaviors that the individual feels compelled to perform) that interfere with social and occupational functioning (Rasmussen and Eisen 1992). Although some OCD patients do not respond adequately to medication, serotonin reuptake inhibitors (SRIs), including SSRIs, are considered first-line treatments for this chronic and often disabling disorder. Double-blind, randomized, controlled studies have shown that these drugs are more effective than placebo in at least a subset of patients, whereas drugs lacking SRI actions are not (Fineberg and Gale 2005). However, there is little consensus on the role of serotonin in OCD or the mechanisms by which SRI drugs decrease obsessions and compulsions (Fineberg and Gale 2005).

There is considerable controversy related to the nature of repetitive behaviors across disorders. Still, individuals with OCD or autism employ certain rituals to maintain order and sameness and experience anxiety when their routines are disrupted. For this reason, exploring the effects of SRIs on the repetitive behavior domain in autism is warranted.

Early studies identified elevated blood levels of 5-HT in autistic individuals (Schain and Freedman 1961), and subsequent literature confirmed that up to 25%–30% of patients with autism have hyperserotonemia (Cook and Leventhal 1996). Researchers have employed a wide variety of methods, including neuroimaging and pharmacological challenges, to continue studying the effects of 5-HT on autistic symptoms. For example, McDougle et al. (1996b) found that adult patients with autism who underwent short-term reduction of tryptophan, a precursor of 5-HT, became less calm and happy and demonstrated overall worsening of autistic behavior with a significant increase in repetitive behaviors such as spinning, rocking, pacing, and hand flapping. Hollander et al. (2000b) found that growth hormone response to sumatriptan, a 5-HT$_{1D}$ receptor agonist, was significantly positively correlated with the severity of repetitive behaviors in autistic adults. In a neuroimaging study, Chugani et al. (1999) compared changes in brain serotonin synthesis capacity over time by using α-[^{11}C]methyl-L-tryptophan and positron emission tomography. They found a significant difference between the autistic and nonautistic groups, suggesting that the development of 5-HT synthesis capacity is disrupted in autistic individuals. Specifically for nonautistic children, 5-HT synthesis capacity is more than 200% of adult values until age 5 years, after which time it decreases toward adult levels. In contrast, children with autism seem to miss this peak in 5-HT synthesis capacity during the toddler years, and their 5-HT synthesis capacity increases slowly between ages 2–15 years to 1.5 times the normal adult values. This has specific implications for treatment of autistic patients under age 5 years.

Although the exact relationship between 5-HT mechanisms and the clinical features of autism has not yet been clearly defined, 5-HT plays a vital role in neurodevelopmental processes such as learning, motor function, and sensory perception, all of which are commonly altered in autistic individuals (Moore et al. 2004). 5-HT's importance in brain development is underscored by evidence that it not only functions as a neurotransmitter but also modulates synaptogenesis (Chugani 2002).

Given the extensive reports supporting abnormalities in the serotonergic system in autism and the results from pharmacogenetic studies using SSRIs, much effort has been made to study the contribution of genetic factors to the etiology of autism. It has been recognized that the pathogenesis of many developmental disorders, including autism, may involve the serotonin transporter gene (*SCL6A4*) (Murphy et al. 2004). This gene, which has short and long alleles, is considered a potential candidate gene for both autism and OCD (McCauley et al. 2004), but there is some debate over whether one of the alleles is more likely to be seen in autism. Cook et al. (1997) found preferential transmission of the short allele of the serotonin transporter gene in autistic individuals and their parents, whereas Klauck et al. (1997) discovered preferential transmission of the long allele of the gene. Of note, Tordjman et al. (2001) did not find that one particular gene variant conveyed an increased likelihood of developing autism; they did discover a correlation between gene variant and severity of autistic behavior, with greater transmission of the short allele in severely impaired individuals and greater transmission of the long allele in individuals with mild to moderate autism.

These data indicate that serotonin plays a role in a number of autism symptoms, with the strongest effects on the repetitive behavior domain. Thus, it follows that SSRIs may ameliorate repetitive, restricted, and ritualistic behaviors in autistic individuals of varying ages and that the study of these medications in this population is warranted.

Serotonin Reuptake Inhibitors: Clomipramine

Clomipramine is a tricyclic antidepressant (TCA) and SRI shown to be effective in disorders with difficult-to-treat repetitive behaviors, such as OCD, trichotillomania (hair pulling), and onychophagia (nail biting) (Leonard et al. 1991; Swedo et al. 1991). In the first controlled investigation of the effect of clomipramine on autistic symptoms, seven patients (6–18 years old) completed a 10-week, double-blind, crossover trial of clomipramine and desipramine, both TCAs (mean dosages of 129 mg/day and 111 mg/day, respectively), following a 2-week, single-blind placebo phase (Gordon et al. 1992). After treatment with clomipramine, subjects showed significant improvement not only in the repetitive and compulsive behaviors but also in other autistic symptoms, including anger and uncooperativeness. Hyperactivity was rated as improved in both drug groups. Side effects of clomipramine included mild sleep disturbance, dry mouth, constipation, and a minor tremor in one patient. Two patients taking desipramine discontinued it during the third week because of adverse behavioral effects.

Gordon et al. (1993) expanded this study to a double-blind comparison of clomipramine, desipramine, and placebo in 24 patients. Following a 2-week, single-blind placebo phase, 12 subjects completed a 10-week, double-blind, crossover comparison of clomipramine and placebo, whereas 12 other patients (including data from the seven patients in the previous pilot study) compared clomipramine and desipramine. The mean dosages at week 5 were 152 mg/day for clomipramine and 127 mg/day for desipramine. Clomipramine was shown to be superior to both desipramine and placebo in ratings of certain autistic symptoms, namely, stereotypies and compulsive, ritualized behavior. There were no differences between desipramine and placebo. Motor hyperactivity was reduced with both drugs but not with placebo. Two patients in the clomipramine group developed cardiac complications: prolongation of the QT interval on electrocardiogram in one patient, and severe tachycardia in the other. One patient taking clomipramine had a grand mal seizure.

In open-label studies of children, adolescents, and adults, clomipramine treatment had a positive effect on overall functioning, with a reduction of compulsive-like symptoms and stereotypies (Brasic et al. 1994; McDougle et al. 1992). These findings differ from those of clomipramine trials in younger children. In an open-label pilot study of seven children (3.5–8.7 years old), all were rated as unchanged compared with baseline at the completion of the study. Adverse events included urinary retention requiring catheterization, increased irritability, and aggression toward self and others (Sanchez et al. 1996). Similarly, five young children who were treated with clomipramine in an open-label trial initially responded but all discontinued the study because of serious adverse events, including serotonin syndrome, a dangerous condition resulting from serotonin excess (Brasic et al. 1998). Together, these studies indicate that clomipramine is effective, but safety issues suggest that it should not be a first-line treatment.

Selective Serotonin Reuptake Inhibitors

Since the use of TCA agents like clomipramine is associated with seizures and cardiotoxicity, many researchers and clinical practitioners have turned to SSRIs, which generally have a better side-effect profile. A number of studies have shown that SSRIs diminish repetitive and ritualistic behaviors and improve social relatedness and language usage, as well as global functioning, in autism. However, these studies have significant limitations, particularly reliance on small samples that include subjects from a broad age range. Study populations include autistic individuals with varying levels of disability, many with comorbid psychiatric disorders and many taking concomitant medications. Some studies follow subjects for only a short period of time, whereas others do not specify their evaluation tools. Despite these limitations, the body of evidence indicates that this class of antidepressants may be helpful to some autistic individuals.

Fluoxetine

Preliminary observations and case reports have shown that fluoxetine alleviates a number of autistic symptoms (Markowitz 1992). In an early case report by Mehlinger et al. (1990), fluoxetine (20 mg every other day) reduced ritualistic behaviors and stereotypies in a 26-year-old female autistic patient, but its efficacy in impaired speech and marked perseveration was unclear. Two case reports that followed described increased tolerance of routine changes but no improvements in language, cognitive, or social functioning (Koshes 1997; Todd 1991). Cook et al. (1992) examined the efficacy of fluoxetine in an open-label trial of 23 autistic children, adolescents, and adults (7–52 years old), as well as in 16 nonautistic patients with mental retardation. Dosages ranged from 20 mg every other day to 80 mg daily. Sixty-five percent of the autistic patients improved in the overall clinical severity of illness and perseverative or compulsive behaviors on Clinical Global Impression (CGI) ratings. Side effects included restlessness, hyperactivity, agitation, decreased appetite, and insomnia, which lessened after dosage reduction or discontinuation. The authors noted that side effects were more common in nonresponders than in responders.

In a retrospective chart review of seven patients (9–20 years old), fluoxetine at a mean dosage of 37.1 mg/day for 1.3–36 months led to significant benefits on four of the five subscales of the Aberrant Behavior Checklist (ABC; Aman et al. 1985), reducing irritability, stereotypy, inappropriate speech, and lethargy (Fatemi et al. 1998). However, it is worth noting that some of the patients received several other medications during the period of treatment with fluoxetine. Side effects reported were transient appetite suppression in two patients, chronic vivid dreams in another patient, and increased hyperactivity in four patients. Increased activity and worsening of hyperactivity were noted in the study as limiting factors for tolerability. Consistent with the previous study, this method and design would require the addition of a placebo control group and blind raters to lessen the chance of bias and expand the assessment of clinical improvement (Hollander et al. 2004).

In a larger open-label study of 37 children (2–7 years old) treated with fluoxetine (doses and titration schedule not reported), 11 of the children had an excellent response on nonstandardized outcome measures: they demonstrated appropriate, responsive language; interacted socially; and had more normal movements (DeLong et al. 1998). Eleven other children had less of a response but still showed improvements in mood, social interaction, and language. The remaining 15 children showed no improvement and the medication was discontinued. The negative responses associated with fluoxetine treatment were hyperactivity, agitation, aggression, and increased obsessive behavior, and the subjects experienced these side effects at different points throughout the study.

In a follow-up study, DeLong et al. (2002) extended the length of time for following the response to fluoxetine treatment to 5–76 months. Also, the sample was expanded to include 129 children (2–8 years old). The study indicated the efficacy of fluoxetine in improved social interaction and communication, a decrease in compulsive and repetitive behaviors, a decrease in problem behaviors, and improvement in global severity. As the authors expected from previous work, treatment response to fluoxetine was positively correlated with familial major affective disorder. Another notable finding was that the children who had an "excellent" or "good" response with fluoxetine treatment came from families with a higher incidence of unusual intellect, talent, or achievement. Tolerance to the drug varied and was limited by behavioral activation and/or irritability or agitation. One group tolerated approximately 8 mg/day, whereas another group tolerated larger dosages of 20 mg/day or 40 mg/day and showed increased response at the higher dosages. In this study, as with several mentioned here, increasing the dose of fluoxetine with the goal of improving social interaction and reducing repetitive behaviors increased the chance of side effects. Although this study supports the usefulness of fluoxetine in treating core symptoms in autism, its limitations include a lack of standardized evaluation tools, unspecified outcome measures, and no placebo control group.

There are few controlled studies with fluoxetine. Our group (Buchsbaum et al. 2001) reported on a 16-week, placebo-controlled, crossover trial of fluoxetine in six autistic adults with a mean age of 30 years. Although three out of the six patients were rated as improved on the CGI Improvement (CGI-I) scale (Guy 1976), all showed improvement on the obsession scale of the Yale-Brown Obsessive Compulsive Scale (Y-BOCS) (Goodman et al. 1989a, 1989b) and the Hamilton Anxiety Rating Scale (Hamilton 1959). We recently published a 20-week, double-blind, placebo-controlled crossover trial of low-dose liquid fluoxetine in 45 children and adolescents (5–16 years old) (Hollander et al. 2005). The study design included two randomized 8-week phases of fluoxetine versus placebo separated by a 4-week washout phase. Patients were free of psychiatric medications for at least 6 weeks prior to beginning the study and remained so throughout the study period. Fluoxetine was begun at a dosage of 2.5 mg/day for the first week, and the dosage was titrated for the next 2 weeks to a maximum of 0.8 mg/kg daily depending on response to treatment and side effects. The mean final total daily dose was 9.9 mg. The results of this trial demonstrated that fluoxetine significantly reduced repetitive behaviors in children and adolescents with autism as measured by the Y-BOCS. In addition, fluoxetine was superior to placebo on the CGI-I, a global composite autism measure that combined the amount of reduction in repetitive behaviors with the overall clinical improvement. When we analyzed the CGI-I scores for improvement of global autism separately, no difference was found between fluoxetine and placebo. However, the CGI-I measure places particular emphasis on social and communication domains, which are less likely to show improvement over an 8-week period than our core target symptom of repetitive behaviors. Overall, fluoxetine was well tolerated; side effects such as diarrhea, weight gain, insomnia, and anxiety were reported more frequently in the fluoxetine group, but they were not severe and were not statistically significant when compared with the placebo group. A total of nine patients required dosage reduction because of activation while taking fluoxetine or placebo: six while taking fluoxetine, two while taking placebo, and one patient in both phases. In addition, the only subject who reported suicidal ideation experienced this effect throughout the entire length of the study, and he had received placebo in the first phase of the study. Accordingly, the frequency and severity of side effects did not reach statistical significance. These data provide an important contribution to the body of research on SSRI treatment of autism and may help guide therapeutic choices in the future.

We recently completed the first double-blind, placebo-controlled fluoxetine trial in adults with autism (E. Hollander, L. Soorya, E. Anagnostou, et al., "Double-Blind Placebo-Controlled Trial of Fluoxetine in Adults With Autism Spectrum Disorders," manuscript in preparation, 2007). During the 12-week study of fluoxetine and placebo, we narrowed our inclusion criteria to adults with a high level of repetitive behavior, as measured by a Y-BOCS score at baseline of 10 or greater on the sum of items 1a5 of the Compulsions subscale. We are looking forward to reporting a successful outcome.

In conclusion, the available evidence suggests that fluoxetine is an efficacious and reasonably well-tolerated treatment for improving repetitive behaviors and global severity in autistic children.

Fluvoxamine

The first placebo-controlled, double-blind study of fluvoxamine in the treatment of adults with autism was a 12-week trial with 30 adults (18–53 years old) (McDougle et al. 1996a). The starting dosage was 50 mg/day, with increases in dosage of 50 mg/day every 3–4 days without exceeding 300 mg/day. The results showed improvements in repetitive thoughts and behavior as measured by the Y-BOCS, reduced aggression as measured by the Brown Aggression Scale (Brown et al. 1996), and increased adaptive functioning as measured by the Vineland Adaptive Behavior Scales (Sparrow et al. 1984). In addition, fluvoxamine was effective in improving social relatedness, particularly language usage, as assessed with the Ritvo-Freeman Real Life Rating Scale (R-F RLRS) (Freeman et al. 1986). Fluvoxamine was well tolerated, with the exception of moderate sedation in two patients and nausea in three patients. These side effects were transient and did not require discontinuation from the study.

On the basis of these positive results, McDougle et al. (2000) conducted a placebo-controlled, double-blind study in 34 children and adolescents (5–18 years old) with autism. They did not find benefits similar to the ones in the adult sample, with the exception of one child who demonstrated improvement. Three patients experienced behavioral activation and discontinued the treatment.

A 10-week open-label study by Martin et al. (2003) in 18 children and adolescents (7–18 years old) assessed the efficacy and tolerability of fluvoxamine, particularly when lower doses and a slower titration were used. Although no significant changes were seen in obsessive-compulsive symptoms or in anxiety-related symptoms in the group overall, eight children (including all four of the females) responded to treatment. The most frequently reported side effects were akathisia, agitation, and sleep difficulties (waking from sleep in the middle of the night), which were all tolerable. However, four subjects experienced behavioral activation that was so severe and persistent even after the dose was lowered that three of the four discontinued the medication. Martin and colleagues also evaluated changes in the level of platelet serotonin, comparing baseline levels with levels at weeks 6 and 10, to determine whether this measurement was associated with each subject's behavioral response. Platelet 5-HT levels have been widely used to assess the degree of SERT blockade in response to SSRIs (Epperson et al. 2001; Muck-Seler et al. 1991; Narayan et al. 1998). In the study by Martin and colleagues, the three full responders all had greater than 90% decline in their 5-HT levels, suggesting that the more robust response requires extensive blockade.

In summary, the evidence supporting the efficacy of fluvoxamine is mixed. Fluvoxamine appears to reduce repetitive thoughts and behaviors in autistic adults, but studies of child and adolescent subjects do not show such promising results. The lack of significant improvement seen in children suggests that the clinical benefits of fluvoxamine may not outweigh the risk of negative effects.

Paroxetine

The SSRI paroxetine has not been well studied in the treatment of autism. Snead et al. (1994) reported that paroxetine was effective in the treatment of self-injurious behavior and anxiety in a 15-year-old male with autism. A later case report by Posey et al. (1999) described the treatment of a 7-year-old male with autism. The researchers found that paroxetine 10 mg/day reduced irritability and preoccupations and improved mood and sleep with no adverse effects.

However, when the dosage was increased to 15 mg/day, the patient developed agitation and insomnia. To date, there have been no larger studies of paroxetine in the treatment of autism.

Citalopram

Namerow et al. (2003) conducted a retrospective chart review of 15 children and adolescents (6–16 years old) with pervasive developmental disorders (PDDs) who were treated with citalopram for 14 to 624 days (mean = 218.8 days). Improvement was measured on the CGI-I. In 10 of the 15 patients, the symptoms that were most responsive to citalopram were those associated with stereotyped patterns of behavior and preoccupation with nonfunctional routines. Seven of the 15 patients showed significant improvement in mood lability, aggression, and irritability. The authors noted that 9 of 10 patients had not responded to prior treatment with other SSRIs. The duration of treatment, but not the amount of citalopram, was correlated positively to response. Only mild side effects, including headaches, sedation, aggression, agitation, and lip dyskinesia, were experienced by five of the patients. Despite the limitations of the study, including an uncontrolled design, the inclusion of patients taking concurrent medications, and a lack of symptom-specific rating scales, the findings indicate that citalopram may be efficacious in the treatment of symptoms associated with autistic disorder. The favorable drug–drug interaction profile suggests a potential advantage of citalopram when used with concomitant psychotropic medications.

Our ongoing multisite study of citalopram (National Institutes of Health [NIH] Studies to Advance Autism Research and Treatment [STAART] Network) is a double-blind, placebo-controlled trial of the efficacy of citalopram in the treatment of children and adolescents (5–17 years old) with autism who demonstrate a high level of repetitive behaviors. This study involves two phases. In Phase 1, subjects are randomly assigned to either the citalopram or placebo group and receive their assigned treatment for 12 weeks. In Phase 2, subjects who show a positive response to citalopram or placebo remain blind to the treatment condition and continue with their assigned treatment for an additional 16 weeks, whereas subjects who fail to respond to placebo in Phase 1 can elect to receive 12 weeks of open-label citalopram treatment. In addition to examining the efficacy of citalopram on autistic behavior, this study intends to evaluate whole blood 5-HT levels and examine the correlation of 5-HT levels with therapeutic response, as well as to gather data on the pharmacogenetics of the children and their families.

Escitalopram

Owley et al. (2005) reported on a clinical trial assessing the safety and efficacy of escitalopram in the treatment of PDDs with a focus on improvements in global severity and irritability. Similar to the citalopram study, this open-label trial demonstrated significant improvement in global functioning on the CGI-I. An added beneficial finding was that 17 of the 28 children were reported to be less irritable on the ABC–Community Version (ABC-CV) Irritability subscale. This study consisted of a forced titration of escitalopram, but the dose was reduced if side effects were noted, as occurred in 18 of the 28 children. The common side effects in the 18 subjects were irritability and hyperactivity. The other 5 children experienced no side effects at the highest dosage (20 mg/day). Fortunately, no suicidal ideation, self-injurious behavior, or sleep disturbances were reported. These positive results warrant further study of escitalopram in children and adults with autism.

Sertraline

To date, only open-label studies of sertraline have been reported. The first of these, by Hellings et al. (1996), examined sertraline treatment in nine mentally retarded adults, five of whom had autistic disorder and other psychiatric comorbidities, including OCD, impulse-control disorders, mood disorder, or psychosis not otherwise specified. The dosage varied from 25 mg/day to 150 mg/day, based on clinical improvement. In eight of the nine patients, there was significant improvement in self-injurious behavior and aggression as measured on the CGI-I. The efficacy of sertraline on compulsive behavior was not studied. Side effects were not reported, aside from worsening skin-picking behavior and increasing agitation in one patient, who subsequently discontinued the medication.

Another case series of sertraline at low doses (25–50 mg/day) reported significant improvement in transition-associated behavioral symptoms in eight of nine children (6–12 years old) with autism (Steingard et al. 1997). Three of the patients showed an initial clinical response, but no additional improvement was observed in the 3–7 months that followed, so sertraline was discontinued. However, six patients maintained the positive progress throughout the follow-up period of several months. Side effects included stomachaches in one child and worsening behavioral symptoms in two children, which occurred when the dosage was increased to 75 mg/day, with the symptoms improving when the dosage was decreased. On the basis of the dose-related adverse behavioral changes in this study and others, smaller doses of sertraline may be optimal for safety and tolerability while still being effective.

The last of the trials to examine the efficacy of sertraline in adults with PDDs (McDougle et al. 1998) was based on the CGI-I, although a number of other behavior rating scales were used as well. The authors found that 24 of the 42 adult subjects were classified as much improved or improved on CGI-I and aggression was decreased. However, there were no statistically significant changes in social or language skills. The adults with autism had more significant responses to sertraline than the adults with Asperger's syndrome or PDD not otherwise specified (PDDNOS). This could in part be caused by the lower functioning of this group at baseline, which gave rise to greater therapeutic response.

Despite the paucity of research on sertraline in autism, open-label studies appear to have found some positive results. These studies should be repeated with a placebo-controlled design to further evaluate the efficacy of this drug.

Serotonin-Norepinephrine Reuptake Inhibitors

Venlafaxine

At low doses, venlafaxine, a mixed serotonin-norepinephrine reuptake inhibitor, was shown to improve repetitive behaviors and restricted interests in children and young adults with autism (Hollander et al. 2000a). This study was limited by its retrospective open-label design, but it did indicate the potential efficacy of venlafaxine.

Mirtazapine

A study on mirtazapine, an antidepressant with both noradrenergic and serotonergic properties, was conducted with an open-label design to evaluate the drug's efficacy and tolerability (Posey et al. 2001). It included 26 subjects (3.8–23.5 years old) with PDDs, 20 of whom had comorbid mental retardation and 17 of whom were taking concomitant psychotropic medications. Improvement was based on the CGI-I and the ABC. The authors noted improvement in a variety of symptoms, including aggression, self-injury, irritability, and hyperactivity, but this improvement was not statistically significant. Also, mirtazapine did not improve social and communication abilities. Three subjects had significant weight gain, but most side effects were transient or mild in severity, and included irritability, sedation, and increased appetite.

Conclusions and Future Directions

Psychopharmacological treatment studies of SSRIs have contributed clinical information that may be useful for dealing with some of the problem behaviors that can interfere with autistic individuals' quality of life. The majority of the studies presented here demonstrate significant improvements in autistic symptomatology, with an emphasis on the compulsive and repetitive behaviors. Unsurprisingly, SSRIs seem to be less effective in treating core symptoms in the areas of language development and social skills than they are in treating repetitive behaviors and transition-related anxiety; these latter symptoms are similar to those seen in OCD, for which SSRI treatment has long been shown to be effective. Some studies have noted improvements in overall global functioning, which may be a direct effect of the medication or a result of the reduction in repetitive behaviors, which allows better functioning across educational and therapeutic settings, with increased learning and participation in activities. Future studies of SSRIs in autism treatment could aim to evaluate the precise impact of these drugs on the social and communication domains.

In addition to efficacy, it is essential to consider the safety and tolerability of these medications (Table 3–1), particularly those used in children. SSRIs generally have a better side-effect profile than clomipramine, but not every patient can tolerate them, and not every patient has enough of a positive response to justify even mild to moderate side effects. Negative effects like activation, hyperactivity, and sleep disturbances are of particular concern in autistic individuals because these individuals may already suffer from a number of behavioral problems. Future studies with or without a placebo control group should monitor side effects in a systematic fashion to ascertain which of the SSRIs might be expected to cause specific side effects in specific populations.

Although the growing number of reports in the literature is encouraging, it is difficult to compare these studies because many are small and uncontrolled, and the subject populations, targeted symptoms, and outcome measures vary widely (Table 3–2). This area of clinical research would benefit tremendously

Table 3–1.   Dosing recommendations and common side effects of selective serotonin reuptake inhibitors (SSRIs) and other antidepressants

Medication	Dosing recommendations	Common side effects	Evidence
Selective serotonin reuptake inhibitors			
Citalopram, escitalopram	Children <40 kg (oral solution): Start with 2.5 mg daily for the first 2 weeks. If no side effects are observed, increase to 5 mg daily for 2 weeks. Increase by 2.5 mg increments to a maximum daily dose of 20 mg. Children >40 kg (oral solution): Start with 2.5 mg daily for the first week. Increase to 5.0 mg daily for the next week. Increase by 2.5 mg increments to a maximum daily dose of 20 mg. Adults: Start with 10 mg daily for the first week. Increase to 20 mg daily for the second week and thereafter. Maximum dose 20–40 mg depending on efficacy and side effects.	Decreased appetite, insomnia, agitation, hyperactivity, restlessness, disinhibition, dry mouth, headache, polyuria, sexual dysfunction, irritability	Child: ++
Fluoxetine	Adults: Start with 10 mg daily for the first week. Increase to 20 mg daily for the second week. Thereafter increase by 20 mg/day weekly to a maximum dosage of 80 mg daily. Children (oral solution): Start with 2.5 mg daily for the first week. Increase by 2.5 mg daily every week while continuing to monitor efficacy and side effects to a maximum dosage of 0.8 mg/kg per day or 20 mg/day.	Decreased appetite, insomnia, agitation, hyperactivity, restlessness, disinhibition, dry mouth, headache, polyuria, sexual dysfunction, irritability	Child: +++

Table 3–1. Dosing recommendations and common side effects of selective serotonin reuptake inhibitors (SSRIs) and other antidepressants (*continued*)

Medication	Dosing recommendations	Common side effects	Evidence
Selective serotonin reuptake inhibitors (*continued*)			
Fluvoxamine	Adults: Start with 50 mg daily. Increase by 50 mg daily every 3–4 days as tolerated, to a maximum dosage of 300 mg daily. Children <40 kg: Start with 12.5 mg daily. Increase by 12.5 mg daily every week to a maximum dosage of 1.5 mg/kg per day. Children >40 kg: Start with 25 mg daily. Increase by 25 mg daily every week to a maximum dosage of 1.5 mg/kg per day.	Decreased appetite, insomnia, agitation, hyperactivity, restlessness, disinhibition, dry mouth, headache, polyuria, sexual dysfunction, irritability	Adult: +++
Sertraline	Adults: Start with 50 mg daily for the first week. Increase by 50 mg daily every week to a maximum dosage of 150–200 mg based on clinical response and side effects. Children: Start with 25 mg daily for the first week. Increase by 25 mg daily every 7–10 days to a maximum dosage of 50–100 mg/day.	Decreased appetite, insomnia, agitation, hyperactivity, restlessness, disinhibition, dry mouth, headache, polyuria, sexual dysfunction, irritability	Adult: ++ Child: ++
Serotonin reuptake inhibitor			
Clomipramine	Adults: Start with 25 mg daily. Increase by 25 mg daily every 4–5 days to a maximum dosage of 150–200 mg/day. Children: Start with 25 mg daily for the first week. Increase by 25 mg daily every 4–5 days to a maximum dosage of 3–5 mg/kg per day or 250 mg/day.	Increased aggression, increased irritability, sedation, ECG changes, urinary retention	Adult: +++ Child: ++

Table 3–1. Dosing recommendations and common side effects of selective serotonin reuptake inhibitors (SSRIs) and other antidepressants *(continued)*

Medication	Dosing recommendations	Common side effects	Evidence
Serotonin-norepinephrine reuptake inhibitors			
Mirtazapine	Start with 7.5 mg daily. Increase by 7.5 mg daily every 1–2 weeks to a maximum dosage of 45 mg daily, depending on improvement of target symptoms and tolerability.	Increased appetite, weight gain, irritability	Adult: ++ Child: ++
Venlafaxine	Start with 12.5 mg daily. Increase gradually in increments of 12.5 mg daily every week based on observed efficacy and tolerability. Maximum total daily dose: 25–50 mg.	Hyperactivity, irritability, aggression, agitation	Adult: + Child: +

Note. += chart reviews and clinical experience; ++= open-label data supporting use; +++= randomized controlled-trial supporting use. ECG= electrocardiogram.

from larger double-blind, placebo-controlled trials with patients selected for specific target symptoms and with outcome measures that accurately reflect improvement.

In addition to these research strategies, studies addressing gender- and age-related differences could be expanded further to clarify therapeutic management and help predict treatment response. Interestingly, Martin et al. (2003) reported that all of the female children included in their study responded to fluvoxamine, suggesting that it may be worthwhile to examine gender differences in treatment response. This would pose significant challenges for recruitment, given the predominance of males affected with autism, but it potentially could aid in establishing predictors of treatment outcome. Fluvoxamine has been shown to have significant efficacy in adults (McDougle et al. 1996a) but the results with this medication have generally been poor in children (Martin et al. 2003; McDougle et al. 1996a). Fluoxetine, citalopram, and escitalopram have been shown to be effective in children and adolescents with varied diagnoses, including autism, Asperger's disorder, and PDDNOS (Hollander et al. 2004; Namerow et al. 2003; Owley et al. 2005, respectively), but data on their effectiveness in adults currently are not available.

Although it is certainly possible that some of these psychiatric drugs would be more effective in children and adolescents than they are in adults because of the course of brain development, it would be worthwhile to examine this possibility in controlled studies. We look forward to reporting the data from our double-blind, placebo-controlled study of fluoxetine in adults with autism (E. Hollander, L. Soorya, E. Anagnostou, et al., "Double-Blind Placebo-Controlled Trial of Fluoxetine in Adults With Autism Spectrum Disorders," manuscript in preparation, 2007). Certainly, evidence that a drug is effective in autistic children and adolescents does not suggest that the drug would be ineffective in autistic adults. Because serotonin synthesis capacity changes with maturation (Chugani et al. 1999), conducting studies comparing prepubertal and postpubertal subjects could be valuable in determining the differences in efficacy of SSRIs in children and adolescents as compared with adults. A large placebo-controlled trial with toddlers and preschool-age children examining the effect of fluoxetine on global functioning is currently under way (NIH STAART Network). This study will also examine whether early treatment with fluoxetine alters the developmental trajectory of children with autism.

Table 3–2.   Studies of selective serotonin reuptake inhibitors (SSRIs) and other antidepressants in autism

Medication	Study	N (age range)	Methodology	Results (areas of improvement)	Side effects
Selective serotonin reuptake inhibitors					
Citalopram	Namerow et al. 2003	15 (6–16 years)	Retrospective chart review	10/15 significantly improved (CGI-I)	Aggression, agitation, headaches, sedation, lip dyskinesia
Escitalopram	Owley et al. 2005	28 (6–17 years)	10-week open-label, retrospective chart review	17/28 significantly improved (ABC-CV, CGI-I) decreased irritability	Irritability, hyperactivity
Fluoxetine	Cook et al. 1992	23 (7–52 years)	Open-label study	65% decreased perseverative/compulsive behaviors, overall clinical severity (CGI-I)	Restlessness, hyperactivity, agitation, decreased appetite, insomnia
	DeLong et al. 1998	37 (2–7 years)	13- to 33-month open-label study	22/37 improvement (languag, social skills; outcomes not described)	Hyperactivity, aggression, increased obsessive behavior

Table 3–2. Studies of selective serotonin reuptake inhibitors (SSRIs) and other antidepressants in autism *(continued)*

Medication	Study	N (age range)	Methodology	Results (areas of improvement)	Side effects
Fluoxetine *(continued)*	Fatemi et al. 1998	7 (9–20 years)	Retrospective chart review	3/7 (Lethargy subscale of ABC-CV)	Hyperactivity, agitation, depression, transient decreased appetite
	Buchsbaum et al. 2001	6 (adult)	16-week placebo-controlled, crossover trial	6/6 significant improvement (Y-BOCS-Obsessions, HARS), 3/6 much improved (CGI-I)	Not described
	DeLong et al. 2002	129 (2–8 years)	5- to 76-month open-label study with discontinuation trials	22/129 excellent response; 67/129 good response; 40/129 fair to poor response (outcome measures not described)	Irritability, agitation
	Hollander et al. 2005	45 (5–16 years)	20-week double-blind, placebo-controlled, crossover study	19/34 significant improvement (CGI-I); significantly decreased repetitive behaviors (Y-BOCS)	Side effects did not differ between fluoxetine and placebo

Table 3–2. Studies of selective serotonin reuptake inhibitors (SSRIs) and other antidepressants in autism *(continued)*

Medication	Study	N (age range)	Methodology	Results (areas of improvement)	Side effects
Selective serotonin reuptake inhibitors (continued)					
Fluvoxamine	McDougle et al. 1996a	30 (18–53 years)	12-week double-blind, placebo-controlled study	Improvement in repetitive thoughts and behaviors (Y-BOCS), decreased aggression (BAS), increased adaptive functioning (Vineland), increased social relatedness (R-F RLRS)	Moderate sedation and nausea
	McDougle et al. 2000	34 (5–18 years)	12-week double-blind, placebo-controlled study	No significant overall improvement (CGI-I)	Behavioral activation
	Martin et al. 2003	18 (7–18 years)	10-week open-label study	No significant overall improvement (CY-BOCS, CGI-I, SCARED)	Sleep difficulties, akathisia/agitation, headaches, decreased appetite, abdominal discomfort, rhinitis; severe behavioral activation (in 4 children)

Table 3–2. Studies of selective serotonin reuptake inhibitors (SSRIs) and other antidepressants in autism *(continued)*

Medication	Study	N (age range)	Methodology	Results (areas of improvement)	Side effects
Sertraline	Hellings et al. 1996	9 (adults)	Open-label study	8/9 decreased self-injurious behavior, aggression (CGI-I)	Agitation
	Steingard et al. 1997	9 (6–12 years)	3–7 month open-label study	6/9 decreased behavioral reactions to "need for sameness" (CGI-I)	Stomachache (one patient)
	McDougle et al. 1998	42 (18–39 years)	12-week open-label study	24/42 improvement (CGI-I); significant improvement (repetitive behaviors, aggression)	Weight gain, anxiety, agitation, headache, anorexia, alopecia, tinnitus

Table 3–2. Studies of selective serotonin reuptake inhibitors (SSRIs) and other antidepressants in autism (*continued*)

Medication	Study	N (age range)	Methodology	Results (areas of improvement)	Side effects
Serotonin reuptake inhibitor					
Clomipramine	Gordon et al. 1992	7 (6–18 years)	10-week double-blind, crossover study of clomipramine and desipramine	Significant improvement for repetitive and compulsive behaviors (modified NIMH OCD scale, CGI-I, autism relevant subscale of CPRS)	Mild sleep disturbance, dry mouth, constipation, minor tremor
	Gordon et al. 1993	24 (6–23 years)	10-week double-blind, crossover study of clomipramine, desipramine, placebo	Decreased compulsive, ritualized behaviors and stereotypies, decreased hyperactivity (both drugs) (modified NIMH OCD scale, CGI-I, autism relevant subscale of CPRS)	Cardiac complications, grand mal seizure (one patient)
	Sanchez et al. 1996	7 (3.5–8.7 years)	5-week open-label study	No changes when compared with baseline (CGI-I)	Urinary retention; increased aggression, irritability, sedation

Table 3–2.   Studies of selective serotonin reuptake inhibitors (SSRIs) and other antidepressants in autism *(continued)*

Medication	Study	*N* (age range)	Methodology	Results (areas of improvement)	Side effects
Serotonin-norepinephrine reuptake inhibitors					
Mirtazapine	Posey et al. 2001	26 (3.8–23.5 years)	4-week to 1-year open-label study	9/26 improvement (CGI-I: aggression, self-injury, irritability, hyperactivity; ABC)	Increased appetite, irritability, transient sedation
Venlafaxine	Hollander et al. 2000a	10 (3–21 years)	Retrospective chart review	6/10 improvement (CGI-I)	Hyperactivity, irritability, restlessness, aggression, inattention, nausea

Note.   ABC-CV = Aberrant Behavior Checklist–Community Version; BAS = Brown Aggression Scale; CGI = Clinical Global Impression; CGI-I = Clinical Global Impression–Improvement; CPRS = Children's Psychiatric Rating Scale; CY-BOCS = Children's Yale-Brown Obsessive Compulsive Scale; HARS = Hamilton Anxiety Rating Scale; NIMH OCD = National Institute of Mental Health obsessive-compulsive disorder; R-F RLRS = Ritvo-Freeman Real-Life Rating Scale; SCARED = Screen for Child Anxiety Related Emotional Disorders; TCA = tricyclic antidepressant; Vineland = Vineland Adaptive Behavior Scales; Y-BOCS = Yale-Brown Obsessive Compulsive Scale.

In conclusion, research shows that antidepressants can be efficacious in reducing symptoms of autism, particularly repetitive and stereotyped behaviors, but antidepressant treatment alone does not offer a complete solution to the complex puzzle of autism. Physicians may consider including these drugs in a comprehensive treatment plan along with behavioral and educational interventions.

References

Aman MG, Singh NN, Stewart AW, et al: The Aberrant Behavior Checklist: a behavior rating scale for the assessment of treatment effects. Am J Ment Defic 5:485–491, 1985

Brasic JR, Barnett JY, Kaplan D, et al: Clomipramine ameliorates adventitious movements and compulsions in prepubertal boys with autistic disorder and severe mental retardation. Neurology 44:1309–1312, 1994

Brasic JR, Barnett JY, Sheitman BB, et al: Behavioral effects of clomipramine on prepubertal boys with autistic disorder and severe mental retardation. CNS Spectr 3:39–46, 1998

Brown K, Atkins MS, Osborne ML, et al: A revised teacher rating scale for reactive and proactive aggression. J Abnorm Child Psychol 24:473–480, 1996

Buchsbaum MS, Hollander E, Haznedar MM, et al: Effect of fluoxetine on regional cerebral metabolism in autism spectrum disorders: a pilot study. Int J Neuropsychopharmacol 4:119–125, 2001

Carrasco JL, Sandner C: Clinical effects of pharmacological variations in selective serotonin reuptake inhibitors: an overview. Int J Clin Pract 59:1428–1434, 2005

Chugani DC: Role of altered brain serotonin mechanisms in autism. Mol Psychiatry 7S2:S16–S17, 2002

Chugani DC, Muzik O, Behen M, et al: Developmental changes in brain serotonin synthesis capacity in autistic and nonautistic children. Ann Neurol 45:287–295, 1999

Cook EH, Leventhal BL: The serotonin system in autism. Curr Opin Pediatr 8:348–354, 1996

Cook EH, Rowlett R, Jaselskis C, et al: Fluoxetine treatment of children and adults with autistic disorder and mental retardation. J Am Acad Child Adolesc Psychiatry 31:739–745, 1992

Cook EH, Courchesne R, Lord C, et al: Evidence of linkage between serotonin transporter and autism. Mol Psychiatry 2:247–250, 1997

DeLong GR, Teague LA, McSwain Kamran MM: Effects of fluoxetine treatment in young children with idiopathic autism. Dev Med Child Neurol 40:551–562, 1998

DeLong GR, Ritch CR, Burch S: Fluoxetine response in children with autistic spectrum disorders: correlation with familial major affective disorder and intellectual achievement. Dev Med Child Neurol 44:652–659, 2002

El Mansari M, Blier P: Mechanism of action of current and potential pharmacotherapies of obsessive-compulsive disorder. Prog Neuropsychopharmacol Biol Psychiatry 30:362–373, 2006

Epperson N, Czarkowski KA, Ward-O'Brien D, et al: Maternal sertraline treatment and serotonin transport in breast-feeding mother-infant pairs. Am J Psychiatry 158:1631–1637, 2001

Fatemi SH, Realmuto GM, Khan L, et al: Fluoxetine in treatment of adolescent patients with autism: a longitudinal open trial. J Autism Dev Disord 28:303–307, 1998

Fineberg NA, Gale TM: Evidence-based pharmacotherapy of obsessive-compulsive disorder. Int J Neuropsychopharmacol 8:107–129, 2005

Freeman BJ, Ritvo ER, Yakota A, et al: A scale for rating symptoms of patients with the syndrome of autism in real life. J Am Acad Child Adolesc Psychiatry 25:130–136, 1986

Goodman WK, Price L, Rasmussen S, et al: The Yale-Brown Obsessive Compulsive Scale. I. Development, use, and reliability. Arch Gen Psychiatry 46:1006–1011, 1989a

Goodman WK, Price L, Rasmussen S, et al: The Yale-Brown Obsessive Compulsive Scale. II. Validity. Arch Gen Psychiatry 46:1012–1016, 1989b

Gordon CT, Rapoport JL, Hamburger SD, et al: Differential response of seven subjects with autistic disorder to clomipramine and desipramine. Am J Psychiatry 149:363–366, 1992

Gordon CT, State RC, Nelson JE, et al: A double-blind comparison of clomipramine, desipramine, and placebo in the treatment of autistic disorder. Arch Gen Psychiatry 50:441–447, 1993

Gorman JM: Mirtazapine: clinical overview. J Clin Psychiatry 60 (suppl 17):9–13, 1999

Guy W: ECDEU assessment manual for psychopharmacology (NIMH Publ No 76–338). Rockville, MD, National Institute of Mental Health, 1976

Hamilton M: The assessment of anxiety states by rating. Br J Med Psychol 32:50–55, 1959

Hellings JA, Kelley LA, Gabrielli WF, et al: Sertraline response in adults with mental retardation and autistic disorder. J Clin Psychiatry 57:333–336, 1996

Hollander E, Kaplan A, Cartwright C, et al: Venlafaxine in children, adolescents, and young adults with autism spectrum disorders: an open retrospective clinical report. J Child Neurol 15:132–135, 2000a

Hollander E, Novotny S, Allen A, et al: The relationship between repetitive behaviors and growth hormone response to sumatriptan challenge in adult autistic disorder. Neuropsychopharmacology 22:163–167, 2000b

Hollander E, Phillips A, King BH, et al: Impact on recent findings on study design of future autism clinical trials. CNS Spectr 9:49–56, 2004

Hollander E, Phillips A, Chaplin W, et al: A placebo controlled crossover trial of liquid fluoxetine on repetitive behaviors in childhood and adolescent autism. Neuropsychopharmacology 30:582–589, 2005

Klauck SM, Poustka F, Benner A, et al: Serotonin transporter (5-HTT) gene variants associated with autism? Hum Mol Genet 6:2233–2238, 1997

Koshes RJ: Use of fluoxetine for obsessive-compulsive behavior in adults with autism. Am J Psychiatry 154:578, 1997

Leonard HL, Lenane MC, Swedo SE, et al: A double-blind comparison of clomipramine and desipramine treatment of severe onychophagia (nail biting). Arch Gen Psychiatry 48:821–827, 1991

Markowitz PI: Effect of fluoxetine on self-injurious behavior in the developmentally disabled: a preliminary study. J Clin Psychopharmacol 12:27–31, 1992

Martin A, Koenig K, Anderson GM, et al: Low-dose fluvoxamine treatment of children and adolescents with pervasive developmental disorders: a prospective, open-label study. J Autism Dev Disord 33:77–85, 2003

McCauley JL, Olson LM, Dowd M, et al: Linkage and association analysis at the serotonin transporter (SLC6A4) locus in a rigid-compulsive subset of autism. Am J Med Genet B Neuropsychiatr Genet 127:104–112, 2004

McDougle CJ, Price LH, Volkmar FR, et al: Clomipramine in autism: preliminary evidence of efficacy. J Am Acad Child Adolesc Psychiatry 31:746–750, 1992

McDougle CJ, Naylor S, Cohen D, et al: A double-blind, placebo-controlled study of fluvoxamine in adults with autistic disorder. Arch Gen Psychiatry 53:1001–1008, 1996a

McDougle CJ, Naylor ST, Cohen DJ, et al: Effects of tryptophan depletion in drug-free adults with autistic disorder. Arch Gen Psychiatry 53:993–1000, 1996b

McDougle CJ, Brodkin ES, Naylor ST, et al: Sertraline in adults with pervasive developmental disorders: a prospective open-label investigation. J Clin Psychopharmacol 18:62–66, 1998

McDougle CJ, Kresch LE, Posey DJ: Repetitive thoughts and behaviors in pervasive developmental disorders: treatment with serotonin reuptake inhibitors. J Autism Dev Disord 30:427–435, 2000

Mehlinger R, Scheftner WA, Poznanski E: Fluoxetine and autism. J Am Acad Child Adolesc Psychiatry 29:985, 1990

Moore ML, Eichner SF, Jones JR: Treating functional impairment of autism with selective serotonin-reuptake inhibitors. Ann Pharmacother 38:1515–1519, 2004

Muck-Seler D, Jakovljevic M, Deanovic Z: Effect of antidepressant treatment on platelet 5-HT content and relation to therapeutic outcome in unipolar depressive patients. J Affect Disord 23:157–164, 1991

Murphy DL, Lerner A, Rudnick G, et al: Serotonin transporter: gene, genetic disorders, and pharmacogenetics. Mol Interv 4:109–123, 2004

Namerow LB, Thomas P, Bostic JQ, et al: Use of citalopram in pervasive developmental disorders. J Dev Behav Pediatr 24:104–108, 2003

Narayan M, Anderson G, Cellar J, et al: Serotonin transporter-blocking properties of nefazodone assessed by measurement of platelet serotonin. J Clin Pychopharmacol 18:67–71, 1998

Narita N, Hashimoto K, Tomitaka S, et al: Interactions of selective serotonin reuptake inhibitors with subtypes of sigma receptors in rat brain. Eur J Pharmacol 307:117–119, 1996

Owley T, Walton L, Salt J, et al: An open-label trial of escitalopram in pervasive developmental disorders. J Am Acad Child Adolesc Psychiatry 44:343–348, 2005

Posey DI, Litwiller M, Koburn A, et al: Paroxetine in autism. J Am Acad Child Adolesc Psychiatry 38:111–112, 1999

Posey DJ, Guenin KD, Kohn AE, et al: A naturalistic open-label study of mirtazapine in autistic and other pervasive developmental disorders. J Child Adolesc Psychopharmacol 11:267–277, 2001

Rasmussen SA, Eisen JL: The epidemiology and differential diagnosis of obsessive compulsive disorder. J Clin Psychiatry 53S:4–10, 1992

Sanchez LE, Campbell M, Small AM, et al: A pilot study of clomipramine in young autistic children. J Am Acad Child Adolesc Psychiatry 35:537–544, 1996

Schain RJ, Freedman DX: Studies on 5-hydroxyindole metabolism in autistic and other mentally retarded children. J Pediatr 58:315–320, 1961

Schroeder SR, Rojahn J, Reese RM: Brief report: reliability and validity of instruments for assessing psychotropic medication effects on self-injurious behavior in mental retardation. J Autism Dev Disord 27:89–102, 1997

Snead RW, Boon F, Presberg J: Paroxetine for self-injurious behavior. J Am Acad Child Adolesc Psychiatry 33:909–910, 1994

Sparrow S, Balla D, Cicchetti DV: Vineland Adaptive Behavior Scales. Circle Pines, MN, American Guidance Service, 1984

Stahl S: Mechanism of action of serotonin selective reuptake inhibitors: serotonin receptors and pathways mediate therapeutic effects and side effects. J Affect Disord 51:215–235, 1998

Steingard RJ, Zimnitzky B, DeMaso DR, et al: Sertraline treatment of transition-associated anxiety and agitation in children with autistic disorder. J Child Adolesc Psychopharmacol 7:9–15, 1997

Swedo SE, Rapoport JL, Leonard HL, et al: Regional cerebral glucose metabolism of women with trichotillomania. Arch Gen Psychiatry 48:828–833, 1991

Todd RD: Fluoxetine in autism (letter). Am J Psychiatry 148:1089, 1991

Tordjman S, Gutknecht L, Carlier M, et al: Role of the serotonin transporter gene in the behavioral expression of autism. Mol Psychiatry 6:434–439, 2001

4

Treatment of Autism With Anticonvulsants and Mood Stabilizers

Evdokia Anagnostou, M.D.

Aaron Jason Fisher, B.A.

Eric Hollander, M.D.

Currently there are no approved medications for the treatment of core and associated symptoms in autism spectrum disorders (ASDs). Selective serotonin reuptake inhibitors (SSRIs) are widely used for the treatment or repetitive behaviors and anxiety, whereas atypical neuroleptics are used for the treatment of irritability and impulsive aggression. However, given the concerns related to weight gain and possible development of metabolic syndrome associated with atypical antipsychotic use, there is an urgency to identify other agents that may

Preparation of the chapter was supported with funding from STAART Autism Center of Excellence Grant No. 5U54 MH06673–02 and the Seaver Foundation.

be useful in the treatment of disruptive behaviors such as irritability, mood instability, and aggression, among other symptoms, in patients with autism. Mood-stabilizing anticonvulsants and other mood stabilizers are promising in that regard, given the high prevalence of comorbid epilepsy and affective disorders in patients with autism.

Comorbid Disorders in Autism

Epilepsy

Epilepsy frequently co-occurs in children and adolescents with autism. The prevalence of seizures in patients with autism varies from 5% to 38.3% in some studies (Tuchman and Rapin 2002). There seems to be a bimodal distribution, with a small peak before age 5 years and a larger peak in adolescence. The increase in risk of epilepsy in autism compared with the general population is primarily driven by the degree of mental retardation and receptive language deficits (Tuchman and Rapin 2002).

There is much controversy about whether the presence of epileptiform abnormalities even in the absence of seizures may contribute to cognitive and language deficits in patients with autism. First, the developing brain may be more susceptible to seizures and epileptiform abnormalities than the mature brain. In addition there is evidence that in certain circumstances epileptiform activity, even in the absence of seizures, may not be benign. *Transient cognitive impairment* is a term used to describe cognitive alterations associated with epileptiform discharges (Aarts et al. 1984). Investigators have demonstrated that up to 50% of patients with epileptiform discharges show cognitive impairment during simultaneous electrical discharges (Shewmon and Erwin 1988a, 1988b). In addition, focal spikes seem to disrupt functional abilities corresponding to the anatomical location of such spikes, such that right-sided discharges are associated with spatial memory deficits, and left-sided discharges are associated with errors in verbal tasks. However, it remains to be seen whether such subclinical epilepsy, thought to contribute to cognitive impairment, responds to treatment.

On the other hand, there exist at least two distinct syndromes in which epileptiform abnormalities are clearly associated with cognitive and behavioral changes and do respond to antiseizure medications. In *electrical status epilepticus during slow-wave sleep* (ESES), epileptiform activity is associated with a variety of cognitive and behavioral abnormalities, including language and motor regression, aggressiveness, deficits in social relatedness, emotional lability, anxiety, and autistic-like features, among others (Galanopoulou et al. 2000; McVicar et al. 2004). Treatment of this syndrome with adrenocorticotropic hormone and/or anticonvulsants leads to resolution of seizures and epileptiform abnormalities and improvement, although rarely complete, in the cognitive/behavioral syndrome (Tassinari et al. 2000). *Landau-Kleffner syndrome* (LKS) is a syndrome of auditory agnosia associated with focal and multifocal spikes or spike-and-wave discharges. LKS occurs in previously developmentally intact children as opposed to ESES, in which developmental abnormalities are often present before the syndrome presents. Seizures may or may not be present. In addition to the receptive language deficits, children with LKS may present with hyperkinesis, irritability, and attention deficits. A few children with LKS and autistic-like regression have been reported in the literature. Treatment with corticosteroids or anticonvulsants is usually successful in resolving seizures and epileptiform discharges provided that no obvious lesion is present, and these agents may improve language and cognitive deficits, although in less than half the patients studied (Beaumanoir 1992).

Language regression also occurs in approximately 30% of children with pervasive developmental disorders (Shinnar et al. 2001; Tuchman and Rapin 1997). Although the precise prevalence of epileptiform abnormalities in these children has been hard to estimate, given that overnight studies are difficult to carry out in this population, it has been suggested that 30%–40% of children with autism and language regression have epileptiform electroencephalograms (EEGs). There is considerable controversy as to whether *autistic regression with epileptiform EEG* (AREE) is on a continuum with LKS and ESES. It is clear that at least in the majority of cases, autism is not an epileptic encephalopathy. The seizures seem to be associated with mental retardation and receptive language deficits that are not universal in patients with autism, and most seizures occur in adolescence much after the onset of autism. Furthermore, it is not possible to clinically distinguish the patients with epileptiform EEGs from those with normal EEGs. It is much more likely that the seizures in AREE are a part of the underline pathophysiology (Tuchman and Rapin 2002). However, the question of whether treatment of subclinical epilepsy in patients with autism may improve some behavioral and cognitive outcomes has not been fully addressed. In addition, the existence of a rare distinct subgroup of children that may have an autistic-like regression secondary to a catastrophic epilepsy or continuous subclinical epileptiform discharges has not been studied.

Affective Disorders

Aggressive and irritable symptoms are main features of both ASDs and bipolar disorder, especially in children (Arnold et al. 2003; Geller et al. 2000). Up to 25% of adults with ASDs have a history of irritability (Allen et al. 2001). Higher functioning individuals with autism may present with symptoms that are mania-like, such as irritability, psychomotor agitation, excessive involvement with pleasurable activities without regard for consequences, labile mood, and grandiosity (Towbin et al. 2005). Elevated rates of affective disorders in first-degree relatives have been reported (Bolton et al. 1998; Piven and Palmer 1999; Sverd 2003), suggesting a possible genetic and neurobiological relation between ASDs and depression, and bipolar and anxiety disorders (DeLong 2004). If this relation does exist, then the use of mood-stabilizing anticonvulsants in this population makes intuitive sense.

Mechanism of Action of Anticonvulsants

Improvements in a variety of symptoms, including epileptic activity, mood instability, aggression, and irritability, have been reported with the use of anticonvulsants in patients with various disorders, including epilepsy, mood disorders, and chronic pain. The question is whether such a wide spectrum of activity is explained by hypothesizing a common pathophysiologic mechanism for these conditions or by assigning multiple modes of action to each of these drugs, or finally whether, considering the chronic nature of such conditions, we should be taking into consideration long-term neuronal molecular alterations caused by both the disease states and the drugs administered (Soderpalm 2002).

The proposed mechanism of action of anticonvulsants falls into three main categories: 1) functional blockade of voltage-sensitive sodium channels (phenytoin, carbamazepine, lamotrigine, valproate), 2) enhancement of inhibitory activity through γ-aminobutyric acid (GABA) (benzodiazepines and barbiturates, but also valproate, vigabatrin, and gabapentin), and 3) inhibition of excitatory glutamatergic transmission (phenobarbital, topiramate, lamotrigine). Several of the drugs mentioned previously could be included in more than one of these categories, and no single common mechanism of action is likely to explain the effect of anticonvulsants across different symptom domains and disorders. Neuronal inhibition, on the other hand, is a common secondary effect, although achieved through separate primary processes. This mechanism of action could explain why such different compounds are effective in such distinct conditions as epilepsy, neuropathic pain, and even mania. However, it cannot explain why it would prevent depressive episodes. In addition, although all anticonvulsants decrease neuronal activity, not all of them are effective against affective lability and irritability. One may need to think of possible common chronic changes to fully understand anticonvulsant effectiveness across such a wide spectrum of disorders. One phenomenon of interest is kindling. *Kindling* refers to a model of epileptogenesis in which intermittent subthreshold electrical stimulations result in the development of generalized seizures and ultimately spontaneous seizures. Kindling is considered to be a nonhomologous analog of psychiatric illness in which the same stimulus may result in progressively increasing physiologic responses (Soderpalm 2002).

From the previous observations, it is possible to hypothesize a role for anticonvulsants in patients with autism both by possibly treating subclinical epilepsy and, even more importantly, by affecting intracellular processes involved in kindling-like models that also may be important for affective instability and irritability/aggression.

Clinical Evidence for Anticonvulsant Efficacy in Autism

Not all anticonvulsant medications have been used in the treatment of patients with ASDs. Valproate, lamotrigine, levetiracetam, carbamazepine, and topiramate have appeared in the literature in association with autism (see Tables 4–1 and 4–2).

Valproate

Valproate is indicated for the treatment of partial or absence seizures and manic episodes associated with bipolar disorder, and for the prevention of migraine headaches. Its main mechanism of action remains unclear, but valproate has been reported to do all of the following (Baf et al. 1994; Costa et al. 2003; Loscher and Vetter 1985):

Table 4–1.   Side effects and recommended monitoring of anticonvulsants and mood stabilizers

Medication	Side effects	Recommended blood monitoring
Valproate	Irritability, restlessness, rash, headaches, weight gain, ataxia, alopecia, gastrointestinal disturbance, hyperammonemic encephalopathy, sedation, thrombocytopenia, polycystic ovarian syndrome, pancreatitis, liver failure, teratogenic effects	Complete blood count (CBC) with platelets, liver function tests (LFTs), valproate levels If there is a change in mental status, then ammonia testing is indicated Therapeutic blood levels: 50–120 μg/mL
Lamotrigine	Dizziness, ataxia, somnolence, headache, diplopia, blurred vision, nausea, vomiting, and rash (Stevens-Johnson syndrome).	None
Levetiracetam	Drowsiness, dizziness, weakness, headache, loss of coordination (e.g., difficulty walking, muscle control), agitation, disinhibition	None
Carbamazepine	Drowsiness, diplopia, headache, ataxia, nausea, vomiting, dizziness, abdominal pain, constipation, diarrhea, loss of appetite, serious rash, hyponatremia, agranulocytosis, hepatic dysfunction	CBC with platelets, LFTs, carbamazepine levels, Therapeutic blood levels: 5–12 μg/mL
Topiramate	Paresthesia, weight decrease, somnolence, anorexia, nausea, weakness, tiredness, drowsiness, dizziness, tingling sensations, dry mouth, constipation, and difficulty with memory	None

Table 4–2.   Target dosing of selected anticonvulsants and mood stabilizers

Medication	Target dosing[a]
Valproate	Children: Start at 125-mg sprinkles, titrate up to clinical efficacy and blood levels 50–120 μg/mL. Usual therapeutic dosage: 20–30 mg/kg/day. Adults: Start at 250 mg, increase by 250 mg/day weekly to clinical significance and blood levels of 50–120 μg/mL.
Lamotrigine[b]	Children: Start at 1 mg/kg/day bid, titrate up slowly to therapeutic effect. Usual maintenance dosage: 2.5–7.5 mg/kg bid. Adults: Start at 50 mg, increase by 50 mg/day weekly to therapeutic effect. Usual maintenance dosage: 150–250 mg bid.
Levetiracetam	Children: Start at 10 mg/kg bid. Increase by 5–10 mg/kg/day weekly to therapeutic effect. Usual maintenance dosage: 30 mg/kg bid. Adults: Start at 500 mg bid. Increase by 500 mg/day weekly to therapeutic effect. Usual maintenance dosage: 3,000 mg/day.
Carbamazepine	Children: Start at 10 mg/kg/day divided bid. Increase by 100 mg/day at weekly intervals until therapeutic effect and blood levels of 5–12 μg/mL. Adults: Start at 200 mg divided bid. Increase by 200 mg/day at weekly intervals until therapeutic effect and blood levels of 5–12 μg/mL.
Topiramate	Children: Start at 1–3 mg/kg/day (12.5–25 mg). Increase by 12.5–25 mg/day weekly to therapeutic effect. Usual maintenance dosage: 2.5–4.5 mg/kg bid. Adults: Start at 25 mg/day. Increase by 25–50 mg/day weekly to therapeutic effect. Usual maintenance dosage: 200 mg bid.

Note.   bid = two times daily.
[a]Patients with renal or liver insufficiency may need adjustment of dosage.
[b]Patients receiving valproate or other enzyme-inducing medication need appropriate adjustments to dosage.

- Potentiate GABA inhibitory effects in the central nervous system (CNS).
- Attenuate N-methyl-D-aspartate–mediated excitation.
- Likely block voltage-dependent sodium channels.
- Possibly influence the serotonin and norepinephrine systems.
- Possibly alter gene expression (*GAD67* and reelin [*RELN*]).

In addition, valproate has been shown to affect second-messenger systems. It decreases cyclic guanosine monophosphate (cGMP) in the cerebellum and increases it in the cortex (Loscher 1993), decreases protein kinase C (Manji et al. 1999), stimulates inositol mono- and biphosphates (Dixon and Hokin 1997), and decreases corticotropin-releasing factor (Stout et al. 2001), all mechanisms that may offer alternative explanations for the mood-stabilizing effect of the drug. Lastly, the drug seems to have some neuroprotective effects, including an increase of the cytoprotective protein Bcl-2 in the CNS (Manji and Chen 2000) and an increase in AP-1 transcription (Chen et al. 1999), which is responsible for the regulation of many cell proteins. Although multiple mechanisms of action have been reported, it is not clear which ones are responsible for the known therapeutic effects.

Evidence for Use in Autism

Multiple studies have demonstrated the efficacy of valproate in treating impulsivity, irritability, and aggression in various populations with psychiatric disorders (Hollander 1999; Hollander et al. 2002, 2003a, 2003b, 2005; Johnson et al. 2003; McElroy et al. 2004; Pallanti et al. 2002). An open-label trial of the efficacy of divalproex in treating ASDs demonstrated improvements in repetitive behaviors, social relatedness, aggression, and mood lability (Hollander et al. 2001). Of interest, all children with epileptiform EEGs in this study were classified as responders. A follow-up double-blind, placebo-controlled pilot study demonstrated efficacy in the treatment of repetitive behaviors (Hollander et al. 2006). In addition, a series of case reports and case series suggests that valproate may be effective in preventing/treating behavioral activation associated with SSRI use in ASDs (Anagnostou et al. 2006; Duggal et al. 2003). Ongoing controlled studies of valproate in autism seem promising for the treatment of irritability and aggression.

Lamotrigine

Lamotrigine is a broad-spectrum agent approved as an adjunctive treatment in adults with partial-onset seizures and for the treatment of generalized seizures associated with Lennox-Gastaut syndrome. In addition there is accumulating evidence to suggest that lamotrigine is an effective mood stabilizer, and multiple clinical trials have documented efficacy in the treatment of bipolar disorder.

The mechanism of action for lamotrigine is not entirely known. Lamotrigine is thought to do the following (Di Martino and Tuchman 2001; Hahn et al. 2004; Moshe et al. 2000; Otsuki et al. 1998; Southam et al. 1998; von Wegerer et al. 1997):

- Modulate ion channels (sodium and calcium), altering neuronal excitability.
- Inhibit the release of glutamate.
- Block serotonin and norepinephrine reuptake at high doses.
- Increase GABA concentrations.

Evidence for Use in Autism

In a large open-label study of lamotrigine in children with epilepsy and various comorbidities, improvements in social engagement, attention, and alertness were reported (Uvebrant and Bauziene 1994). In 8 of the 13 children with autism included in this cohort, improvements were noted in attention, eye contact, irritability, and emotional lability even when there was no improvement in seizures, suggesting a possible specific psychotropic mechanism of action. Similar improvements were noted in a case series of children with Rett's disorder (Uldall 1993). A follow-up double-blind, placebo-controlled trial in children with autistic disorder (Belsito et al. 2001) demonstrated no differences between the subjects who received lamotrigine versus those who received placebo on a variety of measures assessing irritability, hyperactivity, attention, and adaptive outcomes. However, the study was plagued by a very large and unusual placebo response rate. Within the active group, statistically significant improvements were noted in autism core and associated symptoms as measured by the Autism Behavior Checklist and the Aberrant Behavior Checklist. Thus, further larger scale placebo-controlled trials are needed in this area.

Levetiracetam

Levetiracetam is indicated as an adjunctive therapy for the treatment of partial-onset seizures in epileptic patients with or without secondary generalization and is also used for the treatment of myoclonic seizures. It is a novel anticonvulsant with unknown mechanism of action and is chemically unrelated to existing anticonvulsants (Rugino and Samsock 2002). Levetiracetam markedly suppresses kindling development at doses not associated with side effects, and suppression of kindled seizures has been shown to persist even after discontinuation of the medication (Klitgaard and Pitkanen 2003). It is the *S*-enantiomer of piracetam, which is known to be a cognitive enhancer (nootropic) and improves cognition, language, and memory in several neurological conditions including dyslexia and dementia (Genton and Van Vleymen 2000). Although animal models have indicated that levetiracetam may have a less impressive nootropic effect than piracetam, this compound still holds promise.

Evidence for Use in Autism

There has been only one published open-label study of levetiracetam in patients with ASDs (Rugino and Samsock 2002). In the 10 boys with ASD treated in the study, significant improvements were noted in hyperactivity and impulsivity, mood lability, and aggression. The medication was well tolerated. A preliminary trial by our group failed to document global improvement and efficacy in treatment of repetitive behaviors and aggression/irritability (Wasserman et al. 2006). Further randomized trials are needed to further explore any possible behavioral and nootropic effects of levetiracetam.

Topiramate

Topiramate is indicated as monotherapy and adjunctive therapy for the treatment of partial-onset seizures and primary generalized tonic-clonic seizures. It is also approved as a preventive treatment for migraines.

Topiramate is a sulfamate-substituted monosaccharide with multiple mechanisms of action (Guerrinni et al. 2005; Wauquier et al. 1996):

- Blocks voltage-sensitive sodium channels.
- Potentiates $GABA_A$-evoked chloride flux.
- Blocks kainate/2-(α-amino-3-hydroxy-5-methylisoxazole-4-propionic acid (AMPA) glutamate receptors.

- Reduces L-type calcium channel activity.
- Inhibits carbonic anhydrase.

Evidence for Use in Autism

On the basis of an observation that children with epilepsy treated with topiramate lose weight, an open-label study of topiramate in autism was conducted to assess its efficacy in weight reduction in children who had psychotropic medication-induced weight gain (Canitano 2005). Significant weight loss was reported in 2 of 10 children, suggesting that it may be one option for weight control for some children with ASDs and psychotropic-induced weight gain. However, the medication was stopped in three children because of side effects, including agitation, irritability, and hyperactivity. For this reason, and because of cognitive impairments noted in association with this medication in other populations, caution is indicated when prescribing this medication. Larger controlled studies may be of use.

Carbamazepine

Carbamazepine is used for the treatment of simple and complex partial seizures, trigeminal neuralgia, and bipolar affective disorder. As with most other anticonvulsants, the mechanism of action of carbamazepine responsible for its antiepileptic, analgesic, and mood-stabilizing effects is not clear, but its mechanisms of action are as follows (Di Martino and Tuchman 2001; Meldrum 1996; Okada et al. 1998):

- Blocks voltage-sensitive sodium channels.
- Has a bimodal effect on serotonin hippocampal levels.
- Increases GABA receptors in the hippocampus and cortex.

Evidence for Use in Autism

Despite fairly widespread clinical use, there are no studies for the use of carbamazepine in autism. There is, however, a case report of a 20-year-old male with documented normal EEG prior to initiation of carbamazepine who developed generalized tonic-clonic seizures after administration of carbamazepine to treat aggression. Given that there is evidence that several anticonvulsants, especially carbamazepine, may induce or precipitate seizures (Guerrini et al. 1998;

Monji et al. 2004; Yang et al. 2003), caution is indicated when prescribing it to treat behavioral disturbance.

Nonanticonvulsant Mood Stabilizers: Lithium

Lithium carbonate is indicated in the treatment of manic episodes and prevention of subsequent manic and depressive episodes. The specific mechanism of action responsible for its mood-stabilizing effects is unclear, but preclinical studies have shown that lithium does the following:

- Alters sodium transport in nerve and muscle cells.
- Decreases glutamatergic activity.
- Modulates signals affecting the cytoskeleton, contributing to neural plasticity involved in mood recovery and stabilization.
- Adjusts signaling activities regulating second messengers, transcription factors, and gene expression.

The outcome of these effects appears likely to result in limiting fluctuations in activity, contributing to a stabilizing influence and neuroprotective effects.

Evidence for Use in Autism

There are no controlled studies of lithium in patients with autism. A case report of two young children with autism and family history of bipolar disorder treated with lithium noted improvements in aggression and irritability and also in language and social skills (Kerbeshian et al. 1987). In another case report of a child and an adult with autism and comorbid mania-like symptoms, improvements in emotional lability were documented (Steingard and Biederman 1987). Lastly, there have been a series of studies of lithium in developmentally delayed or behaviorally disturbed children. Improvements in aggression and irritability consistently have been reported (Craft et al. 1987; Tyler et al. 1984). However, controlled studies in this area are lacking.

Conclusions

There are several theoretical reasons why anticonvulsants may be useful in the treatment of the symptoms of ASDs. These include the high frequency of epileptiform abnormalities in autism, and the symptoms of affective instability/

irritability, as well as possible phenomena analogous to kindling associated with behavioral disturbances in patients with autism. Data from early pilot studies are very promising. However, large well-controlled studies are required to determine which anticonvulsants are most efficacious and best tolerated in this population. In addition, extensive research is required to further clarify the relationship between epileptiform abnormalities, cognitive function, and ASDs, as well as the role of kindling and possibly other chronic neuronal alterations secondary to the disorder or the medications administered in children and adults with ASDs.

References

Aarts J, Binnie C, Smit A, et al: Selective cognitive impairment during focal and generalized epileptiform EEG activity. Brain 107:293–308, 1984

Allen DA, Steinberg M, Dunn M, et al: Autistic disorder versus other pervasive developmental disorders in young children: same or different? Eur Child Adolesc Psychiatry 10:67–78, 2001

Anagnostou E, Esposito K, Soorya L, et al: Divalproex versus placebo for the prevention of irritability associated with fluoxetine treatment in autism spectrum disorder. J Clin Psychopharmacol 26:444–446, 2006

Arnold LE, Vitiello B, McDougle C, et al: Parent defined target symptoms respond to risperidone in RUPP autism study: customer approach to clinical trials. J Am Acad Child Adolesc Psychiatry 42:1443–1450, 2003

Baf MH, Subhash MN, Lakshmana KM, et al: Sodium valproate induced alterations in monoamine levels in different regions of the rat brain. Neurochem Int 24:67–72, 1994

Beaumanoir A: The Landau-Kleffner syndrome, in Epileptic Syndromes in Infancy, Childhood, and Adolescence, 2nd Edition. Edited by Roger J, Bureau M, Dravet C. London, John Libby, 1992, pp 231–243

Belsito KM, Law PA, Kirk KS, et al: Lamotrigine therapy for autistic disorder: a randomized, double-blind, placebo-controlled trial. J Autism Dev Disord 31:175–181, 2001

Bolton PF, Pickles A, Murphy M, et al: Autism, affective, and other psychiatric disorders: patterns of familial aggregation. Psychol Med 28:385–395, 1998

Canitano R: Clinical experience with topiramate to counteract neuroleptic induced weight gain in 10 individuals with autistic spectrum disorders. Brain Dev 27:228–232, 2005

Chen G, Huang LD, Jiang YM, et al: The mood-stabilizing agent valproate inhibits the activity of glycogen synthase kinase-3. J Neurochem 72:1327–1330, 1999

Costa E, Grayson DR, Guidotti A: Epigenetic downregulation of GABAergic function in schizophrenia: potential for pharmacological intervention? Mol Interv 3:220–229, 2003

Craft M, Ismail IA, Krishnamurti D, et al: Lithium in the treatment of aggression in mentally handicapped patients: a double blind trial. Br J Psychiatry 150:685–689, 1987

DeLong R: Autism and familial major mood disorder: are they related? J Neuropsychiatry Clin Neurosci 16:199–213, 2004

Di Martino A, Tuchman RF: Antiepileptic drugs: affective use in autism spectrum disorders. Pediatr Neurol 25:199–207, 2001

Dixon JF, Hokin LE: The antibipolar drug valproate mimics lithium in stimulating glutamate release and inositol 1,4,5-triphosphate accumulation in brain cortex slices but not accumulation of inositol monophosphates and biphosphates. Proc Natl Acad Sci U S A 94:4757–4760, 1997

Duggal HS, Pathak PC, Coleman CC: Treating selective serotonin reuptake inhibitor-induced behavioral activation with valproate. J Child Adolesc Psychopharmacol 13:113–114, 2003

Galanopoulou AS, Bojko A, Lado F, et al: The spectrum of neuropsychiatric abnormalities associated with electrical status epilepticus in sleep. Brain Dev 22:279–295, 2000

Geller B, Zimerman B, Williams M, et al: Diagnostic characteristics of 93 cases of a prepubertal and early adolescent bipolar disorder phenotype by gender, puberty and comorbid ADHD. J Child Adolesc Psychopharmacol 10:157–164, 2000

Genton P, Van Vleymen B: Piracetam and levetiracetam: close structural similarities but different pharmacological and clinical profiles. Epileptic Disord 2:99–105, 2000

Guerrini R, Belmonte A, Genton P: Antiepileptic drug-induced worsening of seizures in children. Epilepsia 39 (suppl 3):S2–S10, 1998

Guerrini R, Carpay J, Groselj J, et al: Topiramate monotherapy as broad-spectrum antiepileptic drug in a naturalistic clinical setting. Seizure 14:371–380, 2005

Hahn CG, Gyulai L, Baldassano CF, et al: The current understanding of lamotrigine as a mood stabilizer. J Clin Psychiatry 65:791–804, 2004

Hollander E: Managing aggressive behavior in patients with obsessive compulsive disorder and borderline personality disorder. J Clin Psychiatry 60 (suppl 15):38–44, 1999

Hollander E, Dolgoff-Kaspar R, Cartwright C, et al: An open trial of divalproex sodium in autism spectrum disorders. J Clin Psychiatry 62:530–534, 2001

Hollander E, Posner N, Cherkasky S: Neuropsychiatric aspects of aggression and impulse control disorders, in The American Psychiatric Publishing Textbook of Neuropsychiatry and Clinical Neurosciences, 4th Edition. Edited by Yudofsky SC, Hales RE. Washington, DC, American Psychiatry Press, 2002, pp 579–596

Hollander E, Tracy K, Swann A, et al: Divalproex in the treatment of impulsive aggression: efficacy in cluster B personality disorders. Neuropsychopharmacology 28:1186–1197, 2003a

Hollander E, Phillips AT, Yeh CC: Targeted treatments for symptom domains in child and adolescent autism. Lancet 362:732–734, 2003b

Hollander E, Swann A, Coccaro E, et al: Impact of trait impulsivity and state aggression on divalproex versus placebo response in borderline personality disorder. Am J Psychiatry 162:621–624, 2005

Hollander E, Soorya L, Wasserman S, et al: Divalproex sodium vs. placebo in the treatment of repetitive behaviors in autism spectrum disorder. Int J Neuropsychopharmacol 15:209–213, 2006

Johnson BA, Ait-Daoud N, Bowden CL, et al: Oral topiramate for treatment of alcohol dependence: a randomized controlled trial. Lancet 361:1677–1685, 2003

Kerbeshian J, Burd L, Fisher W: Lithium Carbonate in the treatment of two patients with infantile autism and atypical bipolar symptomatology. J Clin Psychopharmacol 7:401–405, 1987

Klitgaard H, Pitkanen A: Antiepileptogenesis, neuroprotection, and disease modification in the treatment of epilepsy: focus on levetiracetam. Epileptic Disord 5 (suppl 1):S9–S16, 2003

Loscher W: Effects of the antiepileptic drug valproate on metabolism and function of inhibitory and excitatory amino acid in the brain. Neurochem Res 18:485–502, 1993

Loscher W, Vetter M: In vivo effects of aminooxyacetic acid and valproic acid on nerve terminal (synaptosomal) GABA levels in discrete brain areas of the rat: correlation to pharmacological activities. Biochem Pharmacol 34:1747–1756, 1985

Manji HK, Chen G: Post-receptor signaling pathways in the pathophysiology and treatment of mood disorders. Curr Psychiatry Rep 2:479–489, 2000

Manji HK, Bebchuk JM, Moore GJ, et al: Modulation of CNS signal transduction pathways and gene expression by mood-stabilizing agents: therapeutic implications. J Clin Psychiatry 60 (suppl 2):27–39, 1999

McElroy SL, Shapira NA, Arnold LM, et al: Topiramate in the long-term treatment of binge-eating disorder associated with obesity. J Clin Psychiatry 65:1463–1469, 2004

McVicar KA, Shinnar S: Landau-Kleffner syndrome, electrical status epilepticus in slow wave sleep, and language regression in children. Ment Retard Dev Disabil Res Rev 10:144–149, 2004

Meldrum BS: Update on the mechanism of action of antiepileptic drugs. Epilepsia 37 (suppl 6):S4–S11, 1996

Monji A, Maekawa T, Yanagimoto K, et al: Carbamazepine may trigger new-onset epileptic seizures in an individual with autism spectrum disorders: a case report. Eur Psychiatry 19:322–323, 2004

Moshe SL: Mechanisms of action of anticonvulsant agents. Neurology 5:S32–S40, 2000

Okada M, Hirano T, Mizuno K: Effects of carbamazepine on hippocampal serotonergic system. Epilepsy Res 31:187–198, 1998

Otsuki K, Morimoto K, Sato K, et al: Effects of lamotrigine and conventional anti-epileptic drugs on amygdala- and hippocampal-kindled seizures in rats. Epilepsy Res 31:101–012, 1998

Pallanti S, Quercioli L, Sood E, et al: Lithium and valproate treatment of pathological gambling: a randomized, single-blind study. J Clin Psychiatry 63:559–564, 2002

Piven J, Palmer P: Psychiatric disorder and the broad autism phenotype: evidence from a family study of multiple incidence autism families. Am J Psychiatry 156:557–563, 1999

Rapin J: Autism: current concepts. N Engl J Med 337:97–104, 1997

Rugino TA, Samsock TC: Levetiracetam in autistic children: an open-label study. J Dev Behav Pediatr 23:225–230, 2002

Shewmon DA, Erwin RJ: The effect of focal interictal spikes on perception and reaction time, I: general considerations. Electroencephalogr Clin Neurophysiol 69:319–337, 1988a

Shewmon DA, Erwin RJ: The effect of focal interictal spikes on perception and reaction time, II: neuroanatomic specificity. Electroencephalogr Clin Neurophysiol 69:338–352, 1988b

Shinnar S, Rapin I, Arnold S, et al: Language regression in childhood. Pediatr Neurol 24:183–189, 2001

Soderpalm B: Anticonvulsants: aspects of their mechanism of action. Eur J Pain 6 (suppl A):3–9, 2002

Southam E, Kirkby D, Higgins GA, et al: Lamotrigine inhibits monoamine uptake in vitro and modulates 5-hydroxytryptamine uptake in rats. Eur J Pharmacol 358:19–24, 1998

Steingard R, Biederman J: Lithium, responsive manic-like symptoms in two individuals with autism and mental retardation. J Am Acad Child Adolesc Psychiatry 26:932–935, 1987

Stout SC, Owens MJ, Lindsey KP, et al: Effects of sodium valproate on corticotropin-releasing factor systems in rat brain. Neuropsychopharmacology 24:624–631, 2001

Sverd J: Psychiatric disorders in individuals with pervasive developmental disorder. J Psychiatr Pract 9:111–127, 2003

Tassinari CA, Rubboli G, Volpi L: Encephalopathy with electrical status epilepticus during slow wave sleep or ESE syndrome including the acquired aphasia. Clin Neurophysiol 111 (suppl 2):S94–S102, 2000

Towbin KE, Pradella A, Gorrindo T, et al: Autism spectrum traits in children with mood and anxiety disorders. J Child Adolesc Psychopharmacol 15:452–464, 2005

Tuchman R, Rapin I: Regression in pervasive developmental disorders: seizures and epileptiform encephalogram correlates. Pediatrics 99:560–566, 1997

Tuchman R, Rapin I: Epilepsy in autism. Lancet Neurol 1:352–358, 2002

Tyler SP, Walsh A, Edwards DE, et al: Factors associated with a good response to lithium in aggressive mentally handicapped subjects. Prog Neuropsychopharmacol Biol Psychiatry 8:751–755, 1984

Uldall P, Hansen FJ, Tonnby B: Lamotrigine in Rett syndrome. Neuropediatrics; 24:339–340, 1993

Uvebrant P, Bauziene R: Intractable epilepsy in children: the efficacy of lamotrigine treatment including non-seizure-related benefits. Neuropediatrics 25:284–289, 1994

von Wegerer J, Hesslinger B, Berger M, et al: A calcium antagonistic effect of the new antiepileptic drug lamotrigine. Eur Neuropsychopharmacol 7:77–81, 1997

Wasserman S, Iyengar R, Chaplin WF, et al: Levetiracetam versus placebo in childhood and adolescent autism: a double-blind placebo-controlled study. Int Clin Psychopharmacol 21:363–367, 2006

Wauquier A, Zhou S: Topiramate: a potent anticonvulsant in the amygdala-kindled rat. Epilepsy Res 24:73–77, 1996

Yang MT, Lee WT, Chu LW, et al: Anti-epileptic drugs-induced de novo absence seizures. Brain Dev 25:51–56, 2003

Treatment of Autism With Antipsychotics

David J. Posey, M.D.

Kimberly A. Stigler, M.D.

Craig A. Erickson, M.D.

Christopher J. McDougle, M.D.

This work was supported in part by Department of Housing and Urban Development Grant B-01-SP-IN-0200 (Dr. McDougle); Research Unit on Pediatric Psychopharmacology–Psychosocial Intervention Grant U10 MH066766 from the National Institute of Mental Health (NIMH), Rockville, MD, to Indiana University (Drs. McDougle, Stigler, and Posey); a Young Investigator Award (Seaver Investigator) from the National Alliance for Research on Schizophrenia and Depression (Dr. Posey); a Daniel X. Freedman Psychiatric Research Fellowship Award (Dr. Stigler); and Career Development Award K23 MH068627 from the NIMH (Dr. Posey).

Mechanism of Action

Most conventional and atypical antipsychotics are potent dopamine receptor antagonists. Atypical antipsychotics differ from conventional antipsychotics in that in addition to blocking dopamine, they most often exhibit antagonism of serotonin (5-hydroxytryptamine) type 2A (5-HT$_{2A}$) receptors. Despite these similarities within each class, the antipsychotics differ in their relative potency of receptor subtype blockade as well as in their side-effect profile.

Rationale for the Use of Antipsychotics in Autism

Antipsychotics are increasingly being used in the treatment of patients with autism. In a recent study of psychotropic drug use in children and adolescents receiving special education for an autism spectrum disorder, antipsychotics were being taken by 69 of 353 students (19.5%) (Witwer and Lecavalier 2005). Much of this use is supported by a growing evidence base of randomized controlled trials of specific conventional and atypical antipsychotics in autism.

The evidence for dopamine's importance in treating patients with autism largely comes from treatment studies. Early research suggested that dopaminergic drugs (e.g., psychostimulants) worsened symptoms of autism (Campbell et al. 1972, 1976) and that dopamine-blocking drugs (e.g., conventional antipsychotics) were associated with improvement in symptoms (reviewed later). Despite these clinical findings, dopaminergic abnormalities have been inconsistently found in studies investigating the neurochemical basis of autism (McDougle et al. 2005a).

Serotonergic abnormalities frequently have been found in various neurochemical studies involving persons with autism (McDougle et al. 2003). Antagonism at 5-HT receptors is thought to underlie the reported advantages of atypical antipsychotics over conventional agents, namely, the reduced propensity to cause extrapyramidal symptoms (EPS) (Pierre 2005). In addition, atypical antipsychotics are generally considered more effective for improving the negative symptoms of schizophrenia (Chouinard et al. 1993). The negative symptoms of schizophrenia (e.g., anhedonia, avolition, apathy) have similarities to the social withdrawal in autism, and therefore risperidone was postulated as possibly having efficacy for treating the underlying social impairment in autism (Fisman and Steele 1996). As will be discussed later, these hopes have not been fully realized.

In this chapter we review studies involving conventional antipsychotics and atypical antipsychotics in the treatment of patients with autism or other pervasive developmental disorders (PDDs). Studies using random assignment to active and control treatments are emphasized. When no randomized controlled trials studying an individual drug have been published, open-label and uncontrolled investigations are discussed. We also review some of the most clinically relevant side effects that arise during treatment with these drugs.

Conventional Antipsychotics

Early Clinical Trials

In the decade spanning 1965–1975, several studies were published that examined the effects of antipsychotics in heterogeneous groups of children that included subjects with autism. Several conventional antipsychotics were studied comparing one active drug with another. Drugs studied included chlorpromazine, trifluoperazine, thiothixene, trifluperidol, fluphenazine, and molindone. Children in these studies were labeled "schizophrenic" or "disturbed" and invariably included some children with "autistic features." Because of the imprecise diagnoses and lack of standardized outcome measures (Campbell et al. 1977), it is difficult to extrapolate these findings to treatment today.

Magda Campbell, who led efforts to investigate these drugs in placebo-controlled trials, chose to study haloperidol in her landmark studies. This choice may have been because of a concern that low-potency antipsychotics were associated with a higher risk of adverse cognitive effects and sedation. Haloperidol was also noted to be faster acting (Faretra et al. 1970) and associated with less EPS (Engelhardt et al. 1973) than another high-potency antipsychotic, fluphenazine.

Haloperidol

In Campbell's first study, children (ages 2.6–7.2 years) with autism were randomly assigned to receive haloperidol or placebo in combination with one of two different language training groups (response-contingent reinforcement and noncontingent reinforcement) (Campbell et al. 1978). The optimal dosage of haloperidol was 1.7 mg/day. Haloperidol was associated with significant improvement in withdrawal and stereotypy in children 4.5 years and older as assessed by the Children's Psychiatric Rating Scale (CPRS; Fish 1985).

The combination of haloperidol and response-contingent reinforcement was associated with acceleration of acquisition of imitative speech, suggesting that haloperidol might have some beneficial effects on learning when combined with behavioral treatment. Sedation was frequent (12 of 20 subjects) and dose related. An acute dystonic reaction occurred in two children. No adverse effects on cognition were detected with a standard cognitive battery. A subsequent replication study had similar findings (Cohen et al. 1980).

The effects of haloperidol on learning were next assessed in a 12-week double-blind, crossover study of 40 autistic children (ages 2.3–6.9 years) randomly assigned to receive haloperidol-placebo-haloperidol or placebo-haloperidol-placebo (4 weeks in each treatment phase) (Anderson et al. 1984). The optimal dosage of haloperidol was 1.1 mg/day. Significant improvement was seen on the Clinical Global Impression (CGI) Scale (Guy 1976) as well as the CPRS in areas of withdrawal, stereotypies, hyperactivity, abnormal object relations, fidgetiness, negativism, angry affect, and lability of affect. On a discrimination learning task, haloperidol was associated with positive effects on learning. In a multiple regression analysis, verbal developmental level and haloperidol (and not level of maladaptive behavior) significantly accounted for the variance in learning. This finding suggested that haloperidol, at optimal doses, may have positive effects on attention unrelated to its ability to decrease maladaptive behavior. Excessive sedation and irritability were the most common adverse events, and acute dystonic reactions occurred in 11 children. A subsequent study found comparable results for behavioral improvement but was not able to replicate the effect on discrimination learning (Anderson et al. 1989).

The efficacy of haloperidol over 6 months was examined in 60 children (ages 2.3–7.9 years) with autistic disorder (Perry et al. 1989). Previous responders to haloperidol were enrolled in the study and randomly assigned to receive 6 months of either continuous or discontinuous (5 days on/2 days off) administration of haloperidol. After 6 months of haloperidol treatment, subjects were given placebo for 4 weeks. The mean dosage of haloperidol was 1.2 mg/day. Significant improvement was seen on the CPRS (fidgetiness, withdrawal, unspontaneous relation to examiner, other speech deviances, and stereotypies), and 56% were rated as "much improved" on the CGI. Three children developed dyskinesias during haloperidol treatment, whereas nine others developed dyskinesias upon medication withdrawal; all dyskinesias were reversible. Improvement was maintained over the course of the 6-month treatment. There was no difference between continuous and discontinuous administration of haloperidol. After discontinuation, 35 (59%) patients were rated as worse on the CGI. Discriminant analyses of variables important in clinical deterioration found higher dose, greater improvement while taking haloperidol, and more severe behavioral problems to be characteristic of the group that worsened when haloperidol was discontinued.

Because of the high frequency of dyskinesias, tardive and withdrawal dyskinesias were followed prospectively in 118 autistic children (ages 2.3–8.2 years) with no history of seizure disorder, preexisting dyskinesias, or identifiable cause for their autism. Subjects were assigned to cycles of 6 months of haloperidol treatment followed by 4 weeks of placebo (Campbell et al. 1997). If haloperidol was still clinically indicated following one cycle of treatment, then subsequent treatment cycles took place. Dyskinesias developed in 40 children (33.9%), although the majority of the dyskinesias were due to medication withdrawal and were reversible. In a subgroup of 10 children receiving a haloperidol at a higher dosage (average=3.4 mg/day) at study exit (compared with 2.0 mg/day for the overall group), 9 (90%) developed dyskinesias. In another subgroup of 9 children who developed tardive dyskinesia, females were overrepresented. Pre- and perinatal complications were also more frequent in those who developed dyskinesias (Armenteros et al. 1995).

Pimozide

In a multicenter, double-blind, placebo-controlled crossover study, pimozide was found to be as efficacious as haloperidol in the treatment of 87 children (ages 6–13 years) with behavioral problems, including 34 with "autistic disturbance" (Naruse et al. 1982). Subjects were treated for 8 weeks in each treatment phase. The dosage of pimozide ranged from 1 to 9 mg/day. Assessment of efficacy was based on parent and therapist rating scales, as well as general impression. "Sleepiness" was significantly more frequent with both pimozide and haloperidol compared with placebo.

Current Role of Conventional Antipsychotics in the Treatment of Autism

In summary, multiple studies have found haloperidol efficacious for improving a variety of behavioral symptoms in young children with autism. There is less robust evidence for the efficacy of the other conventional antipsychotics.

Haloperidol treatment frequently leads to acute dystonic reactions, withdrawal dyskinesias, and tardive dyskinesia. This high risk of EPS has limited the use of these medications to patients with the most treatment-refractory conditions. When treatment with haloperidol is undertaken, low doses and shorter durations of haloperidol treatment should be considered to limit the risk of tardive dyskinesia, which is associated with higher cumulative doses.

Atypical Antipsychotics

Published Reports and Trials

The atypical antipsychotics have largely replaced haloperidol and other conventional antipsychotics in the treatment of autism in the United States. In this section we review the most commonly prescribed atypical antipsychotics (clozapine, risperidone, olanzapine, quetiapine, ziprasidone, aripiprazole) in the United States. We also discuss amisulpride, an atypical antipsychotic that has not been approved in the United States, and amoxapine, an antidepressant that has properties comparable to those of atypical antipsychotics. In addition, a controlled add-on study of cyproheptadine (a $5\text{-}HT_{2A}$ receptor antagonist) to haloperidol is reviewed in this section because $5\text{-}HT_{2A}$ receptor blockade is a central property of most atypical antipsychotics.

Clozapine

To date, only letters to the editor have been published describing the use of clozapine in treating persons with autism. In the first of these, three children with autism and marked hyperactivity, fidgetiness, or aggression were treated for up to 8 months, with dosages ranging from 200 to 450 mg/day (Zuddas et al. 1996). Two of the three children showed sustained improvement, although the third had a return of symptoms to baseline levels after an initial response. In another report, a 17-year-old male with autism and severe mental retardation showed a significant reduction in signs of "overt tension," hyperactivity, and repetitive motions in response to clozapine 275 mg/day during a 15-day hospitalization (Chen et al. 2001). In the third report, a 32-year-old man with autism and profound mental retardation showed marked improvement of aggressiveness and social interaction after 2 months of treatment with clozapine 300 mg/day (Gobbi and Pulvirenti 2001). The patient's symptoms had been refractory to numerous prior medication trials, and the patient had been admitted to the hospital frequently for self-injurious, aggressive, and destructive behavior. The patient showed progressive improvement over a 5-year period.

The lack of any additional studies of clozapine in autism might reflect concern regarding the risk of agranulocytosis. The need for weekly white blood cell count monitoring is a huge drawback in children with autism given their notable difficulty tolerating phlebotomy. In addition, the risk of seizures with clozapine (especially at high doses) should be considered in light of a high prevalence of seizure disorders in persons with autism.

Risperidone

Shortly after the approval of risperidone in 1993, several case reports and open-label trials appeared reporting marked benefits of this medication in the treatment of disruptive behaviors in autism (for a review, see Posey and McDougle 2000). In this section we focus on the three placebo-controlled trials of risperidone in autism published to date and their relevance to clinical treatment.

The first placebo-controlled trial of risperidone in the treatment of autism involved 31 adults (mean age=28.1 years) with autism or PDD not otherwise specified (McDougle et al. 1998). Risperidone (mean dosage=2.9 mg/day) was significantly more efficacious than placebo, with 8 of 14 (57%) subjects being categorized as responders on the CGI versus none of 16 in the placebo group. Specifically, risperidone was efficacious for reducing interfering repetitive behavior as well as aggression toward self, others, and property. Improvement was also seen in measures of anxiety and depression. Significant differences between risperidone and placebo were not captured on scales measuring social relatedness to people and language. Thirteen of 15 (87%) subjects randomly assigned to receive risperidone had at least one adverse effect, although this included only mild, transient sedation in 5 subjects, compared with 5 of 16 (31%) subjects given placebo (agitation in all 5 cases). Weight gain occurred in a minority (2 of 14 [14%]) of risperidone-treated subjects and was significantly less than that reported in the pediatric trials discussed below.

A double-blind, placebo-controlled study of risperidone in children and adolescents with autism was completed by the Research Units on Pediatric Psychopharmacology (RUPP) Autism Network (McCracken et al. 2002). A total of 101 children (mean age=8.8 years) were randomly assigned to receive 8 weeks of risperidone or placebo. At baseline, all patients had significant irritability, aggression, or self-injury as rated by an Aberrant Behavior Checklist

(ABC; Aman et al. 1985) Irritability subscale score of 18 or greater. Treatment with risperidone for 8 weeks (mean dosage = 1.8 mg/day) resulted in a 57% reduction in the Irritability subscale score of the ABC as compared with a 14% decrease in the placebo group. Sixty-nine percent of the risperidone-treated subjects versus 12% of those given placebo were categorized as treatment responders. Risperidone was associated with an average weight gain of 2.7 kg as compared with 0.8 kg with placebo. Drooling was more commonly reported with risperidone than with placebo, but standardized measures of acute and tardive EPS were not significantly different between groups.

The RUPP study also examined the other four subscales of the ABC: social withdrawal, stereotypy, hyperactivity, and inappropriate speech. Risperidone led to greater reduction in all these behaviors, but the reductions in social withdrawal and inappropriate speech were only significant at the $P =$ 0.03 level, which was considered insignificant following a Bonferroni correction for multiple analyses. To further analyze the efficacy of risperidone on the core symptoms of autism, McDougle et al. (2005b) examined secondary outcome measures that included a modified Ritvo-Freeman Real Life Rating Scale (R-F RLRS) (Freeman et al. 1986) and modified Children's Yale-Brown Obsessive Compulsive Scale (CY-BOCS) (Scahill et al. 1997). On the R-F RLRS, significant improvement was seen on the following subscales: Sensory Motor Behaviors, Affectual Reactions, Sensory Responses. However, there was not significant change on the Social Relationship to People or the Language subscales. Risperidone was more efficacious than placebo in reducing interfering repetitive behavior on the CY-BOCS.

A companion study to the initial 8-week acute risperidone trial by the RUPP Autism Network has also been completed (RUPP Autism Network 2005). In this study, 63 subjects who responded to 8 weeks of acute treatment continued taking open-label risperidone for an additional 4 months. During this open-label continuation phase, the mean risperidone dose remained stable, and there was no clinically significant worsening of target symptoms. Five (8%) subjects discontinued the drug because of loss of efficacy, and one discontinued the drug because of adverse effects. Subjects gained an average of 5.6 kg of body weight during the total 6-month course of risperidone treatment. Thirty-two subjects who continued to be classified as responders after the 16-week extension were then randomly assigned to continue to take risperidone versus gradual substitution with placebo (over the course of 3 weeks). Ten of 16

(62.5%) subjects randomly assigned to receive placebo relapsed compared with 2 of 16 (12.5%) subjects who continued taking risperidone, suggesting that risperidone treatment beyond 6 months is needed to prevent relapse. This relapse with drug withdrawal has also been confirmed in another placebo-controlled discontinuation study of risperidone in patients with PDDs (see Troost et al. 2005).

A second multicenter, placebo-controlled study of risperidone in children with PDDs has been conducted in Canada (Shea et al. 2004). In this study, 79 children (mean age = 7.5 years) were randomly assigned to receive either risperidone (mean dosage = 1.2 mg/day) or placebo for 8 weeks. No specific entry criteria other than a diagnosis of PDD and a Childhood Autism Rating Scale (CARS) (Schopler et al. 1980) score of less than 30 were reported. However, the average baseline ABC Irritability subscale score of 20 suggests that these children were, on average, highly symptomatic at study entry. Risperidone was associated with a 64% reduction in ABC Irritability versus 31% in the placebo group. On the CGI, 21 of 40 (53%) risperidone-treated subjects were "much" or "very much improved" compared with 7 of 39 (18%) placebo-treated subjects. Significant improvement ($P<0.05$) was seen on all subscales of the ABC but were of greatest magnitude for Irritability and Hyperactivity. Social withdrawal decreased by 63% in the risperidone group compared with 40% for placebo ($P<0.01$). Weight gain following 8 weeks of risperidone was 2.7 kg compared with 1.0 kg for placebo. EPS as measured by standardized rating scales were equal in both groups.

The two studies of risperidone in children with autism produced similar results in terms of efficacy and adverse events. These studies eventually led to U.S. Food and Drug Administration (FDA) approval of risperidone for the treatment of irritability in children and adolescents with autism. In addition, there is evidence that risperidone is efficacious for hyperactivity, repetitive behavior, and perhaps social withdrawal in children with PDDs who exhibit high levels of baseline irritability.

Olanzapine

Three prospective open-label trials of olanzapine in PDDs have been published. In a 12-week study of olanzapine (mean dosage 7.8 mg/day; range = 5–20 mg/day) in children, adolescents, and adults (age range = 5–42 years) with autism and other PDDs, 6 of 8 (75%) patients who entered a 12-week open-label trial were judged to be responders on the basis of the CGI (Potenza et al. 1999). Significant improvements in overall symptoms of autism, motor restlessness/hyperactivity, social relatedness, affectual reactions, sensory responses, language usage, self-injury, aggression, irritability or anger, anxiety, and depression were observed. Significant changes in repetitive behaviors did not occur for the group. The drug was well tolerated, with the most significant adverse effects being increased appetite and weight gain in 6 patients. The mean weight for the group increased 8.4 kg during the course of the 12-week trial.

In another open-label study, 12 children with autism (mean age=7.8 years) were randomly assigned to 6 weeks of open-label treatment with olanzapine or haloperidol (Malone et al. 2001). Mean final dosages were 7.9 mg/day for olanzapine and 1.4 mg/day for haloperidol. Five of 6 (83%) subjects in the olanzapine group and 3 of 6 (50%) in the haloperidol group were rated as responders. Weight gain from baseline to the end of treatment was significantly higher in the olanzapine group (mean=4.1 kg) compared with the haloperidol group (mean=1.5 kg).

In a third study, 25 children (mean age=11.2 years) with PDDs were treated with olanzapine (mean dosage=10.7 mg/day) for 3 months (Kemner et al. 2002). In contrast to the other two studies, olanzapine was effective in only 3 (12%) subjects. The reason for the lower response rate is unclear but could have been due to the relatively low level of disruptive behavior at baseline. In this study, the mean ABC Irritability subscale score was 11, which is low compared with the baseline values in the two studies of risperidone in children (18 and 20, respectively). The other two olanzapine investigations discussed above had a specific entry criterion based on degree of disruptive behavior.

Quetiapine

Four open-label studies or case series have reported on the use of quetiapine in treating PDDs. In the first of these, six children and adolescents (ages 6–15 years) with autism were treated with quetiapine (mean dosage=225 mg/day) during a 16-week open-label trial (Martin et al. 1999). Quetiapine was poorly tolerated by four subjects who terminated early because of sedation (n=3) or a seizure (n=1). The two subjects who finished the study were classified as responders on the CGI. Increased appetite and weight gain were also reported. The investigators concluded that quetiapine was poorly tolerated and generally ineffective in this diagnostic group.

Another open-label trial of quetiapine in patients with PDDs enrolled nine adolescents (ages 12–17 years) with autism (Findling et al. 2004). Subjects were treated with quetiapine (mean dosage=292 mg/day) for 12 weeks. Six of the nine subjects completed the trial. Two of the nine (22%) subjects were judged responders on the CGI. Two subjects discontinued quetiapine early because of sedation and increased agitation/aggression, respectively. Overall, adverse effects reported for the group included sedation, weight gain, agitation, and aggression.

Retrospective studies published recently have been slightly more optimistic as to the efficacy of quetiapine in patients with PDDs. In one case series, 20 patients (ages 5–28 years) were treated with quetiapine (mean dosage=249 mg/day) over an average duration of follow-up of 60 weeks (range=4–180 weeks) (Corson et al. 2004). Eight of 20 (40%) patients were judged responders to quetiapine based on a CGI performed at the time of clinic visits. Adverse effects occurred in 50% of patients but only led to drug discontinuation in 15% of cases.

In another case series, quetiapine (mean dosage=477 mg/day) was effective in treating 6 of 10 (60%) patients (ages 5–19 years) with PDDs as judged by the CGI (Hardan et al. 2005). Significant improvement was also found on the Conduct, Hyperactivity, and Inattention subscales of the Conners' Parent Rating Scale (Goyette et al. 1978). Adverse effects were mild and included sedation, sialorrhea, and weight gain.

At first glance, the response rate in these uncontrolled studies is lower than that reported for risperidone. The highest response rate in any of these studies was 60%. In the study by Hardan et al. (2005), somewhat higher doses of quetiapine were reached compared with the other three studies. Controlled trials of quetiapine would be needed to more accurately determine its efficacy and appropriate dosing in the treatment of autism and other PDDs.

Ziprasidone

Two published studies have examined the effectiveness of ziprasidone in PDDs. In one study, ziprasidone (mean dose=59 mg/day) was associated with "much" or "very much" improvement on the CGI in 6 of 12 (50%) children and adolescents (mean age=11.6 years) with PDDs following an average duration of treatment of 14 weeks (McDougle et al. 2002). Improvement was seen in symptoms of aggression, agitation, and irritability. Transient sedation was the most common side effect. No cardiovascular side effects were observed. On average, patients lost weight during treatment with ziprasidone, but the weight loss could have been secondary to being switched from other drugs that had been causing excessive weight gain. Mean change in body weight for the group was -5.8 ± 12.5 lbs. (range$=-35$ to 6 lbs.). Five patients lost weight, 5 had no change, 1 gained weight, and 1 had no follow-up weight measurement beyond the baseline measure.

In the second study, 10 adults with autism and mental retardation living in a residential setting were switched to ziprasidone from other atypical antipsychotics (clozapine, risperidone, quetiapine), most commonly because of excessive weight gain (Cohen et al. 2004). By 6 months after the switch, they had lost a significant amount of weight that averaged 9.5 lbs. The changes in maladaptive behavior were not significantly different, and they reported that 6 patients had improved, 1 was unchanged, and 3 had decompensated. The FDA has raised concerns about the potential for QTc interval prolongation with ziprasidone on electrocardiography. Therefore, the drug should not be given to individuals with cardiac disease or who take other medications that can prolong the QTc interval unless carefully monitored.

Aripiprazole

Aripiprazole is the newest atypical antipsychotic available in the United States. This drug differs from other atypical antipsychotics in that it is a *partial* dopamine D_2 and 5-HT_{1A} agonist in addition to being a 5-HT_{2A} antagonist (Burris et al. 2002). In one case series, five patients (mean age$=12.2$ years) received aripiprazole (mean dosage$=12$ mg/day) for an average duration of 13 weeks (Stigler et al. 2004a). Five (100%) subjects were deemed responders on the basis of the CGI. Significant improvement was noted in a variety of interfering behavioral symptoms, including aggression, self-injury, and irritability. Aripiprazole was well tolerated. No acute EPS or changes in heart rate or blood pressure were recorded. Two of the five subjects experienced mild transient somnolence. There was a reduction in average weight, but this weight loss may have been secondary to discontinuing a prior atypical antipsychotic drug that had been causing significant weight gain.

Amisulpride

Amisulpride is an atypical antipsychotic that is not available in the United States but is commonly prescribed in the United Kingdom and elsewhere for the treatment of schizophrenia. It is associated with a relatively low incidence of weight gain in adults but is frequently associated with hyperprolactinemia (McKeage and Plosker 2004). One randomized, double-blind trial of amisulpride focused on the role that dopamine function may play in autism (Dollfus et al. 1992). In this crossover study, nine patients with autism, hyperactivity, and severe mental retardation were treated with 4 weeks of amisulpride and bromocriptine (a dopamine agonist) separated by a 6-week placebo phase. In this small study, amisulpride was not associated with significant improvement on standardized rating scales.

Amoxapine

Amoxapine is an antidepressant that is both a norepinephrine reuptake inhibitor and a dopamine antagonist. Clinical and preclinical studies have found amoxapine to have similarities to atypical antipsychotics in terms of its receptor pharmacology and clinical efficacy (Apiquian et al. 2005). There has been only one report of the use of amoxapine in the treatment of autism (Craven-Thuss and Nicolson 2003). In this report, two children (ages 9 and 10 years) with autism were treated with amoxapine (100 mg/day and 150 mg/day, respectively) over the course of several weeks and showed improvement in agitation, aggression, hyperactivity, and anxiety. However, the epileptogenic potential of amoxapine (Coccaro and Siever 1985), especially in overdose, may be a limiting factor in this diagnostic group, in which individuals are at higher risk for seizure disorders.

Cyproheptadine

Cyproheptadine is not an antipsychotic but is a potent $5\text{-}HT_{2A}$ antagonist. In a double-blind, placebo-controlled trial (Akhondzadeh et al. 2004), 40 children (ages 3–11 years) with autism were randomly assigned to receive haloperidol plus cyproheptadine or haloperidol plus placebo during the course of an 8-week study. In combination with haloperidol, cyproheptadine was more efficacious than placebo in terms of reducing ABC and CARS scores. The rates of EPS, increased appetite, and other side effects were comparable in both groups, but the study may have been underpowered to detect these differences. This study is interesting especially in the absence of any double-blind studies that have directly compared atypical antipsychotics with conventional ones.

Current Role of Atypical Antipsychotics in the Treatment of Autism

Atypical antipsychotics are one of the most commonly prescribed drug classes in the treatment of patients with autism, owing in part to the growing evidence base documenting efficacy. Atypical antipsychotics have largely replaced the conventional antipsychotics in most community surveys (Witwer and Lecavalier 2005). Despite their popularity, atypical antipsychotics can cause a number of significant side effects that need to be considered when using these medications in persons with autism.

Side Effects

Weight Gain

Weight gain is one of the most troublesome side effects of atypical antipsychotics when these medications are used in children and adolescents (Stigler et al. 2004b). It is especially concerning because obesity can set the stage for the development of serious medical problems including diabetes, hyperlipidemia, and cardiovascular disease.

The available published evidence suggests that weight gain is greatest for clozapine and olanzapine and least for ziprasidone and aripiprazole (Stigler et al. 2004b). The weight gain occurring with risperidone and quetiapine appears to be intermediate. However, it should be emphasized that this assessment is based on average weight gain. There are some individuals who do not gain excessive weight while taking these drugs and others who gain weight even while taking weight-neutral atypical antipsychotics.

Children may be at greatest risk for this side effect, but little research has been done comparing weight gain between children and adults (Fedorowicz and Fombonne 2005). In a study of children with autism from the RUPP Autism Network, weight gain was most prominent during the first 8 weeks of treatment and decelerated over the subsequent 4 months of risperidone treatment (Martin et al. 2004). In this study, serum leptin levels at 8 weeks did not predict weight gain at the end of the study, suggesting that elevated leptin is likely not a cause for atypical antipsychotic–induced weight gain in this population.

Given the likelihood for these medications to cause weight gain, it is very important to educate patients and their families about this adverse effect. In addition, regular monitoring of weight also appears reasonable. Given that weight gain can precede the development of diabetes and hyperlipidemia, periodic monitoring of fasting blood glucose and lipid profiles appears reasonable as well.

Antipsychotic-induced weight gain is usually associated with increased appetite and increased food intake rather than a large change in underlying metabolic activity (Gothelf et al. 2002). Therefore, efforts aimed at reducing food intake (or increasing physical activity) are reasonable. If weight gain occurs with an atypical antipsychotic, switching to another atypical antipsychotic that is less likely to promote weight gain may be one option (Cohen et al. 2004; McDougle et al. 2002; Stigler et al. 2004a), but there have been no prospective studies that have examined this approach in children.

There are no good antidotes for the weight gain secondary to antipsychotics. If efforts to curb food intake or increase physical activity and/or switching to a more weight-neutral drug are unsuccessful, the addition of a second drug (e.g., topiramate, dextroamphetamine) that might have an added benefit of weight loss could be considered. However, the efficacy of this strategy has not been proved (Werneke et al. 2002), and there are limited data examining these approaches in children. These additional drugs might be considered if there are other symptoms present that require another drug (e.g., a seizure disorder requiring an anticonvulsant; persistent hyperactivity requiring a psychostimulant). However, the clinician must bear in mind that these drugs may bring new side effects of their own.

Hyperprolactinemia

The RUPP Autism Network measured serum prolactin in their studies of risperidone in children with autism (Anderson et al. 2007). Prolactin measurements were obtained at baseline, 8 weeks, 6 months, and 18 months. Risperidone was associated with a fourfold increase in prolactin at 8 weeks, but prolactin levels tended to be less elevated at 6 and 18 months. For those subjects treated with risperidone for 18 months, the prolactin level was 25.3 ± 15.6 ng/mL (compared with 10.4 ± 10.1 ng/mL at baseline). Interestingly, despite elevations in serum prolactin levels, there were no reported side effects or changes on physical exam (e.g., gynecomastia, galactorrhea) that one typically associates with hyperprolactinemia. However, the absence of such changes could be secondary to the subject sample, which was predominantly male and prepubertal.

These subjects may be less likely to experience these side effects than postpubertal females. Similar findings for prolactin have been found in using risperidone to treat children and adolescents with disruptive behavior disorders (Findling et al. 2003).

Given the unknown significance of hyperprolactinemia, it would be important to discuss this side effect with patients and families and inform them that it has been associated with significant problems, including gynecomastia, amenorrhea, and osteoporosis. In addition, the likelihood of increased prolactin varies among different antipsychotics. The risk appears to be highest for risperidone but lower for other atypical antipsychotics (Haddad and Wieck 2004). This may factor into the decision making around prescribing, especially in the context of overt side effects.

Extrapyramidal Symptoms

EPS are common when using haloperidol in the treatment of children with autism. Fortunately, the available data suggest that the atypical antipsychotics are less likely to cause EPS. In the studies of risperidone done by the RUPP Autism Network (McCracken et al. 2002), standardized measures of acute EPS (the Simpson-Angus Extrapyramidal Side Effects Scale [Simpson and Angus 1970]) and tardive dyskinesia (the Abnormal Involuntary Movement Scale [National Institute of Mental Health 1985]) were not different between risperidone and placebo (Aman et al. 2005). Indeed, overall rates of any side effect elicited by a structured checklist that could have been EPS were low and often comparable to those seen with placebo. The one exception to this was drooling, which was more commonly reported in children treated with risperidone ($P=0.04$). Research is needed on the frequency of EPS with other atypical antipsychotics in this diagnostic population. In addition, currently available studies have not addressed the long-term risk of tardive dyskinesia.

Summary

Both haloperidol and risperidone have been shown to be efficacious for treating several of the behavioral symptoms associated with autism. The current role of haloperidol is limited because of the risk of EPS, especially tardive dyskinesia. Because of this, atypical antipsychotics are more commonly used today in treating persons with autism. Despite the efficacy of risperidone, in deciding whether to prescribe this drug, the clinician must factor in the side

Table 5–1. Commonly prescribed atypical antipsychotics and their use in patients with autism

Medication	Starting dosage range (mg/day)[a]	Effective dosage range (mg/day)[b]	Dosing frequency	Side-effect considerations	Monitoring considerations	Published evidence supporting use
Risperidone	0.25–0.5	0.5–6	qd–tid	Weight gain, EPS/TD, hyperprolactinemia, sedation[c]	Weight, BMI, fasting glucose and lipid profile, AIMS, prolactin	+++
Olanzapine	2.5–5	5–40	qd–tid	Weight gain, EPS/TD, hyperprolactinemia,[d] sedation[c]	Weight, BMI, fasting glucose and lipid profile, AIMS	++
Quetiapine	25–50	75–800	qd–tid	Weight gain, EPS/TD, hyperprolactinemia,[d] sedation[c]	Weight, BMI, fasting glucose and lipid profile, AIMS	++
Ziprasidone	20–40	20–160	qd–tid	Weight neutral,[e] EPS/TD, QT prolongation, hyperprolactinemia[d]	Weight, BMI, fasting glucose and lipid profile, AIMS, ECG[f]	++
Aripiprazole	2.5–5	5–30	qd–bid	Weight neutral,[e] EPS/TD	Weight, BMI, fasting glucose and lipid profile, AIMS	+

Note. Dosage recommendations are based on both review of published literature and clinical experience. + =single case series; ++ =multiple open-label trials and/or case series; +++ =two randomized controlled trials. AIMS=Abnormal Involuntary Movement Scale; bid=two times daily; BMI=body mass index; ECG=electrocardiogram; EPS=extrapyramidal symptoms; qd=once a day; TD=tardive dyskinesia; tid=three times daily.
[a]Lower starting doses are most appropriate for younger children and higher doses for older adolescents and adults. [b]Wide dose range reflects individual variation in both target symptoms and responsiveness. [c]Sedation can occur with any atypical antipsychotic, but is most common with these drugs. [d]Hyperprolactinemia is less frequently reported, more transient, or only apparent at the highest doses of these drugs. [e]Weight gain may occasionally occur with these drugs, especially in children with developmental disorders, but is less frequent compared with other atypical antipsychotics. [f]ECG monitoring may be considered in children given the lack of available safety data in this age group.

effects, especially weight gain, hyperprolactinemia, and the possibility of tardive dyskinesia. Suggested dosing guidelines for the five most commonly prescribed atypical antipsychotics used in treating autism, as well as their side-effects and monitoring considerations, are shown in Table 5–1.

Conclusions

Despite risperidone's efficacy for reducing behavioral symptoms, it is unclear whether this agent (or any other atypical antipsychotic) improves any of the core symptoms of autism. Further studies of these drugs in nonirritable children with autism or studies using other measures of social impairment might be informative. It also remains to be determined whether atypical antipsychotics other than risperidone are effective in the treatment of disruptive behavior in autism. Both short- and long-term efficacy studies of other drugs are needed in this population. The long-term significance of hyperprolactinemia, as well as the long-term risk of tardive dyskinesia, needs to be determined in either prospectively defined cohorts or via larger controlled studies of longer duration. Finally, further research that informs the clinical management of weight gain occurring with these drugs when used in autism is needed. Areas of interest might include identifying patients who are genetically more susceptible to this side effect as well as determining the best approach to management (e.g., diet/exercise, drug switching, pharmacological treatments).

References

Akhondzadeh S, Erfani S, Mohammadi R, et al: Cyproheptadine in the treatment of autistic disorder: a double-blind placebo-controlled trial. J Clin Pharm Ther 29:145–150, 2004

Aman MG, Singh NN, Stewart AW, et al: The Aberrant Behavior Checklist: a behavior rating scale for the assessment of treatment effects. Am J Ment Defic 89:485–491, 1985

Aman MG, Arnold LE, McDougle CJ, et al: Acute and long-term safety and tolerability of risperidone in children with autism. J Child Adolesc Psychopharmacol 15:869–884, 2005

Anderson GM, Scahill L, McCracken JT, et al: Effects of short- and long-term risperidone treatment on prolactin levels in children with autism. Biol Psychiatry 61:545–550, 2007

Anderson LT, Campbell M, Grega DM, et al: Haloperidol in treatment of infantile autism: effects on learning and behavioral symptoms. Am J Psychiatry 141:1195–1202, 1984

Anderson LT, Campbell M, Adams P, et al: The effects of haloperidol on discrimination learning and behavioral symptoms in autistic children. J Autism Dev Disord 19:227–239, 1989

Apiquian R, Fresan A, Ulloa RE, et al: Amoxapine as an atypical antipsychotic: a comparative study vs risperidone. Neuropsychopharmacology 30:2236–2244, 2005

Armenteros JL, Adams PB, Campbell M, et al: Haloperidol-related dyskinesias and pre- and perinatal complications in autistic children. Psychopharmacol Bull 31:363–369, 1995

Burris KD, Molski TF, Xu C, et al: Aripiprazole, a novel antipsychotic, is a high-affinity partial agonist at human dopamine D2 receptors. J Pharmacol Exp Ther 302:381–389, 2002

Campbell M, Fish B, David R, et al: Response to triiodothyronine and dextroamphetamine: a study of preschool schizophrenic children. J Autism Child Schizophr 2:343–358, 1972

Campbell M, Small A, Collins P, et al: Levodopa and levoamphetamine: a crossover study in young schizophrenic children. Curr Ther Res Clin Exp 19:70–86, 1976

Campbell M, Geller B, Cohen IL: Current status of drug research and treatment with autistic children. J Pediatr Psychol 2:153–161, 1977

Campbell M, Anderson LT, Meier M, et al: A comparison of haloperidol and behavior therapy and their interaction in autistic children. J Am Acad Child Psychiatry 17:640–655, 1978

Campbell M, Armenteros JL, Malone RP, et al: Neuroleptic-related dyskinesias in autistic children: a prospective, longitudinal study. J Am Acad Child Adolesc Psychiatry 36:835–843, 1997

Chen NC, Bedair HS, McKay B, et al: Clozapine in the treatment of aggression in an adolescent with autistic disorder (letter). J Clin Psychiatry 62:479–480, 2001

Chouinard G, Jones B, Remington G, et al: A Canadian multicenter placebo-controlled study of fixed doses of risperidone and haloperidol in the treatment of chronic schizophrenic patients. J Clin Psychopharmacol 13:25–40, 1993

Coccaro EF, Siever LJ: Second generation antipsychotics: a comparative review. J Clin Pharmacol 25:241–260, 1985

Cohen IL, Campbell M, Posner D, et al: Behavioral effects of haloperidol in young autistic children: an objective analysis using a within-subjects reversal design. J Am Acad Child Adolesc Psychiatry 19:665–677, 1980

Cohen SA, Fitzgerald BJ, Khan SR, et al: The effect of a switch to ziprasidone in an adult population with autistic disorder: chart review of naturalistic, open-label treatment. J Clin Psychiatry 65:110–113, 2004

Corson AH, Barkenbus JE, Posey DJ, et al: A retrospective analysis of quetiapine in treatment of pervasive developmental disorders. J Clin Psychiatry 65:1531–1536, 2004

Craven-Thuss B, Nicolson R: Amoxapine in the treatment of interfering behaviors in autism (letter). J Am Acad Child Adolesc Psychiatry 42:515–516, 2003

Dollfus S, Petit M, Menard JF, et al: Amisulpride versus bromocriptine in infantile autism: a controlled crossover comparative study of two drugs with opposite effects on dopaminergic function. J Autism Dev Disord 22:47–60, 1992

Engelhardt DM, Polizos P, Waizer J, et al: A double-blind comparison of fluphenazine and haloperidol in outpatient schizophrenic children. J Autism Child Schizophr 3:128–137, 1973

Faretra G, Dooher L, Dowling J: Comparison of haloperidol and fluphenazine in disturbed children. Am J Psychiatry 126:1670–1673, 1970

Fedorowicz VJ, Fombonne E: Metabolic side effects of atypical antipsychotics in children: a literature review. J Psychopharmacol 19:533–550, 2005

Findling RL, McNamara NK, Gracious BL, et al: Quetiapine in nine youths with autistic disorder. J Child Adolesc Psychopharmacol 14:287–294, 2004

Findling RL, Kusumakar V, Daneman D, et al: Prolactin levels during long-term risperidone treatment in children and adolescents. J Clin Psychiatry 64:1362–1369, 2003

Fish B: Children's Psychiatric Rating Scale (scoring). Psychopharmacol Bull 21:753–764, 1985

Fisman S, Steele M: Use of risperidone in pervasive developmental disorders: a case series. J Child Adolesc Psychopharmacol 6:177–190, 1996

Freeman BJ, Ritvo ER, Yakota A, et al: Scale for rating symptoms of patients with the syndrome of autism in real life. J Am Acad Child Adolesc Psychiatry 25:130–136, 1986

Gobbi G, Pulvirenti L: Long-term treatment with clozapine in an adult with autistic disorder accompanied by aggressive behavior (letter). J Psychiatry Neurosci 26:340–341, 2001

Gothelf D, Falk B, Singer P, et al: Weight gain associated with increased food intake and low habitual activity levels in male adolescent schizophrenic inpatients treated with olanzapine. Am J Psychiatry 159:1055–1057, 2002

Goyette CH, Conners CK, Ulrich RF: Normative data on revised Conners Parent and Teacher Rating Scales. J Abnorm Child Psychol 6:221–236, 1978

Guy W: ECDEU assessment manual for psychopharmacology (NIMH Publ No 76–338). Rockville, MD, National Institute of Mental Health, 1976

Haddad PM, Wieck A: Antipsychotic-induced hyperprolactinaemia: mechanisms, clinical features and management. Drugs 64:2291–2314, 2004

Hardan AY, Jou RJ, Handen BL: Retrospective study of quetiapine in children and adolescents with pervasive developmental disorders. J Autism Dev Disord 35:387–391, 2005

Kemner C, Willemsen-Swinkels SH, de Jonge M, et al: Open-label study of olanzapine in children with pervasive developmental disorder. J Clin Psychopharmacol 22:455–460, 2002

Malone RP, Cater J, Sheikh RM, et al: Olanzapine versus haloperidol in children with autistic disorder: an open pilot study. J Am Acad Child Adolesc Psychiatry 40:887–894, 2001

Martin A, Koenig K, Scahill L, et al: Open-label quetiapine in the treatment of children and adolescents with autistic disorder. J Child Adolesc Psychopharmacol 9:99–107, 1999

Martin A, Scahill L, Anderson GM, et al: Weight and leptin changes among risperidone-treated youths with autism: 6-month prospective data. Am J Psychiatry 161:1125–1127, 2004

McCracken JT, McGough J, Shah B, et al, Research Units on Pediatric Psychopharmacology Autism Network: Risperidone in children with autism and serious behavioral problems. N Engl J Med 347:314–321, 2002

McDougle CJ, Holmes JP, Carlson DC, et al: A double-blind, placebo-controlled study of risperidone in adults with autistic disorder and other pervasive developmental disorders. Arch Gen Psychiatry 55:633–641, 1998

McDougle CJ, Kem DL, Posey DJ: Case series: use of ziprasidone for maladaptive symptoms in youths with autism. J Am Acad Child Adolesc Psychiatry 41:921–927, 2002

McDougle CJ, Posey DJ, Potenza MN: Neurobiology of serotonin function in autism, in Autism Spectrum Disorders. Edited by Hollander E. New York, Marcel Dekker, 2003, pp 199–220

McDougle CJ, Erickson CA, Stigler KA, et al: Neurochemistry in the pathophysiology of autism. J Clin Psychiatry 66 (suppl 10):9–18, 2005a

McDougle CJ, Scahill L, Aman MG, et al: Risperidone for the core symptom domains of autism: results from the study by the autism network of the Research Units on Pediatric Psychopharmacology. Am J Psychiatry 162:1142–1148, 2005b

McKeage K, Plosker GL: Amisulpride: a review of its use in the management of schizophrenia. CNS Drugs 18:933–956, 2004

Naruse H, Nagahata M, Nakane Y, et al: A multi-center double-blind trial of pimozide (Orap), haloperidol and placebo in children with behavioral disorders, using cross-over design. Acta Paedopsychiatr 48:173–184, 1982

National Institute of Mental Health: Abnormal Involuntary Movement Scale (AIMS). Psychopharmacol Bull 21:1077–1080, 1985

Perry R, Campbell M, Adams P, et al: Long-term efficacy of haloperidol in autistic children: continuous versus discontinuous drug administration. J Am Acad Child Adolesc Psychiatry 28:87–92, 1989

Pierre JM: Extrapyramidal symptoms with atypical antipsychotics: incidence, prevention, and management, Drug Saf 28:191–208, 2005

Posey DJ, McDougle CJ: The pharmacotherapy of target symptoms associated with autistic disorder and other pervasive developmental disorders. Harv Rev Psychiatry 8:45–63, 2000

Potenza MN, Holmes JP, Kanes SJ, et al: Olanzapine treatment of children, adolescents, and adults with pervasive developmental disorders: an open-label pilot study. J Clin Psychopharmacol 19:37–44, 1999

Research Units on Pediatric Psychopharmacology Autism Network: Risperidone treatment of autistic disorder: longer-term benefits and blinded discontinuation after 6 months. Am J Psychiatry 162:1361–1369, 2005

Scahill L, Riddle MA, McSwiggin-Hardin M, et al: Children's Yale-Brown Obsessive Compulsive Scale: reliability and validity. J Am Acad Child Adolesc Psychiatry 36:844–852, 1997

Schopler E, Reichler RJ, DeVellis RF, et al: Toward objective classification of childhood autism: Childhood Autism Rating Scale (CARS). J Autism Dev Disord 10:91–103, 1980

Shea S, Turgay A, Carroll A, et al: Risperidone in the treatment of disruptive behavioral symptoms in children with autistic and other pervasive developmental disorders. Pediatrics 114:E634–E641, 2004

Simpson GM, Angus JW: A rating scale for extrapyramidal side effects. Acta Psychiatr Scand 212:11–19, 1970

Stigler KA, Posey DJ, McDougle CJ: Case report: aripiprazole for maladaptive behavior in pervasive developmental disorder. J Child Adolesc Psychopharmacol 14:455–463, 2004a

Stigler KA, Potenza MN, Posey DJ, et al: Weight gain associated with atypical antipsychotic use in children and adolescents: prevalence, clinical relevance, and management. Pediatr Drugs 6:33–44, 2004b

Troost PW, Lahuis BE, Steenhuis MP, et al: Long-term effects of risperidone in children with autism spectrum disorders: a placebo discontinuation study. J Am Acad Child Adolesc Psychiatry 44:1137–1144, 2005

Werneke U, Taylor D, Sanders T: Options for pharmacological management of obesity in patients treated with atypical antipsychotics. Int Clin Psychopharmacol 17:145–160, 2002

Witwer A, Lecavalier L: Treatment incidence and patterns in children and adolescents with autism spectrum disorders. J Child Adolesc Psychopharmacol 15:671–681, 2005

Zuddas A, Ledda MG, Fratta A, et al: Clinical effects of clozapine on autistic disorder (letter). Am J Psychiatry 153:738, 1996

Cholinesterase Inhibitor Therapy in Patients With Autism Spectrum Disorders

Michael G. Chez, M.D.

Carolyn Coughlin

Matthew Kominsky

Research to date has found no single unifying anatomical pathology for autism spectrum disorders. However, recent neuroimaging studies suggest asymmetries and thickening of white matter in the prefrontal cortex (Herbert et al. 2003, 2004). In addition, postmortem studies in autistic adult brains have found thickened frontal lobes as well as abnormal neurons in the limbic and temporal lobes that interconnect to the prefrontal cortex (Bauman and Kemper 1988, 1994). Clinically, neuropsychological data support defects in behavior of autistic patients that imply frontal lobe dysfunction (Ozonoff et al. 1991, 1994).

The clinical observation of frontal symptoms of apraxic behavior and per-severation led to clinical trials using anticholinesterase medications in 1999 (Chez et al. 2000). In 2001, anatomical research was published to support the hypothesis that cholinergic mechanisms may be abnormal in the autistic brain (Perry et al. 2001). Perry and colleagues described finding significant reduction in frontal nicotinic receptors and parietal muscarinic receptors in samples of autistic individuals versus healthy control subjects. Subsequent clinical studies with open-label and double-blind prospective studies and retrospective open-label studies have been published (Chez et al. 2001, 2003; Hardan and Handen 2002; Hertzman 2003). In this chapter we review the clinical experience with cholinesterase inhibitors to treat patients with autism.

History of Cholinesterase Inhibitors

The first anticholinesterase agent was found in the Calabar bean *(Physostigma venenosum),* with subsequent isolation of a crystalline alkaloid known as phys-ostigmine in 1864 (Giacobini 2000). The agent physostigmine has been used to further develop both treatment and toxins for the past 140 years. The toxicity of excessive cholinesterase inhibition through the autonomic parasympathetic nervous system was found to be blocked by atropine. Subsequently, development of less radical inhibitors of acetylcholinesterase was done to safely increase levels of acetylcholine (ACh) without the lethal effects seen when cardiovascular and parasympathetic peripheral side effects occurred.

Selective agents that act within the central nervous system were subsequently developed. The first drug to be produced was tacrine, followed by rivastigmine and donepezil. Whereas rivastigmine acts on the central nervous system cho-linesterases butyrylcholinesterase (BuChE) and acetylcholinesterase (AChE), donepezil acts preferentially on central AChE. Galantamine is another centrally acting AChE inhibitor (AChE-I) derived from plants.

Rivastigmine and donepezil are considered irreversible cholinesterase inhibitors. Their half-lives differ clinically, with rivastigmine lasting 8–12 hours and donepezil lasting 5–9 days. The difference between these drugs is in their effect in Alzheimer's disease. Whereas plaque formation may be altered by butyrylcholine (BuCh) levels, this probably is not as significant a mechanism in autism. The effect on AChE-I is probably the main effect of both drugs. Galantamine is reversible when binding to the AChE receptor. This leads again to debate about which type of drug is more effective. Although both reversible and irreversible types increase ACh, there is in theory a greater chance of antigenicity to the irreversibly bound receptors versus the reversible receptors. The irreversible types may offer more constant effect on available ACh.

The three agents that have central preference for AChE-I activity that are clinically available for human use are donepezil, rivastigmine, and galantamine. They are all approved for treatment of Alzheimer's disease by the U.S. Food and Drug Administration (FDA) but have not yet been approved for pediatric use. Pediatric use has been reported for Down's syndrome and Tourette's syndrome, as well as autism (Kishnani et al. 1999, Riback 2001).

Cholinergic Mechanisms in Autism

In the human brain AChE is far more abundant than BuChE. Cholinergic neurons synthesize ACh, whereas cholinoceptive neurons contain either muscarinic or nicotinic receptors that are responsive to ACh. Cholinergic ACh-rich neurons have synaptic swelling contacting cholinoceptive neurons. In Alzheimer's disease, loss of cholinergic neurons in the basal forebrain is posited as the basis for the clinical effect of cholinesterase inhibitor action that allows increased ACh to reach the nicotinic and muscarinic receptor cells. In autism the histological findings that have been described by Perry and colleagues (2001) actually show deficits in the cholinoceptive sites, with decreased nicotinic receptors in the prefrontal cortex as well as decreased muscarinic cholinergic receptors in the parietal cortex.

Perry and colleagues looked at cholinergic receptor subtypes in the autistic adult brain as well as in control subjects without autism who either were normally developing or had mental retardation. The cerebral cortical forebrain levels of AChE were normal in autistic samples, as were M_2 muscarinic receptor subtypes. However, the number of cortical M_1 receptors was up to 30% lower compared with control subjects, wirh significant levels of decreased activity reached in the parietal regions. Both the parietal and frontal cortex showed significant reduction in nicotinic α and β receptors in the patients with autism. The basal forebrain did not show the nicotinic receptor differences but interestingly did show three times the elevation of brain-derived neurotrophic factor (BDNF), which suggests the possibility of injury to the basal forebrain in these autistic samples. These findings suggested to Perry and colleagues that cholinergic manipulation may have a therapeutic effect in autism. Independently of their research, early clinical usage had already started (Chez et al. 2000, 2001).

In addition to neuronal activity, AChE may be involved, with neuronal plasticity having a separate role from the hydrolysis of ACh. The fact that neuronal plasticity may be impaired in autism also may be a potential factor in cholinesterase inhibitor therapy. Although the main focus is on ACh activity, BuCh activity does cluster in both the limbic regions and glial cells but not in cerebral cortical neurons (Giacobini 2000). Glial activity for AChE differs from cortical AChE in catalytic properties such as pH effects and inhibitor sensitivities. The role of glial cells in neuronal inflammation may play a role in autism and affect neuronal growth. This activity theoretically may be influenced by the levels of glial cholinesterase activity. This area of research has not been investigated in autism to date.

Treatment Experience With Cholinesterase Inhibitors in Autism

Clinical trials with cholinesterase inhibitors in autism have been limited to three drugs—donepezil, rivastigmine, and galantamine—and consist mostly of open-label trials, with only one double-blind study to date. Table 6–1 lists a summary of these trials and the level of evidence of the usefulness of these agents. There is obviously a very limited power to these studies and a paucity of appropriately placebo-controlled published data.

The drug used most in published reports has been donepezil. First published as open-label trials (Chez et al. 2000), research was subsequently followed up by a double-blind study (Chez et al. 2001, 2003) involving 43 children with autism spectrum disorders (either autism or pervasive developmental disorder as defined by DSM-IV-TR [American Psychiatric Association 2000] criteria). The dosage of donepezil was 2.5 mg/day in this study, as determined from previous pediatric open-label experience. Outcome measures included the Childhood Autism Rating Scale (CARS; Schopler et al. 1988), Gardner's Receptive (ROWPVT) and Expressive (EOWPVT) One-Word Picture Vocabulary Test (Gardner 2000a, 2000b), and clinician global assessment of the patients. Gains were noted to be significant after the 12-week prospective study, with trends noted by 6 weeks. Gains were seen in decreased severity of autistic behaviors, and

Table 6–1. Cholinesterase therapies and evidence of effectiveness in the treatment of patients with autism spectrum disorders

Medication	Dosage	Study	N (age group)	Length of study (weeks)	Study methodology	Measurement tools
Donepezil	2.5–5 mg/day	Chez et al. 2000	39 (pediatric)	12	Open label, retrospective	CARS, CGI, OWPVT
Donepezil	2.5–5 mg/day	Chez. et al. 2003	43 (pediatric)	12	Placebo controlled, prospective	CARS, CGI, EOWPVT, ROWPVT
Donepezil	5 mg/day	Harden and Handen 2002	8 (pediatric and adolescent)	12	Open label, prospective	ABC, CGI
Galantamine	4–12 mg/day	Hertzman 2003	3 (adult)	Not fixed	Open label, retrospective	CGI
Rivastigmine	0.2–0.5 mg bid	Chez. et al. 2004	32 (pediatric)	12	Open label, prospective	CARS, CGI, Conners, GARS, EOWPVT, ROWPVT

Note. ABC=Aberrant Behavioral Checklist; bid=twice daily; CARS=Childhood Autism Rating Scale; CGI=Clinical Global Impression scale; Conners=Conners' Parent Rating Scale (for attention-deficit/hyperactivity disorder; EOWPVT=Expressive One-Word Picture Vocabulary Test; GARS=Gilliam Autism Rating Scale; ROWPVT=Receptive One-Word Picture Vocabulary Test.

in receptive and expressive speech, compared with the placebo group. This finding was similar to the finding of a prior open-label study by the same researchers. Another small retrospective open-label trial with donepezil was performed (Hardan and Handen 2002). This study had only 8 patients (mean age=11 years vs. 6.8 years in the Chez double-blind study) and assessed efficacy with the Aberrant Behavior Checklist (ABC; Aman et al. 1985) and the Clinical Global Impression (CGI) Scale (Guy 1976). Improved behavior in irritability and hyperactivity was significant for 50% of the patients, but speech and stereopathies were unchanged. However, the ABC is designed to measure speech changes, and this may explain the fact that no change in outcome was found for this small group. Mild lethargy and gastrointestinal discomfort were noted in this group.

Of 283 patients treated with either donepezil, rivastigmine, or galantamine, 20.3% had no change, and side effects observed included nausea or gastrointestinal distress (3.9%), irritability (18.4%), sleep disturbance (5.3%), and urinary accidents (2.4%) (M.G.Chez, unpublished data, 2005).

Rivastigmine was studied in autistic children as an open-label prospective study (Chez et al. 2004). The results were determined for outcome using the CARS, Gilliam Autism Rating Scale (GARS; Gilliam 1995), the ROWPVT, EOWPVT, and the Conners' Parent Rating Scale for attention-deficit/hyperactivity disorder (ADHD) (Conners 1989). Thirty-two children with autism or pervasive developmental disorders by DSM-IV (American Psychiatric Association 1994) criteria were studied (mean age=6.9 years). Significant improvements were noted at the conclusion of 12 weeks of treatment in the CARS score improvement, EOWPVT, and Conners' Parent Rating Scale for ADHD. A trend that did not quite reach statistical significance was noted for the ROWPVT. The dosage ranged from 0.4–0.8 mg twice daily. Rivastigmine side effects were very similar to the side effects found with donepezil, including irritability and gastrointestinal nausea or loose stools. About one-third of the patients experienced these side effects to a degree that would limit treatment compliance.

Galantamine experience is limited to one published report in three adults with autism (Hertzman 2003). Dosages of galantamine ranged from 4 to 12 mg/day maximum, with increased verbal fluency noted in two of the three patients by observer impression. No standardized testing was done. The patient who worsened also had not responded to a trial of donepezil. Unpublished data are also available in a small group of children treated with galantamine who showed slight improvement in receptive language but less robust response than with either rivastigmine or donepezil (M. G. Chez, unpublished data, 2005).

The overall impression of the therapeutic use of these drugs is that some clinical benefit to the core symptoms of autism can be obtained in observed improvement in communication or behavior. Donepezil has the most data in the limited published literature. Results of ongoing double-blind studies with donepezil are pending at the time of this publication. Further follow-up research regarding the findings of Perry and colleagues has not been done to clarify sites of pharmacological intervention for these cholinergic enhancing drugs. Recommendations to widely use these therapies at this time cannot be made based on evidence-based clinical medicine. However, more double-blind results, especially with donepezil, may eventually lead to donepezil or similar drugs becoming another option for symptomatic treatment of autism traits. Research to date suggests no life-threatening side effects in the use of these drugs in children with autism spectrum disorders.

Conclusions

Evidence suggests that cholinergic receptor types are decreased throughout the frontal and parietal cerebral cortex in patients with autism. This may reflect an underlying predisposition based on abnormal brain development or reflect acquired damage to the brain that alters the receptors. Enhancement of levels of ACh by cholinesterase inhibitors has been studied clinically in adults and children with autism. Results are mixed, but overall they suggest some language and behavioral improvements. However, a fairly high rate of side effects have been noted in clinical use. Therefore judicious individual assessment based on a patient's clinical features should be done before initiating a trial of cholinesterase inhibitors for autism. No global recommendation for treatment can be concluded from the available data at this time. Further investigation is needed into the underlying pathology of autism and the significance of cholinergic receptor deficits as well as more controlled and double-blind, placebo-controlled studies in the use of cholinesterase inhibitors in the treatment of patients with autism.

References

Aman MG, Singh NN, Stewart AW, et al: The Aberrant Behavior Checklist: a behavior rating scale for the assessment of treatment effects. Am J Ment Defic 89:485–491, 1985

American Psychiatric Association: Diagnostic and Statistical Manual of Mental Disorders, 4th Edition. Washington, DC, American Psychiatric Association, 2000

American Psychiatric Association: Diagnostic and Statistical Manual of Mental Disorders, 4th Edition. Text Revision. Washington, DC, American Psychiatric Association, 1994

Bauman ML, Kemper TL: Limbic and cerebellar abnormalities: a finding in early infantile autism (abstract). Neurology 47:369, 1988

Bauman ML, Kemper TL: Neuroanatomic observations of the brain in autism, in The Neurobiology of Autism. Edited by Bauman ML, Kemper TL. Baltimore, MD, Johns Hopkins University Press, 1994

Chez MG, Nowinski CV, Buchanan CP: Donepezil use in children with autistic spectrum disorders. Ann Neurol 48:541, 2000

Chez MG, Tremb R, Nowinski CV, et al: Double-blinded placebo-controlled Aricept study in children with autistic spectrum disorder (abstract). Ann Neurol 49:S95–S96, 2001

Chez MG, Buchanan TM, Becker M, et al: Donepezil hydrochloride: a double-blind study in autistic children. J Pediatr Neurol 1:83–88, 2003

Chez MG, Aimonovitch M, Buchanon T, et al: Treating autistic spectrum disorders in children: utility of the cholinesterase inhibitor rivastigmine Tartrate. J Child Neurol 19:165–169, 2004

Conners CK: Conners' Parent Rating Scale. North Tonawanda, NY, Multi-Health Systems Inc, 1989

Gardner MF: Expressive One-Word Picture Vocabulary Test. Novato, CA, Academic Therapy Publications, 2000a

Gardner MF: Receptive One-Word Picture Vocabulary Test. Novato, CA, Academic Therapy Publications, 2000b

Giacobini E: Cholinesterases and Cholinesterase Inhibitors. London, Martin Dunitz, 2000

Gilliam JE: Gilliam Autism Rating Scale. Austin, TX, Pro-Ed, 1995

Guy W: ECDEU assessment manual for psychopharmacology (NIMH Publ No 76–338). Rockville, MD, National Institute of Mental Health, 1976

Hardan AY, Handen BL: A retrospective open trial of adjunctive donepezil in children and adolescents with autistic disorder. J Child Adolesc Psychopharmacol 12:237–241, 2002

Herbert MR, Ziegler DA, Deutsch CK, et al: Dissociations of cerebral cortex, subcortical and cerebral white matter volumes in autistic boys. Brain 126 (part 5):1182–1192, 2003

Herbert MR, Ziegler DA, Makris N, et al: Localization of white matter volume increase in autism and developmental language disorder. Ann Neurol 55:530–540, 2004

Hertzman M: Galantamine in the treatment of adult autism: a report of three clinical cases. Int J Psychiatry Med 33395–398, 2003

Kishnani PS, Sullivan JA, Walter BK, et al: Cholinergic therapy for Down's syndrome. Lancet 353:1064–1065, 1999

Ozonoff S, Pennington BF, Rogers SJ: Executive function deficits in high-functioning autistic individuals: relationship to theory of mind. J Child Psychol Psychiatry 32:1081–1103, 1991

Ozonoff S, Strayer D, McMahon W, et al: Executive function abilities in autism and Tourette's syndrome: an information processing approach. J Child Psychol Psychiatry 35:1015–1032, 1994

Perry EK, Lee ML, Martin-Ruiz CM, et al: Cholinergic activity in autism: abnormalities in the cerebral cortex and basal forebrain. Am J Psychiatry 158:1058–1066, 2001

Riback PS: Donepezil for tics in Tourette syndrome (abstract). Ann Neurol 50: S117, 2001

Schopler E, Reichler RJ, Renner BR: The Childhood Autism Rating Scale (CARS). Los Angeles, CA, Western Psychological Services, 1988

Stimulants and Nonstimulants in the Treatment of Hyperactivity in Autism

Yann Poncin, M.D.

Lawrence Scahill, M.S.N., Ph.D.

DSM-IV advises against a diagnosis of attention-deficit/hyperactivity disorder (ADHD) when a pervasive developmental disorder (PDD) is present (American Psychiatric Association 2000). However, symptoms of hyperactivity, distractibility, and impulsiveness are common reports in children with PDDs (Tsai 1996; Volkmar and Klin 2005). Indeed, a high percentage of children in PDD clinics are diagnosed with ADHD before the diagnosis of a PDD (V.K. Jensen et al. 1997). In an early report, Rutter et al. (1967) observed a 43% rate of hyperkinesis in a sample of 63 children with "infantile psychosis." This former diagnostic category likely included children who would be diagnosed with autistic disorder today (Volkmar and Klin 2005). Ghaziuddin

Support for this work comes from National Institute of Mental Health Grant N01MH70009 (Dr. Scahill).

et al. (1998) found that among consecutive referrals for Asperger's disorder, over one-third of the 35 subjects met criteria for ADHD. More recently, Yoshida and Uchiyama (2004) set aside the DSM-IV diagnostic convention and examined the frequency of ADHD in a group of 53 clinically ascertained children with so-called high-functioning PDDs (defined as autism, Asperger's disorder, or PDD not otherwise specified [PDDNOS], and IQ >70). The study sample was derived from a larger group of 520 children ages 7–15 years and was ascertained over a 6-month period from a general outpatient child psychiatry service. Using the ADHD Rating Scale (DuPaul et al. 1998) completed by parents and teachers, direct observation, and a clinical interview, the researchers identified 68% ($n=36$) children with ADHD. In a review of clinic records from a specialized clinic for neuropsychological testing, 16 of 27 (59%) of the children with PDDNOS or autism met the criteria for ADHD (Goldstein and Schwebach 2004). Although these studies involved selected samples, the high frequency of ADHD symptoms in these case series strongly suggests that this symptom domain warrants assessment in children with PDDs.

Careful examination of clinically ascertained samples of children with ADHD also reveals a high percentage of PDDs in children referred and diagnosed with ADHD (Clark et al. 1999; Dyck et al. 2001; Luteijn et al. 2000). Furthermore, the neuropsychological profile in children with high-functioning forms of PDD has features in common with children with ADHD (Geurts et al. 2004). In a controlled comparison of executive function deficits in children with ADHD, high-functioning PDDs, and control subjects, Geurts et al. (2004) showed that children with ADHD and PDDs shared several deficits in common, although children with PDDs had impairment across more neuropsychological domains. Although somewhat controversial, the overlap of ADHD and PDDs is embodied in the European diagnosis known as deficits in attention, motor control, and perception (DAMP) (Gillberg 2003). Thus, despite the convention of making the diagnosis of ADHD or a PDD—but not both—there are common features in clinical and cognitive profiles. This raises a fundamental question about whether approaches to the pharmacological treatment of ADHD are appropriate for children with PDDs accompanied by an ADHD clinical profile.

Parent surveys on medication use in PDD samples provide insight into clinical practice. These surveys suggest that clinicians are convinced that ADHD symptoms are appropriate targets for medication. For example, in a study of a group of 109 children with high-functioning PDDs, Martin et al. (1999) found stimulants were prescribed for 20% of respondents (only antidepressants were prescribed for a higher percentage of respondents). Aman et al. (2005) reviewed medication trends in the treatment of autism over a 10-year period in the state of North Carolina. The investigators observed a nearly 50% rise in the use of medication from 1993 to 2000. Stimulants were the second most commonly used class of medication after antidepressants. Inspection of these data suggests a doubling in the rate of stimulant use from 6% to 13.8% over the decade.

In view of these community survey data and the frequent occurrence of hyperactivity and inattention in children with PDDs, some investigators argue that the exclusion of ADHD in children with PDDs should be reconsidered (Ghaziuddin et al. 1992; Holtmann et al. 2005; Tsai 1996; Yoshida and Uchiyama 2004). Others maintain, however, that empirical data necessary to delineate ADHD as a separate diagnosis in children with PDDs are inadequate (Volkmar and Klin 2005).

Since the late 1950s, several theories about the etiology of ADHD have been advanced. These theories include the dysregulation of norepinephrine and dopamine circuits resulting in deficits in attention, executive function, attention, impulse control, and motor regulation (Arnsten and Li 2005; Nigg 2005). Both genetics and environmental exposures may play a role in these deficits (Bradshaw and Sheppard 2000; Smalley et al. 2005). Whether these etiologies apply to the ADHD picture in children with PDDs is unknown (Dyck et al. 2001; Geurts et al. 2004; Luteijn et al. 2000; Ozonoff and Jensen 1999; Roeyers et al. 1998; Smalley et al. 2005). What is clear is that there are common features as well as differences in ADHD and PDDs. For clinicians and families faced with planning treatment for children with PDDs accompanied by hyperactivity, distractibility, and impulsiveness, the question is whether interventions that are effective for ADHD are also effective for similarly affected children with PDDs. In this chapter we examine the evidence for pharmacotherapy in children and adolescents with PDDs accompanied by hyperactivity, distractibility, and impulsiveness. We begin with a review of the evidence on the use of stimulants in the treatment of PDDs. This is followed by an examination of nonstimulants for these target symptoms in PDDs.

Stimulants

Mechanism of Action

The stimulants, which consist of methylphenidate, dexmethylphenidate, D-amphetamine, and *d,l*-amphetamine, have been used for the treatment of hyperactivity and inattention ever since Charles Bradley (1937) reported success with Benzedrine in the treatment of impulsive children. Both methylphenidate and amphetamine block the reuptake of dopamine and, to a lesser extent, norepinephrine. Amphetamine stimulates the release of newly synthesized dopamine. By contrast, methylphenidate promotes release of stored dopamine (Pliszka 2005). Frontal and subcortical circuits, which play a central role in attention, motor planning, and impulse control, are mediated by dopamine and norepinephrine. Evidence from neuroimaging studies suggests that dysregulation of these circuits plays a role in ADHD. Thus, the mechanism of stimulant medications appears to be relevant to the pathophysiology of ADHD (Pliszka 2005).

Although the role of dopamine and norepinephrine has been examined in ADHD, parallel findings in children with PDDs and ADHD have not been documented.

Evidence in the Treatment of ADHD

Hundreds of controlled studies have demonstrated the effect of stimulants in ADHD in both children and adults (Ford et al. 2003). The Multimodal Treatment Study of Children With ADHD (MTA Cooperative Group 1999, 2004) showed that methylphenidate is effective for both short-term and intermediate-term benefits in typically developing children with ADHD. The study showed that careful medication management by an expert was superior to comprehensive behavioral treatment alone and community care, which consisted primarily of methylphenidate.

Finally, careful medication management alone by experts in the research centers was equivalent on ADHD outcomes compared with behavioral treatment in combination with the same careful medication management in the same research centers. Although equivalent, both medication managed by experts and combined treatment with medication and behavioral intervention were superior to behavioral treatment alone and community care (P. S. Jensen et al. 2001; MTA Cooperative Group 1999). The superiority of well-managed methylphenidate treatment over community care suggests that community care is effective but not optimal.

Evidence in the Treatment of Hyperactivity and Inattention in PDDs

In contrast, the benefits of stimulants for hyperactivity in children with PDDs are far less supported by research data. Early reports suggested that stimulants were generally ineffective and associated with adverse events—especially irritability and stereotypies (Campbell 1975; Campbell and Cohen 1978). However, sample sizes were small, and subject selection was not always clear. Indeed, there have been only a few placebo-controlled trials involving developmentally disabled populations. Most of these studies involved children with mental retardation—either PDD status was not reported or the subjects did not have a PDD diagnosis (see Aman et al. 2003 for a detailed review). As of the time of this writing, there have been only three double-blind, placebo-controlled trials exploring the stimulant treatment of ADHD-like symptoms in patients with PDDs (Handen et al. 2000; Quintana et al. 1995; Research Units on Pediatric Psychopharmacology [RUPP] Autism Network 2005a). All three of these studies compared methylphenidate with placebo.

Quintana et al. (1995) conducted a double-blind, placebo-controlled crossover study with two methylphenidate dose levels in 10 children with autism. The subjects showed modest but significant improvement without severe side effects. There was no statistical difference between the two methylphenidate doses, and unlike studies of methylphenidate in mental retardation, there was no relationship between IQ and response.

Handen et al. (2000) conducted a double-blind, placebo-controlled, crossover study of methylphenidate (0.3 or 0.6 mg/kg) in 13 children with autism and symptoms of ADHD. They found that 8 subjects responded positively based on a 50% decrease in the Conners' Parent Rating Scale for ADHD. Three of the children were unable to complete one of the methylphenidate doses because of adverse events. They concluded that methylphenidate can be effective in children with autism and ADHD symptoms, but patients with autism seem particularly susceptible to side effects, including social withdrawal and irritability, especially when the medication is used at higher doses.

The vulnerability to adverse effects from stimulants is supported by the retrospective chart review of 195 children and adolescents with PDDs treated with stimulants in a specialty clinic for children with PDDs (Stigler et al. 2004). Using doses ranging from 2.5 to 80 mg (mean dose = 12.5 mg) for methylphenidate and 2.5 to 45 mg (mean dose = 10.4 mg) for L-amphetamine/D-amphetamine, these investigators reported limited benefit for stimulants. Moreover, the stimulants were poorly tolerated. Adverse effects often lead to discontinuation. Agitation was the most common adverse effect; irritability, dysphoria, aggression, and dyspepsia were also common.

Acknowledging the inadequate guidance for clinicians on the use of stimulants in children with PDDs accompanied by hyperactivity, the RUPP Autism Network (2005a) conducted a multisite study in 72 children with PDDs and ADHD. To be included in the study, children had to be between age 5 and 14 years, have a mental age of at least 18 months, meet criteria for a PDD (PDDNOS, Asperger's disorder, or autistic disorder), and have at least a moderate level of hyperactivity. The protocol included a 7-day test-dose phase, during which the children were treated openly with the three dose levels of immediate-release methylphenidate and placebo for 2 days each. Children who tolerated all doses of methylphenidate during the test dose were enrolled in a 4-week, double-blind, crossover trial of placebo and three methylphenidate dose levels in random order. The medication was administered in identically appearing capsules three times per day (breakfast, noon, and 4 P.M.); the 4 P.M. dose of active drug was roughly half the strength of the morning dose. The median morning dose levels of methylphenidate were 0.125 mg/kg, 0.25 mg/kg, and 0.6 mg/kg. The primary outcome measure was the Aberrant Behavior Checklist (ABC; Aman et al. 1985) Hyperactivity subscale rated by parents and teachers. Using specific criteria for positive response (improvements on parent and teacher measures and global ratings by a blinded clinician), subjects were treated for an additional 8 weeks with the best dose to evaluate the durability of the short-term results.

Parent ratings showed improvement compared with placebo, ranging from 12% for the low dose and 20% for the medium and highest dose levels (effect size = 0.3–0.05). Teacher ratings also showed modest improvement, ranging from 12% to 17% (effect size = 0.25–0.35). Thirty-five of the 72 patients enrolled showed a positive response to a least one dose of methylphenidate (RUPP Autism Network 2005a). Neither age, nor IQ, nor diagnosis had a significant moderating effect on parent- or teacher-rated ABC Hyperactivity subscale scores. These results indicate that both the magnitude of response and the likelihood of positive response are lower in hyperactive children with PDDs compared with typically developing children with ADHD. In the MTA study, for example, approximately 75% of children treated in the research centers showed a positive response to methylphenidate, and the magnitude of improvement on ADHD outcome measures was 50% on average (MTA Cooperative Group 1999).

Results of the RUPP study also suggest that children with PDDs are at higher risk for adverse events compared with typically developing children with ADHD. Considering the test-dose period and the crossover phase, the rate of study termination because of adverse events was 18% (13 of 72) compared with 1.3% in the MTA study. Irritability was the most common reason to exit the study (this may be similar to the agitation described by Stigler et al. 2004). Other adverse effects included appetite suppression, insomnia, increased stereotypies, and tics.

Summary of the Evidence and Recommendations

Taken together, the results of the RUPP study (2005a) indicate that methylphenidate can be an effective treatment for children with PDDs and ADHD. However, the magnitude of response is likely to be small to moderate. Attempts to enhance the response by pushing the dose are likely to encounter unacceptable adverse events. The use of a test dose may help identify the tolerable dose, which can then be evaluated for efficacy (Di Martino et al. 2004). As with typically developing children with ADHD, use of parent and teacher ratings to monitor progress is recommended.

Alpha-Adrenergic Agonists

Mechanism of Action

The α_2-adrenergic agonists clonidine and guanfacine were developed for the treatment of hypertension and later used in psychiatry for various indications. α_2-Adrenergic agonists decrease the firing of presynaptic noradrenergic receptors in the locus coeruleus. This reduced firing by locus coeruleus neurons turns down norepinephrine function, which is presumed to reduce arousal and hyperactivity. Presynaptic α_{2a} receptors may also modulate dopamine neurotransmission, and this effect may contribute to improving inattention (Newcorn et al. 2003). In a series of animal studies, Arnsten and colleagues have shown that guanfacine also has postsynaptic effects via long axons projecting from the locus coeruleus to prefrontal cortex (Arnsten and Li 2005). This more direct effect on prefrontal function may contribute to decreased distractibility, impulsiveness, and overactivity. Guanfacine also has a longer duration of action and is less sedating than clonidine.

Evidence in the Treatment of ADHD

The α-adrenergic agonists have been used to treat children with tics and/or ADHD for over two decades (Cohen et al. 1979). The multisite study conducted by the Tourette's Syndrome Study Group (2002) showed that clonidine was superior to placebo, equal to methylphenidate, and additive when combined with methylphenidate in children with ADHD and tic disorders. In a pilot study of 34 children with ADHD and tic disorders, guanfacine was found to be superior to placebo for tics and on teacher ratings of ADHD symptoms (Scahill et al. 2001). These studies showed that the magnitude of effect for clonidine and guanfacine is likely to be smaller than the large effects observed with the stimulants in ADHD. The α_2-adrenergic agonists may also exert greater effects on hyperactive-impulsive symptoms and less effect on symptoms of inattention.

The evidence for the α_2-adrenergic agonists in PDDs is more limited. Jaselskis et al. (1992) conducted a double-blind, placebo-controlled, crossover study with clonidine in eight boys with autistic disorder accompanied by significant inattention, impulsiveness, and hyperactivity. All eight subjects had unsuccessful treatment with antipsychotics, methylphenidate, or desipramine. Each treatment phase was 6 weeks in duration. At doses ranging from 4 to 10 μg/kg per day, clonidine led to improvement on the teacher and parent ratings of hyperactivity. Six of the eight subjects continued with open-label treatment after the double-blind phase. Of these, four relapsed within a few months, and only two subjects continued on clonidine for up to a year. Sedation was a common side effect.

Another double-blind, placebo-controlled, crossover study examined the transdermal clonidine patch (dosage range=0.1–0.3 mg/day) in nine males ages 5–33 years (Fankhauser et al. 1992). Clonidine delivered this way led to significant, but modest, improvement on the Clinical Global Impression (CGI) scale for overactivity (Guy 1976). Common adverse effects included sedation and fatigue along with redness and itching under the patch. A measurable decrease in systolic blood pressure was observed, but there were no complaints or other signs of hypotension.

To get preliminary results on efficacy and safety of guanfacine, Posey and colleagues conducted a retrospective chart review in 80 children (ages 3–18 years) with PDDs (Posey et al. 2004). Based on the CGI Improvement (CGI-I) scale, 20 of 75 subjects (27%) were rated much improved or very much improved on hyperactivity. In addition to the problem of retrospective rating of benefit, the target symptoms and duration of treatment (from 7 to 1,700 days) varied in these children. Thus, it is difficult to assess these results. The average medication dosage was 2.6 mg/day given in divided doses (two or three times per day). Adverse effects included transient sedation (31%) and irritability (6.3%).

The RUPP Autism Network conducted an open-label trial of guanfacine in 25 children with PDDs and ADHD (Scahill et al. 2006). This pilot trial was conducted in tandem with the RUPP methylphenidate study (RUPP Autism Network 2005a). Children who were excluded from the study because of a recent history of failed treatment with methylphenidate or those who did not show improvement in the RUPP methylphenidate study were invited to participate in the guanfacine trial. The 23 boys and 2 girls had a mean age of 9 (± 3.14) years and a parent-rated baseline ABC Hyperactivity score of 31.3 (± 8.89). After 8 weeks of treatment, the parent-rated ABC Hyperactivity subscale score improved by 40% to 18.9 (± 10.37) (effect size=1.4). The teacher-rated ABC Hyperactivity subscale score decreased by 25%, from 29.9 (± 9.12) at baseline to 22.3 (± 9.44) at endpoint (effect size=0.83). Despite the suggested large effects, only 12 children (48%) were rated as much improved or very much improved on the CGI-I scale. At dosages ranging from 1.0 to 3.0 mg/day given in two or three divided doses, common adverse effects included irritability, sedation, sleep disturbance (insomnia or midsleep awakening), and constipation. Irritability led to discontinuation in four subjects. There were no significant changes in pulse, blood pressure, or electrocardiogram (ECG). These results suggest that guanfacine may be useful for the treatment of hyperactivity in children with PDDs, but large-scale, placebo-controlled studies are needed.

Summary of the Evidence and Recommendations

Taken together, the data on the use of clonidine and guanfacine to treat ADHD-like symptoms in children with PDDs are insufficient to guide practice. Even at low doses, clonidine may be associated with unacceptable sedation. As in other populations, parents should be educated about the potential for rebound hypertension upon abrupt discontinuation of clonidine, although this is probably less likely to be a problem with guanfacine. Guanfacine also appears to be less likely to cause sedation, although midsleep awakening can present a problem for clinical management. The usual dosage of guanfacine ranged from 1.0 to 3.0 mg/day divided in two or three doses. Problems such as midsleep awakening can be managed by adjusting the time and distribution of doses. Medical monitoring of clonidine and guanfacine includes assessment of blood pressure, especially during the dose adjustment phase. Consensus is lacking on the need for more specific cardiac monitoring such as ECGs, with some guidelines recommending baseline and periodic monitoring (Dulcan 1997) and others, including the American Heart Association, indicating that ECG monitoring is not necessary (Gutgesell et al. 1999).

Antidepressants

Mechanism of Action

Most antidepressant medications in current use block the reuptake of norepinephrine, serotonin, or both. A notable exception is the novel antidepressant bupropion, which blocks reuptake of norepinephrine and dopamine (Stahl et al. 2004). In the treatment of patients with ADHD, most attention has been on bupropion and the specific norepinephrine reuptake inhibitor desipramine. By contrast, selective serotonin reuptake inhibitors (SSRIs) do not appear to be relevant for the treatment of ADHD. Atomoxetine, a selective norepinephrine reuptake inhibitor, is not used in the treatment of depression. Animal data also indicate that atomoxetine increases dopamine in the prefrontal cortex (Swanson et al. 2006).

Evidence in the Treatment of ADHD

Atomoxetine is the only nonstimulant drug that is approved for the treatment of ADHD. Bupropion and desipramine have each demonstrated significant benefits over placebo on ADHD outcomes in more than one randomized trial (see Rains and Scahill 2006 for a review of these studies). In general, the magnitude of effect of these medications is less than that observed with the stimulants. Thus, atomoxetine and bupropion are considered second-line agents in the treatment of patients with ADHD. Because of concerns about cardiac conduction abnormalities, many clinicians are reluctant to use desipramine in children.

Evidence in the Treatment of Hyperactivity and Inattention in PDDs

Atomoxetine and bupropion have not been studied in children with PDDs. There are a few trials with the tricyclic antidepressants, including desipramine and clomipramine. Gordon et al. (1993) observed a significant decrease in hyperactivity in their 10-week, double-blind, crossover study of clomipramine, desipramine, and placebo. The 24 subjects ranged in age from 6 to 23 years. Clomipramine and desipramine were superior to placebo and equal to each other on a clinician rating of hyperactivity. The mean dosage was 4.3 mg/kg per day for clomipramine and 4 mg/kg per day for desipramine. One subject had a seizure while on clomipramine; irritability and temper outbursts were more common with desipramine.

In a three-phase crossover study, Remington et al. (2001) compared haloperidol, clomipramine, and placebo in 36 subjects ranging in age from 10 to 36 years (mean age = 16.3 years). Each treatment phase was 6 weeks in duration followed by a 1-week washout. Clomipramine was associated with small improvement (11% drop on the ABC Hyperactivity subscale; see Table 7–1). By contrast, haloperidol was significantly better than placebo, with a 27% improvement on the hyperactivity subscale). Adverse effects were common during the clomipramine phase and included fatigue, insomnia, tachycardia, nausea, diaphoresis, and decreased appetite. Twelve subjects withdrew from the clomipramine phase because of "behavioral problems." It is not clear whether these were newly emerging or worsening behavioral problems or simply a continuation of ongoing behavioral problems. In addition to the burden of blood level and ECG monitoring, these results suggest that clomipramine does not have an important role to play in the treatment of ADHD in children with PDDs.

Amantadine

Mechanism of Action

Amantadine has multiple pharmacological actions as evidenced by its use as an antiviral agent and as a treatment for Parkinson's disease. The beneficial effects in Parkinson's disease are presumed to be a result of its dopamine-releasing effects, which also may contribute to its effects on behavior. Amantadine is also an *N*-methyl-D-aspartate antagonist. It is this mechanism that has prompted interest in the treatment of autism, because dysregulation of the glutamatergic system has been proposed to play a role in the neurobiology of autism (King et al. 2001).

Evidence in the Treatment of ADHD

The role of amantadine in the treatment of ADHD has not been evaluated.

Evidence in the Treatment of Hyperactivity and Inattention in PDDs

In a 4-week randomized clinical trial of 39 subjects (ages 5–19 years), King et al. (2001) reported a 22% drop in ABC Hyperactivity subscale scores in the amantadine group (from 29.4 at baseline to 23 at endpoint) compared with a 6% increase in the placebo group (from 32.7 at baseline to 35.6 at endpoint). This difference between drug and placebo was not statistically significant. The starting dosage of liquid amantadine was 2.5 mg/kg per day, and the dosage was increased to 2.5 mg/kg twice daily by week 3. The most common adverse effect was insomnia. A major limitation of this study is the wide range of hyperactivity of the sample at baseline (from 16 to 46 on the ABC Hyperactivity subscale), which suggests that subjects with lower scores have little room for improvement.

Summary of the Evidence and Recommendations

Further study with amantadine or other medications in this class (e.g., memantine) is warranted before specific recommendations can be made.

Naltrexone

Mechanism of Action

Naltrexone is an opiate antagonist that has Food and Drug Administration indications for the treatment of alcohol and opioid dependence. The endogenous opioids may play a role in the modulation of several behaviors, including motor activity, memory, learning, reward, and social interaction. Interest in naltrexone was prompted by early studies showing higher levels of β-endorphins in children with autism, which was presumed to be related to dysfunction of the pineal-hypothalamic-pituitary-adrenal axis (Buitelaar 2003). The potential relevance of opioid antagonists for the treatment of ADHD has not been articulated.

Evidence in the Treatment of ADHD

The efficacy and safety of naltrexone for the treatment of ADHD have not been evaluated.

Evidence in the Treatment of Hyperactivity in PDDs

Naltrexone has been proposed as a treatment for autism for well over a decade (Campbell et al. 1989). The proposed indications have included self-injurious behavior and communication deficits (Scahill and Martin 2005). Although most of these proposed applications have not been supported by placebo-controlled trials, a few studies observed benefits in hyperactivity in children with autism (see below). Despite examination in several placebo-controlled studies, however, the magnitude of effect is modest.

Campbell et al. (1993) conducted a 3-week double-blind, placebo-controlled trial in 41 children between the ages of 3 and 8 years. On a clinician measure of hyperactivity, naltrexone was superior to placebo. The results of this study prompted others to replicate the findings. Willemsen-Swinkels et al. (1996) conducted a 4-week double-blind, placebo-controlled, crossover study in 23 children with autism ages 3–7 years. Most children were treated with a 20-mg capsule given in the morning (mean dose = 1 mg/kg per day). Outcome measures included ABC and CGI rated by parents and teachers. The results are difficult to interpret because ABC subscales scores are not presented. Five of 20 children with complete data were rated as much improved on the CGI by parents and teachers (though there was not complete agreement on which children showed a positive response).

This same group of investigators then enrolled 6 of the 7 children considered positive responders in a 6-month open-label continuation study using the same dosage (approximately 20 mg/day) (Willemsen-Swinkels et al. 1999). Hyperactivity levels remained approximately the same at 6 months, suggesting the continued efficacy of naltrexone in the treatment-responsive group. Noting that most parents did not elect to continue treatment with naltrexone at the end of the 6-month study, the investigators did not strongly endorse the use of naltrexone for hyperactivity.

Kolmen et al. (1995, 1997) conducted a pair of randomized, double-blind, placebo-controlled, crossover trials in a combined sample of 24 children with autism. The studies enrolled children ages 3–8 years, 21 boys and 3 girls. No threshold score for hyperactivity was required for entry. Each treatment arm was approximately 14 days; the dose of naltrexone was 1 mg/kg per day given in a single morning dose. There was a 37.5% decrease from baseline on the Conners' rating scale, but this change was not significantly different from that seen with placebo. On the Conners' Teacher Questionnaire, there was no evidence of improvement on the active drug. Common side effects included drowsiness and loss of appetite.

Summary of the Evidence and Recommendations

Although well tolerated, the results of these studies do not strongly support the use of naltrexone for the treatment of hyperactivity in children with autism. If other interventions have been unsuccessful, a trial of naltrexone may be considered. The starting dosage of naltrexone in the trials discussed above ranged from 12.5 to 25 mg/day, with an increase to 25–50 mg in the first week (target dosage approximately 1 mg/kg per day).

Antipsychotics

Antipsychotics have a long history of use in the treatment of children with PDDs (see Chapter 5, "Treatment of Autism With Antipsychotics," for a detailed review). Few antipsychotic trials in children with PDDs have focused on hyperactivity as the target symptom. In this section we review briefly studies that measured the impact of antipsychotic medication on hyperactivity. These data may be useful for the comparing the magnitude of effect on hyperactivity for the antipsychotic drugs with that of other medications reviewed previously in this chapter.

Evidence in the Treatment of Hyperactivity and Inattention in PDDs

Several controlled studies conducted by Campbell and colleagues have shown that haloperidol is effective for hyperactivity (Anderson et al. 1984, 1989; Campbell and Cohen 1978; Cohen et al. 1980). The drawbacks of haloperidol in these studies have also been well documented (Campbell et al. 1997).

The RUPP Autism Network (2002) conducted a multisite, randomized, placebo-controlled trial of risperidone in 101 children with autistic disorder accompanied by severe tantrums, aggression, or self-injurious behavior. Although the primary outcome measure was the Irritability subscale of the ABC, the impact on the ABC Hyperactivity subscale was also examined. After 8 weeks of treatment with an average dosage of 1.8 mg/day, the Hyperactivity subscale showed a decline of 47% (from 31.8 at baseline to 17 at endpoint) with risperidone compared with 15% (from 32.3 at baseline to 27.6 at endpoint) with placebo (effect size= 1.0). These gains in hyperactivity were stable over a 4-month extension phase (RUPP Autism Network 2005b). Similar findings with risperidone were reported in an open-label study conducted by Troost et al. (2005) and in a short-term, placebo-controlled study by Shea et al. (2004). Clearly, these effects on hyperactivity are of greater magnitude than the effects of other classes of drugs reviewed previously in this chapter.

Olanzapine was evaluated in a 3-month open-label study of 25 children ages 6–16 years (Kemner et al. 2002). The mean ABC Hyperactivity subscale score declined by 34% (from 16.9 at baseline to 11.2 at endpoint). Use of the other atypical antipsychotics is documented only in case reports, small case series, or retrospective studies, which provide limited information.

Although the occurrence of neurological side effects is lower with the atypical antipsychotics compared with traditional agents, weight gain and related metabolic complications are emerging as salient issues (Martin et al. 2004; Newcomer 2005). Given these concerns, the use of atypical antipsychotics for hyperactivity should not be considered a first-line treatment. On the other hand, if the hyperactivity were accompanied by significant disruptive behavior, explosive behavior, or aggression, the use of a potent drug such as risperidone would be appropriate. There is some evidence that risperidone may have additive effects when used in combination with stimulants (Aman et al. 2004).

Table 7–1. Studies showing improvement on the Hyperactivity subscale of the parent-rated Aberrant Behavior Checklist (Aman et al. 1985)

Author/year	Drug	N	Design	Age range, years	Baseline	Endpoint	Percent change[a]
King et al. 2001	Amantadine	39	Placebo-controlled	5–19	29.4 (NR)	23 (NR)	22
Remington et al. 2001	Clomipramine	36	Placebo-controlled, crossover	10–36	26 (NR)	23 (NR)	11
Remington et al. 2001	Haloperidol	36	Placebo-controlled, crossover	10–36	26 (NR)	19 (NR)	27
RUPP 2002	Risperidone	101	Placebo-controlled	5–17	31.8 (9.6)	17.0 (9.7)	47
Shea et al. 2004	Risperidone	79	Placebo-controlled	5–12	27.3 (9.7)	12.4 (NR)	55
RUPP 2005a	Methylphenidate	66	Placebo-controlled, crossover	5–14	33.2 (8.7)	17.2 (9.9)	34[b]
Scahill et al. 2006	Guanfacine	25	Open	5–14	29.9 (9.1)	22.3 (9.4)	25

Note.   NR = not reported; RUPP = Research Units on Pediatric Psychopharmacology Autism Network.
[a]No correction for placebo.
[b]Percent change on the best dose for each subject.

Conclusions

As shown in Table 7–1, the results of these studies indicate that methylphenidate, when given at its optimal dose, is moderately effective in reducing hyperactivity in children with PDDs. Findings from the RUPP Autism Network (2005a) study show that pushing the dose of methylphenidate to levels commonly used in typically developing children with ADHD often results in unacceptable adverse effects. Risperidone shows a medium to large effect on hyperactivity. However, prudent use of this drug suggests that it should be reserved for children with high levels of hyperactivity in the presence of tantrums, aggression, or self-injurious behavior. Amantadine may warrant additional study for cases in which hyperactivity is clearly the target symptom, because the variability in the sample in this published report may have limited detection of benefit. Clomipramine does not appear effective for this indication in children with PDDs. To establish the benefits of guanfacine in children with PDDs and ADHD, a larger placebo-controlled study is needed.

References

Aman MG, Singh NN, Stewart AW, et al: The Aberrant Behavior Checklist: a behavior rating scale for the assessment of treatment effects. Am J Ment Defic 89:485–491, 1985

Aman MG, Buican B, Arnold LE: Methylphenidate treatment in children with borderline IQ and mental retardation: analysis of three aggregated studies. J Child Adolesc Psychopharmacol 13:29–40, 2003

Aman MG, Binder C, Turgay A: Risperidone effects in the presence/absence of psychostimulant medicine in children with ADHD, other disruptive behavior disorders, and subaverage IQ. J Child Adolesc Psychopharmacol 14:243–254, 2004

Aman MG, Lam KS, Van Bourgondien ME: Medication patterns in patients with autism: temporal, regional and demographic influences. J Child Adolesc Psychopharmacol 15:116–126, 2005

American Psychiatric Association: Diagnostic and Statistical Manual of Mental Disorders, 4th Edition, Text Revision. Washington, DC, American Psychiatric Association, 2000

Anderson LT, Campbell M, Grega DM, et al: Haloperidol in the treatment of infantile autism: effects on learning and behavioral symptoms. Am J Psychiatry 141:1195–1202, 1984

Anderson LT, Campbell M, Adams P, et al: Effects of haloperidol on discrimination learning and behavioral symptoms in autistic children. J Autism Dev Disord 19:227–239, 1989

Arnsten AF, Li BM: Neurobiology of executive functions: catecholamine influences on prefrontal cortical functions. Biol Psychiatry 57:1377–1384, 2005

Bradley C: The behavior of children receiving benzedrine. Am J Psychiatry 94:577–585, 1937

Bradshaw JL, Sheppard DM: The neurodevelopmental frontalstriatal disorders: Evolutionary adaptiveness and anomalous lateralization. Brain Lang 73:297–320, 2000

Buitelaar JK: Miscellaneous compounds: beta-blockers and opiate antagonists, in Pediatric Psychopharmacology: Principles and Practice. Edited by Martin A, Scahill L, Charney DS, et al. New York, Oxford University Press, 2003, pp 353–362

Campbell M: Pharmacotherapy in early infantile autism. Biol Psychiatry 10:399–423, 1975

Campbell M, Cohen I: Treatment of infantile autism. Compr Ther 4:33–37, 1978

Campbell M, Overall JE, Small AM, et al: Naltrexone in children: an acute open dose range tolerance trial. J Am Acad Child Adolesc Psychiatry 28:200–206, 1989

Campbell M, Anderson LT, Small AM, et al: Naltrexone in autistic children: behavioral symptoms and attentional learning. J Am Acad Child Adolesc Psychiatry 32:1283–1291, 1993

Campbell M, Armenteros JL, Malone RP, et al: Neuroleptic-related dyskinesias in autistic children: a prospective, longitudinal study. J Am Acad Child Adolesc Psychiatry 36:835–843, 1997

Clark T, Feehan C, Tinline C, et al: Autistic symptoms in children with attention deficit-hyperactivity disorder. Eur Child Adolesc Psychiatry 8:50–55, 1999

Cohen DJ, Young JG, Nathanson JA, et al: Clonidine in Tourette's syndrome. Lancet 2:551–553, 1979

Cohen IL, Campbell M, Posner D, et al: Behavioral effects of haloperidol in young autistic children: an objective analysis using a within-subjects reversal design. J Am Acad Child Psychiatry 19:665–677, 1980

Di Martino A, Melis G, Cianchetti C, et al: Methylphenidate for pervasive developmental disorders: safety and efficacy of a single test dose and ongoing therapy: an open pilot study. J Child Adolesc Psychopharmacol 14:207–218, 2004

Dulcan M: Practice parameters for the assessment and treatment of children, adolescents, and adults with attention-deficit hyperactivity disorder. American Academy of Child and Adolescent Psychiatry. J Am Acad Child Adolesc Psychiatry 36 (suppl 10):85S–121S, 1997

DuPaul GJ, Anastopoulos AD, Power TJ, et al: Parent ratings of attention-deficit/hyperactivity disorder symptoms: factor structure and normative data. J Psychopathol Behav Assess 20:83–102, 1998

Dyck MJ, Ferguson K, Shochet IM: Do autism spectrum disorders differ from each other and from non-spectrum disorders on emotion recognition tests? Eur Child Adolesc Psychiatry 10:105–116, 2001

Fankhauser MP, Karumanchi VC, German ML, et al: A double-blind, placebo-controlled study of the efficacy of transdermal clonidine in autism. J Clin Psychiatry 53:77–82, 1992

Ford RE, Greenhill LL, Posner K: Stimulants, in Pediatric Psychopharmacology: Principles and Practice. Edited by Martin A, Scahill L, Charney DS, et al. New York, Oxford University Press, 2003, pp 255–263

Geurts HM, Verte S, Oosterlaan J, et al: How specific are executive functioning deficits in attention deficit hyperactivity disorder and autism? J Child Psychol Psychiatry 45:836–854, 2004

Ghaziuddin M, Tsai L, Alessi N: ADHD and PDD: J Am Acad Child Adolesc Psychiatry 31:567, 1992

Ghaziuddin M, Weidmer-Mikhail E, Ghaziuddin N: Comorbidity of Asperger syndrome: a preliminary report. J Intellect Disabil Res 42 (part 4):279–283, 1998

Gillberg C: Deficits in attention, motor control, and perception: a brief review. Arch Dis Child 88:904–910, 2003

Goldstein S, Schwebach AJ: The comorbidity of pervasive developmental disorder and attention deficit hyperactivity disorder: results of a retrospective chart review. J Autism Dev Disord 3:329–339, 2004

Gordon CT, State RC, Nelson JE, et al: A double-blind comparison of clomipramine desipramine, and placebo in the treatment of autistic disorder. Arch Gen Psychiatry 50:441–447, 1993

Gutgesell H, Atkins D, Barst R, et al: AHA Scientific Statement: cardiovascular monitoring of children and adolescents receiving psychotropic drugs. J Am Acad Child Adolesc Psychiatry 38:1047–1050, 1999

Guy W: ECDEU assessment manual for psychopharmacology (NIMH Publ No 76–338). Rockville, MD, National Institute of Mental Health, 1976

Handen BL, Johnson CR, Lubetsky M: Efficacy of methylphenidate among children with autism and symptoms of attention-deficit hyperactivity disorder. J Autism Dev Disord 30:245–255, 2000

Holtmann M, Bolte S, Poustka F: ADHD, Asperger syndrome, and high-functioning autism. J Am Acad Child Adolesc Psychiatry 44:1101, 2005

Jaselskis CA, Cook EH Jr, Fletcher KE, et al: Clonidine treatment of hyperactive and impulsive children with autistic disorder. J Clin Psychopharmacol 12:322–327, 1992

Jensen PS, Hinshaw SP, Swanson JM, et al: Findings from the NIMH Multimodal Treatment Study of ADHD (MTA): implications and applications for primary care providers. J Dev Behav Pediatr 22:60–73, 2001

Jensen VK, Larrieu JA, Mack KK: Differential diagnosis between attention-deficit/hyperactivity disorder and pervasive developmental disorder not otherwise specified. Clin Pediatr 36:555–561, 1997

Kemner C, Willemsen-Swinkels SH, de Jonge M, et al: Open-label study of olanzapine in children with pervasive developmental disorder. J Clin Psychopharmacol 22:455–460, 2002

King BH, Wright DM, Handen BL, et al: Double-blind, placebo-controlled study of amantadine hydrochloride in the treatment of children with autistic disorder. J Am Acad Child Adolesc Psychiatry 40:658–665, 2001

Kolmen BK, Feldman HM, Handen BL, et al: Naltrexone in young autistic children: a double-blind, placebo-controlled crossover study. J Am Acad Child Adolesc Psychiatry 34:223–231, 1995

Kolmen BK, Feldman HM, Handen BL, et al: Naltrexone in young autistic children: replication study and learning measures. J Am Acad Child Adolesc Psychiatry 36:1570–1578, 1997

Luteijn EF, Serra M, Jackson S et al: How unspecified are disorders of children with a pervasive developmental disorder not otherwise specified? A study of social problems in children with PDD-NOS and ADHD. Eur Child Adolesc Psychiatry 9:168–179, 2000

Martin A, Scahill L, Klin A, et al: Higher functioning pervasive developmental disorders: rates and patterns of psychotropic drug use. J Am Acad Child Adolesc Psychiatry 38:923–931, 1999

Martin A, Scahill L, Anderson G, et al: Weight and leptin changes among risperidone-treated youths with autism: 6-month prospective data. Am J Psychiatry 161:1125–1127, 2004

MTA Cooperative Group: A 14-month randomized clinical trial of treatment strategies for attention-deficit/hyperactivity disorder. Multimodal Treatment Study of Children With ADHD. Arch Gen Psychiatry 56:1073–1086, 1999

MTA Cooperative Group: National Institute of Mental Health Multimodal Treatment Study of ADHD follow-up: changes in effectiveness and growth after the end of treatment. Pediatrics 113:762–769, 2004

Newcomer JW: Second-generation (atypical) antipsychotics and metabolic effects: a comprehensive literature review. CNS Drugs 19 (suppl 1):1–93, 2005

Newcorn JH, Schulz KP, Halperin JM: Adrenergic agonists: clonidine and guanfacine, in Pediatric Psychopharmacology: Principles and Practice. Edited by Martin A, Scahill L, Charney DS, et al. New York, Oxford University Press, 2003, pp 264–273

Nigg JT: Neuropscyhologic theory and findings in attention-deficit/hyperactivity disorder: the state of the field and salient challenges for the coming decade. Biol Psychiatry 57:1424–1435, 2005

Ozonoff S, Jensen J: Brief report: specific executive function profiles in three neurodevelopmental disorders. J Autism Dev Disord 29:171–177, 1999

Pliszka SR: The neuropsychopharmacology of attention-deficit/hyperactivity disorder. Biol Psychiatry 57:1385–1390, 2005

Posey DJ, Puntney JI, Sasher TM, et al: Guanfacine treatment of hyperactivity and inattention in pervasive developmental disorders: a retrospective analysis of 80 cases. J Child Adolesc Psychopharmacol 14:233–241, 2004

Quintana H, Birmaher B, Stedge D, et al: Use of methylphenidate in the treatment of children with autistic disorder. J Autism Devel Disord 25:283–294, 1995

Rains A, Scahill L: Non-stimulant medications in children with ADHD. J Child Adolesc Psychiatric Nursing 19:44–47, 2006

Remington G, Sloman L, Konstantareas M, et al: Clomipramine versus haloperidol in the treatment of autistic disorder: a double-blind, placebo-controlled, crossover study. J Clin Psychopharm 21:440–444, 2001

Research Units on Pediatric Psychopharmacology Autism Network: Randomized, controlled, crossover trial of methylphenidate in pervasive developmental disorders with hyperactivity. Arch Gen Psychiatry 62:1266–1274, 2005a

Research Units on Pediatric Psychopharmacology Autism Network: Risperidone treatment of autistic disorder: longer-term benefits and blinded discontinuation after 6 months. Am J Psychiatry 162:1361–1369, 2005b

Roeyers H, Keymeulen H, Buysse A: Differentiating attention-deficit/hyperactivity disorder from pervasive developmental disorder not otherwise specified. J Learn Disabil 31:565–571, 1998

Research Units on Pediatric Psychopharmacology (RUPP) Autism Network: Risperidone in children with autism and serious behavioral problems. N Engl J Med 347:314–321, 2002

Rutter M, Greenfield D, Lockyear L: A five to fifteen year follow-up study of infantile psychosis. II. Social and behavioural outcome. Br J Psychiatry 113:1183–1199, 1967

Scahill L, Martin A: Psychopharmacology, in Handbook of Autism and Pervasive Developmental Disorders, Volume 2: Assessment, Interventions, and Policy, 3rd Edition. Edited by Volkmar F, Paul R, Klin A, et al. Hoboken, NJ, Wiley, 2005, pp 1102–1117

Scahill L, Chappell PB, Kim YS, et al: A placebo-controlled study of guanfacine in the treatment of children with tic disorders and attention deficit hyperactivity disorder. Am J Psychiatry 158:1067–1074, 2001

Scahill L, Aman MG, McDougle CJ, et al: An open prospective trial of guanfacine in children with pervasive developmental disorders. J Child Adolesc Psychopharmacol 16:589–598, 2006

Shea S, Turgay A, Carroll A, et al: Risperidone in the treatment of disruptive behavioral symptoms in children with autistic and other pervasive developmental disorders. Pediatrics 114:E634–E641, 2004

Smalley SL, Loo SK, Yang MH, et al: Toward localizing genes underlying cerebral asymmetry and mental health. Am J Med Genet B Neuropsychiatr Genet 135:79–84, 2005 [erratum: Am J Med Genet B Neuropsychiatr Genet 136:107, 2005]

Stahl SM, Pradko JF, Haight BR, et al: A review of the neuropharmacology of bupropion, a dual norepinephrine and dopamine reuptake inhibitor. Prim Care Companion J Clin Psychiatry 6:159–166, 2004

Stigler KA, Desmond LA, Posey DJ, et al: A naturalistic retrospective analysis of psychostimulants in pervasive developmental disorders. J Child Adolesc Psychopharmacol 14:49–56, 2004

Swanson CJ, Perry KW, Koch-Krueger S, et al: Effect of the attention deficit/hyperactivity disorder drug atomoxetine on extracellular concentrations of norepinephrine and dopamine in several brain regions of the rat. Neuropsychopharmacolgy 50:755–760, 2006

Tourette's Syndrome Study Group: Treatment of ADHD in children with tics: a randomized controlled trial. Neurology 58:527–536, 2002

Troost PW, Lahuis BE, Steenhuis MP, et al: Long-term effects of risperidone in children with autism spectrum disorders: a placebo discontinuation study. J Am Acad Child Adolesc Psychiatry 44:1137–1144, 2005

Tsai LY: Brief report: comorbid psychiatric disorders of autistic disorder. J Autism Dev Disord 26:159–163, 1996

Volkmar FR, Klin A: Issues in the classification of autism and related conditions, in Handbook of Autism and Pervasive Developmental Disorders, Volume 1: Diagnosis, Development, Neurobiology, and Behavior, 3rd Edition. Edited by Volkmar F, Paul R, Klin A, et al. Hoboken, NJ, Wiley, 2005, pp 5–41

Willemsen-Swinkels SHN, Buitelaar JK, van Engeland H: The effects of chronic naltrexone treatment in young autistic children: a double-blind placebo-controlled crossover study. Biol Psychiatry 39:1023–1031, 1996

Willemsen-Swinkels SH, Buitelaar JK, van Berckelaer-Onnes IA, et al: Brief report: six months continuation treatment in naltrexone-responsive children with autism: an open-label case-control design. J Autism Dev Disord 29:167–169, 1999

Yoshida Y, Uchiyama T: The clinical necessity for assessing attention deficit/hyperactivity disorder (AD/HD) symptoms in children with high-functioning pervasive developmental disorder (PDD). Eur Child Adolesc Psychiatry 13:307–314, 2004

8

Applied Behavior Analysis in the Treatment of Autism

Tristram Smith, Ph.D.

Dennis Mozingo, Ph.D.

Daniel W. Mruzek, Ph.D.

Jennifer R. Zarcone, Ph.D.

Several professional organizations identify behavioral or applied behavior analysis (ABA) intervention as the treatment of choice for individuals with autism spectrum disorders (ASDs) (Maine Administrators of Services for Children with Disabilities 2000; New York State Department of Health, Early Intervention Program 1999). Similarly, Lilienfeld (2005) noted that although a large and

Preparation of this manuscript was supported in part by National Institutes of Health Grant U54 MH066397 to the University of Rochester (Phenotype and Genotype of Autism). The authors thank Jennifer Katz for reviewing drafts of the manuscript.

growing number of scientifically questionable treatments are available for ASDs, research indicates that ABA is the most efficacious intervention. Other reviews call attention to important limitations in research on ABA but concur that it has the most extensive scientific backing (Lord et al. 2002).

ABA is perhaps best known as an intervention for ASDs, but more generally it is an applied science and profession of service delivery that addresses a variety of socially significant issues, including typical and special education, behavioral medicine, clinical psychology and psychiatry, and performance in business and industry (Bailey and Burch 2005; Sulzer-Azaroff and Mayer 1991). ABA emphasizes careful assessment of how environmental events influence the behavior of an individual. The assessment includes contextual factors such as the classroom or other settings in which a behavior occurs; motivational variables such as hunger, thirst, or need for information; antecedent events for a behavior such as instructions or greetings from another person; and consequences that either increase or decrease the likelihood that the behavior will occur again in the future. Consequent events that increase behavior are called *reinforcers;* consequent events that decrease behavior are said to result in *extinction.*

Assessment leads to the design, implementation, and (further) evaluation of environmental modifications to change behaviors. In intervention for individuals with ASDs, these behaviors include language and communication, social and play skills, cognitive and academic skills, motor skills, independent living skills, and problem behavior (Smith et al. 2007). Behaviors are usually measured from direct observations that are repeated on multiple occasions with the same individual over time. In addition, acceptability of interventions and outcomes to consumers and caregivers is regarded as essential (Wolf 1978) and is frequently ascertained from ratings or other assessment procedures.

Although focusing on environmental events, ABA practitioners recognize that ASDs are biological disorders, and they consider research on genetic and neurological etiologies to be necessary for the continued development of effective intervention (Smith et al. 2007). However, they also posit that the biological functioning in individuals with autism leads them to be ill-fitted to typical environments (Bijou and Ghezzi 1999; Lovaas and Smith 1989). For this reason, they view environmental modifications as likely to be effective in helping individuals with ASDs make behavior changes that improve their functioning and quality of life, and they have developed an array of interventions to achieve these goals, as is discussed later in this chapter.

Although other interventions such as psychotropic medications are also validated scientifically, ABA is unique in that the same methodology is used routinely for both research and clinical applications. This methodology is largely one of single-subject research design in which individuals serve as their own control subjects, and interventions are evaluated for each person to which they are applied. Typically, the design involves comparing a baseline phase in which individuals receive no intervention to one or more intervention phases, with data collected continuously through all phases.

An example is the *alternating treatment design.* In this design, intervention is implemented on alternate days or sessions; on the other days, there is no intervention. This design is used when the effects of an intervention are expected to occur within single days or sessions. When an intervention might take longer to have an impact, an alternative is the *reversal design,* in which a baseline of several sessions, days, or weeks is followed by an intervention, followed by a return to the baseline phase, and so on. Another approach is the *multiple baseline design,* which involves having two or more baseline phases that are of varying lengths and then applying treatment to one baseline at a time (Bailey and Burch 2002). In these designs, if the behavior improves relative to the baseline phase each time that the intervention is introduced, one can conclude that the treatment may have produced this improvement. If the behavior does not improve, the intervention is refined or changed.

Although single-subject methodologies were developed by ABA practitioners, their applications extend to non-ABA interventions. For example, single-subject designs have been used to assess the efficacy of psychotropic medication (Zarcone et al. 2004) as well as popular but unsubstantiated interventions such as sensory integrative therapy (Smith et al. 2005), auditory integration training (Mudford et al. 2000), and facilitated communication (Jacobson et al. 2005). Thus, in addition to overseeing ABA interventions, ABA practitioners can contribute to evaluations of other interventions received by individuals with ASDs.

Research on Applied Behavior Analysis and Models of Service Delivery

Numerous single studies indicate that ABA methods are effective in improving communication (Goldstein 2002), social skills (McConnell 2002), and management of problem behavior (Horner et al. 2002). Research also has been conducted on the effects of combining ABA methods into an intervention program or model. Table 8–1 summarizes some of the main models for delivering ABA interventions to individuals with ASDs. Some models are comprehensive, designed to address all areas of need, whereas others are directed toward a more circumscribed, specific set of goals.

Early Intensive Behavioral Intervention

One comprehensive approach is early intensive behavioral intervention (EIBI). EIBI is characterized by 20–40 hours per week of treatment for 2 or more years, beginning before age 5 years. EIBI involves carefully structured, one-on-one, and small-group interventions based on a broad curriculum that emphasizes communication, social skills, cognition, and pre-academic skills (e.g., imitation, matching, letter and number concepts) (Leaf and McEachin 1999). Once children reach school age, they may continue participation in behaviorally based educational approaches and/or more traditional special or regular education techniques to address areas of ongoing need, as described later in the subsection "Other Applied Behavior Analysis Models."

In a seminal study that used matched control groups and multiple pretreatment and follow-up measures, Lovaas (1987) reported an average gain of 20 IQ points for 19 children with autism participating in 40 hours per week of EIBI for 2 years or more. The treatment initially took place in children's homes, with a focus on highly structured one-on-one instruction. As children progressed, treatment focused on promoting social interaction and entering children into community settings such as schools. Nine children from the EIBI group (47%) achieved average intellectual functioning and were subsequently enrolled in general education classrooms. In contrast, IQ scores of children in two control groups (i.e., a group receiving only 10 hours of behavioral intervention and a group receiving other types of intervention) remained virtually unchanged, with only 1 child out of 40 demonstrating intellectual functioning in the normal range. A follow-up study (McEachin et al. 1993) determined that the intellectual and academic gains of the original EIBI group remained stable several years after treatment up to, on average, 13 years of age. Subsequent studies have yielded smaller gains than those reported by Lovaas (1987) but confirm that EIBI may increase scores on standardized tests of intelligence, language, and adaptive behavior (Smith 1999). Although these studies, including

Table 8–1. Some models of applied behavior analysis (ABA) service delivery

Type of service	Example	Description
Comprehensive intervention		
Early intensive behavioral intervention	UCLA Young Autism Project (Lovaas 1987)	40 hours per week of individual, in-home intervention based on a comprehensive curriculum for children with autism spectrum disorders (ASDs) who begin treatment before age 4 years
ABA classrooms	Princeton Child Development Institute (McClannahan and Krantz 1997)	25 hours per week in a self-contained classroom with ABA interventions administered individually or in small groups for school-age children with autism
Occupational and residential supports	Eden Model (Holmes 1997)	Residential facility with ABA intervention for self-help and vocational skills
Supported inclusion	LEAP Preschool (Strain and Cordisco 1994)	15 hours per week of intervention, emphasizing peer-mediated social skills training in a preschool classroom containing both children with ASDs and typically developing children
Skills-focused models		
Individual treatment	Communication: Picture Exchange Communication System (Bondy and Frost 2001)	Two service providers working together to teach an individual with an ASD to select pictures and give them to a communication partner to indicate wants or needs
	Self-management: Contingency contracting (Mruzek et al. 2007)	Written contract developed collaboratively with high-functioning children with ASDs to reduce problem behavior
	Academics: Direct Instruction reading (Engelmann et al. 1988)	Structured ABA curriculum for teaching reading skills individually or in groups

Table 8–1. Some models of applied behavior analysis (ABA) service delivery *(continued)*

Type of service	Example	Description
Skills-focused models *(continued)*		
Parent training	Parent-delivered pivotal response training (Schreibman and Koegel 2005)	Instruction to parents on creating opportunities to teach their children with ASDs in the context of everyday activities
Staff/teacher training	Behavioral skills training for teachers (Sarokoff and Sturmey 2004)	Didactic instruction and in vivo supervision for teachers on the use of structured teaching procedures
Peer tutoring	Peer-mediated social skills training (Odom et al. 1999)	Teaching peers to serve as tutors to help individuals with ASDs increase their social interactions

Note.   LEAP = Learning Experiences: An Alternative Program for Preschoolers and Parents.

the 1987 Lovaas report, have methodological weaknesses, most notably nonrandom assignment of participants to treatment groups, the body of scientific evidence indicates EIBI may be very effective as an intervention for autism.

In addition to the EIBI model developed by Lovaas and colleagues, there are a number of other EIBI models (Handleman and Harris 2001). Some, such as *Learning Experiences: An Alternative Program for Preschoolers and Parents* (LEAP; Strain and Cordisco 1994), take place at school rather than home. LEAP includes preschool services in which children with ASDs are integrated with typically developing peers and the parents of the children with ASDs are given extensive training. Interventions strongly emphasize promoting social skills using ABA teaching methods. An uncontrolled follow-up study indicated that six children who entered LEAP between the ages of 30 and 53 months maintained their behavioral and developmental gains at age 10 years (Strain and Hoyson 2000). Another model is *pivotal response treatment* (PRT), which aims to teach pivotal responses that, when acquired, improve performance across numerous skill areas (Koegel and Koegel 2006). A number of studies have documented short-term effects of PRT, but data on long-term outcomes are currently unavailable. PRT may be provided to preschool-age children or to older children with ASDs.

Some findings suggest that ABA-based early intervention may be more effective than alternative approaches. Notably, Howard et al. (2005), compared 14 months of EIBI to two other interventions: 1) intensive, "eclectic" autism treatment (30 hours per week of one-on-one and one-on-two instruction) that includes TEACCH (Treatment and Education of Autistic and Related Communication-Handicapped Children) methodology (Schopler 1997), sensory integrative therapy (Bundy et al. 2002), and some ABA; and 2) nonintensive public special education. Participants were carefully matched (but not randomly assigned) to groups. Although the groups did not differ significantly on any pretreatment measure, the EIBI group demonstrated an average increase of 31 points in IQ (59 at intake and 90 at follow-up), whereas participants in the other two treatments showed an average increase of only 9 points. The EIBI group also made greater gains in scores on language and adaptive behavior measures. Thus, intensity of treatment in the absence of consistently applied ABA strategies and techniques was not sufficient for treatment effectiveness in this study.

Because of the intensity of EIBI, concerns have been raised about the feasibility of implementing it in community settings. Although one study of community-based treatment yielded disappointing results (Bibby et al. 2002), others suggest that it may be effective if close supervision is provided. For example, Sallows and Graupner (2005) found that treatment run by parents who received approximately 6 hours of expert consultation per month for 4 years yielded outcomes similar to those of clinic-directed treatment.

Other Applied Behavior Analysis Models

Although EIBI was developed for toddlers and preschoolers with autism, and thus is appropriate for that age group, there are also comprehensive ABA models for older children and adults with ASDs throughout the lifespan. These programs take place in specialized classrooms, residences, or occupational settings. They differ from EIBI in that they place less emphasis on intensive, individualized, structured teaching and focus more on facilitating participation in group activities and fostering the ability to complete tasks independently (without direct supervision). Research shows that persons with ASDs in these programs learn many new skills (McClannahan et al. 2002). Still, little information is available on long-term outcomes such as whether graduates of the programs succeed afterward in less specialized settings.

Specific skills models may involve working directly with persons with ASDs in a particular area (e.g., social interaction) or training parents, peers, or service providers to implement ABA interventions. Training may take place at the home, in an inclusive education program or community setting, or at a specialized school or job site. It typically includes instruction on characteristics of ASDs, assistance with identifying skills to teach, guided practice in applying ABA methods, direction on how to collect data on the effects of intervention, and establishment of a system for communication and collaboration between the intervention setting and home. The amount of training varies depending on the needs of the trainees and the individual with autism but often consists of a training workshop that lasts several days, followed by 1–2 hours per week of ongoing consultation. This consultation is gradually reduced as the trainees become proficient in applying ABA methods appropriate for the individual with ASD. Many studies document that with training, parents, peers, and educators can become proficient at implementing ABA interventions under supervision of a professional ABA practitioner (Sarokoff and Sturmey 2004). Again, however, little information is available on long-term outcomes.

Applied Behavior Analysis Providers

ABA is often provided by paraprofessionals and other nonspecialists who work under the supervision of a professional ABA practitioner, called a *behavior analyst*. To ensure treatment quality, it is important that the behavior analyst possess appropriate qualifications, which include 1) recognition as a board-certified behavior analyst (BCBA) or a master's or doctoral degree with a specialty in behavior analysis, 2) completion of a 1-year internship in providing ABA for individuals with ASDs under the supervision of a BCBA or similarly qualified professional who specializes in this area, and 3) adherence to *Guidelines for Responsible Conduct for Behavior Analysts* (Autism Special Interest Group 2004; Bailey and Burch 2005; Behavior Analyst Certification Board 2004). The Behavior Analyst Certification Board maintains a list of BCBAs and their contact information on their Web site (www.bacb.com). Although many BCBAs work with populations other than individuals with ASDs, the list may be a useful resource for locating ABA practitioners (Bailey and Burch 2005).

Applied Behavior Analysis Intervention Methods

ABA intervention models, whether comprehensive or skills focused, typically incorporate a variety of teaching methods (see Table 8–2), rather than relying on any one technique. Practitioners select from these techniques to develop an individualized intervention plan and modify the plan based on data regarding an individual's progress. Comprehensive models and methods that involve intensive individual instruction such as imitation training and discrete trial teaching may be especially appropriate for younger or more delayed individuals with ASDs. Skills-focused models and methods such as modeling and self-management may be best suited for older and higher functioning individuals such as those with Asperger's disorder.

Social, Play, and Leisure Skills

Imitation often is one of the first behaviors to be addressed in ABA interventions for social skills because the ability to imitate a verbal or physical action is an important prerequisite for learning more complex skills. ABA interventions to teach imitation usually involve one-on-one instruction in which increasingly complex imitation goals are introduced systematically. This approach can result

Table 8–2.   Examples of empirically validated interventions for skill development and problem behaviors for individuals with autism spectrum disorders (ASDs)

Behavior(s)	Type of intervention	Examples
Social, play, and leisure skills	Imitation training	One-on-one adult-directed instruction (Young et al. 1994)
	Peer tutoring	Didactic instruction from peers on turn taking, asking and answering social questions, and other social skills (Laushey and Heflin 2000)
	Modeling (in vivo and video)	Models of prosocial or play behavior (Charlop-Christy et al. 2000)
	Application to classrooms	Intervention by all classmates (Kamps et al. 1994), scripted social interactions (Krantz and McClannahan 1993)
Communication	Discrete trial instruction	Speech sounds, discriminations between different words and language forms (Smith 2001)
	Incidental teaching	Used to teach language elaboration, language during natural routines/activities (McGee et al. 1983)
	Augmentative communication	Sign language (Layton 1988)
Daily living and occupational skills	Task analysis training	Dressing, brushing teeth, food preparation, pedestrian skills (Matson et al. 1996)
Problem behavior	Functional communication training	Teaching/reinforcing appropriate verbal responses that serve the same function as the problem behavior (Durand and Carr 1992)
	Differential reinforcement	Teaching and reinforcing activities incompatible (e.g., toy play) with target problem behavior; reinforcement of other behaviors alternative to or incompatible with problem behavior (Eason et al. 1982; Lindberg et al. 1999)

Table 8–2. Examples of empirically validated interventions for skill development and problem behaviors for individuals with autism spectrum disorders (ASDs) *(continued)*

Behavior(s)	Type of intervention	Examples
Self-management	Activity schedules	Teaching individuals with ASDs to follow pictorial schedules of leisure and self-help activities without monitoring from an adult (McClannahan and Krantz 1999)
	Contingency contracting	Written contract developed collaboratively with high-functioning children with ASDs to reduce problem behavior (Mruzek et al. 2007)

in generalized imitation to new models (Young et al. 1994) and may set the stage for improvement in other areas of cognitive and social development considered critical to autism intervention, including joint attention, spontaneous speech, and social initiations (Ingersoll and Schreibman 2006; Rogers and Bennetto 2000; Whalen et al. 2006). However, additional research is needed to determine whether such improvement is associated with general gains in reciprocal social interaction (e.g., ability to form close, age-appropriate friendships).

Once an individual has mastered basic imitation skills, other social skills can be taught by either adults or peer tutors. The use of peers is often preferable because peers may be less intrusive than adults in settings such as play groups, and skills that are learned from peers may be more likely to generalize to typical social situations that individuals encounter outside of training (Weiss and Harris 2001). Simply being in proximity of a peer without some other intervention is probably not sufficient to produce increases in social interaction (Myles et al. 1993). However, just asking the peer to play with the individual with an ASD can be effective, as can directing peers to provide didactic instruction in areas such as turn taking, looking at the speaker, getting attention from others, and giving answers to questions (Laushey and Heflin 2000). Peers who are the same age as or are slightly younger than the individual with an ASD may be more effective as tutors than older peers (Lord and Hopkins 1986). Videotaping peers or adults as they model appropriate social or play behavior has also been shown to be effective and may in fact be more beneficial than in vivo modeling (Charlop-Christy et al. 2000).

Although peer-mediated strategies produce immediate gains in social skills, generalizing these gains to new situations and maintaining them over time pose a challenge (Stahmer et al. 2003). Strategies that may improve generalization and maintenance include teaching individuals with ASDs to self-monitor their responses to others (Koegel et al. 1992), involving an entire class in implementing interventions (Kamps et al. 1992), providing scripts or cues of social interactions that the child can use across a variety of peers or situations (Krantz and McClannahan 1993), or using strategies to expand on social initiations that some individuals with ASDs spontaneously direct toward peers (Kennedy and Shukla 1995).

Teaching specific play and leisure skills to individuals with ASDs overlaps substantially with social skills training because play situations are often social in nature. In addition, many individuals with ASDs have a restricted repertoire of activities that are of interest to them, and they may lack age-appropriate symbolic and sociodramatic play skills (Baron-Cohen 1987). Thus, several behavioral interventions focus on increasing novel or creative responses in children with ASDs such as using modeling activities (Stahmer et al. 2003) or giving systematic reinforcement when the child varies the sequence of activities during games rather than repeating the same sequence (Miller and Neuringer 2000).

Most of these interventions were developed for preschool- and school-age children with ASDs. Given that social demands change across the lifespan, it is unclear how effective the interventions are for adolescents and adults with ASDs. Research on interventions for these individuals has been fairly limited, although some encouraging findings have been described. For example, investigators have reported success in teaching adolescents or adults with ASDs to request help and to respond appropriately to such requests (Farmer-Dougan 1994; Harris et al. 1990). Interactive computer programs may give opportunities for individuals with ASDs of all ages to learn and practice social skills such as recognizing and responding to facial expressions displayed by others (Pioggia et al. 2005).

Another important subpopulation that has received relatively little scientific study comprises children with high-functioning autism or Asperger's disorder. Peer tutoring may be effective for this group (Kamps et al. 1994; Thiemann and Goldstein 2004). Providing social skills training in a clinic is another potentially beneficial intervention (Barry et al. 2003), although generalization across peers and settings may occur more readily when the training is conducted within the context of the classroom. Self-monitoring and contingency contracting also have been reported to be successful (Mruzek et al. 2007).

Communication

Establishing basic communication skills in children with ASDs before age 5 years may result in positive, long-term effects (McEachin et al. 1993). One approach that has been used extensively with preschool- and school-age children with ASDs is *discrete trial instruction,* which is characterized by 1) one-on-one interaction between the practitioner and the child in a distraction-free environment, 2) clear and concise instructions from the practitioner, 3) highly specific procedures for prompting correct responses and fading these prompts, and

4) immediate reinforcement for correct responses. Discrete trial instruction is especially useful for teaching new forms of behavior (e.g., new speech sounds) and new discriminations between stimuli (e.g., responding differentially to different words) (Smith 2001).

An additional method for increasing language skills is incidental teaching, which involves using daily or commonly occurring events to promote language within everyday contexts. Incidental teaching situations arise from an individual's motivation or desire for something. For example, a child's reaching for a cookie at snack time may present an opportunity for an adult to teach requesting or to require increasingly elaborate requests. Because incidental teaching occurs within a natural context, it may promote generalization of skills to new situations to a greater extent than discrete trial instruction (McGee et al. 1983). However, individuals cannot generalize skills unless they have first learned them, and some individuals with ASDs may learn skills more rapidly from discrete trial instruction than from incidental teaching (Kok et al. 2002). Thus, a combination of discrete trial instruction and incidental teaching is often recommended (Smith 2001).

ABA interventions may focus on helping individuals with ASDs use spoken language or augmentative and alternative communication systems such as speech-output devices, sign language, or selection of photographs or pictures to indicate wants or needs (Bondy and Frost 2001). The availability of a variety of communication systems may facilitate identifying a means of communication that best meets an individual's needs.

Enhancing an individual's communication skills concurrently may decrease problem behavior. Functional communication training is an approach in which instructors teach or reinforce a functionally equivalent communicative response that can replace problem behavior (Carr and Durand 1985). For example, an individual with an ASD may learn to make a verbal request for a preferred object or activity instead of displaying aggression and apply this new skill across settings (Durand and Carr 1992).

One of the core concerns with teaching communication skills to children with ASDs is that it often involves prompting children and contriving situations with the goal of making a response more likely. Spontaneous language continues to be one of the primary deficits in children with ASDs even after successful language training has resulted in a variety of verbal responses (Bodfish 2004). As with other social behaviors, there has been increased focus on teaching and reinforcing communicative initiations and training for generalization across a variety of people and situations (Yoder and Warren 1999).

Repetitive Behaviors, Circumscribed Interests, and Other Problem Behaviors

Persons with ASDs engage in a variety of repetitive and problem behaviors that may impede learning or interfere with daily living skills. In some cases, their behaviors may pose a danger to themselves or others, or such behaviors may disrupt the environment. The behaviors that have received the most attention are repetitive or stereotypic behaviors, aggression, and self-injurious behavior.

The physiologic and environmental factors that are associated with the behaviors are examined for each individual, using a process called *functional assessment, functional behavioral assessment,* or *functional analysis.* ABA practitioners hypothesize that problem behavior is often a learned response that is inadvertently reinforced by environmental events such as attention from others or opportunities to access preferred activities (Iwata et al. 2002). Understanding the role of these events can assist in designing interventions. For example, if an individual engages in disruptive behavior to gain attention, a target for treatment might be to ignore the problem behavior when it occurs and teach the individual to recruit attention through a simple request.

Several methods have been developed for conducting functional assessments. The most straightforward approach is simply to use checklists such as the Motivation Assessment Scale (Durand and Crimmins 1988) and Questions About Behavioral Function (Matson and Vollmer 1995) to ask caregivers why they believe that an individual engages in problem behavior. Interviews that include open-ended questions such as the Functional Assessment Interview (O'Neill et al. 1997) can provide more extensive information. Alternatively, direct observation of the individual in his or her everyday environment can be performed to help identify relationships between the occurrence of problem behavior and environmental events that occur immediately before or after the behavior. Finally, experimental functional analysis can be conducted in which the antecedents and consequences for problem behavior are systematically introduced and withdrawn in a clinical, home, or school setting (Iwata et al. 1994).

Research on problem behavior indicates that, in addition to having higher rates of repetitive behaviors than individuals with other developmental disabilities, individuals with ASDs may be more likely to engage in self-injurious behavior, property destruction, and aggression (McClintock et al. 2003). Individuals with ASDs also may be more likely than other individuals to display problem behavior to escape demands, prevent an interruption in repetitive activities (Reese et al. 2003), or gain access to repetitive activities (Fisher et al. 1998b).

Evaluation of the function of stereotypic or repetitive behavior has indicated that repetitive behavior (in individuals both with and without autism) often occurs at high rates regardless of environmental factors (Fisher et al. 1998a). A few studies, however, have shown that repetitive behavior can be affected by environmental factors such as escape from demands and attempts to access preferred activities (Kennedy et al. 2000). Additionally, repetitive behavior may increase under conditions that provoke anxiety (Woods and Miltenberger 1996), when an unfamiliar person is present (Runco et al. 1986), or during certain activities such as music or gym class (Cuvo et al. 2001; Patel et al. 2000). The availability of competing activities such as toys (either novel or familiar) can significantly decrease the behavior, particularly when individuals are taught how to participate appropriately in these activities (Eason et al. 1982) and are given prompts and reinforcement for doing so (Lindberg et al. 1999).

Daily Living, Community, and Vocational Skills

Individuals with ASDs may have limited self-help skills, including dressing themselves, preparing food independently, and maintaining personal hygiene. In addition, they often have difficulty with community activities at locations such as church, stores, and restaurants. Adolescents and adults may have difficulty developing vocational skills that can result in long-term employment. These difficulties may be more subtle in individuals with high-functioning autism or Asperger's disorder but are still likely to be present.

Matson et al. (1996) reported that the daily living skills most commonly targeted for treatment in individuals with ASDs were dressing, brushing teeth, food preparation, and community skills (e.g., crossing the street). Techniques such as task analysis, which involves breaking down a complex behavior into small steps, and the use of visual schedules, in which steps of an activity are displayed in separate pictures or photographs, appear to be especially useful. Several studies have focused on ABA interventions for establishing appropriate community behaviors, but generalization of skills outside of the training context has been inconsistent (Haring et al. 1987). ABA curricula have been developed to teach academic and vocational skills; these curricula are based on a task analysis of the skills and involve developing the skills in a series of carefully planned, small steps (Engelmann et al. 1988). However, evaluations of the effectiveness of these curricula for individuals with ASDs have been infrequent; hence, this is an area that merits further research.

Manuals and Curriculum Guides

Commercially available curriculum guides or manuals describe ABA models of service delivery and treatment methods, although only one (Lovaas 1981) has been used to guide treatment in research studies (e.g., Lovaas 1987). Several other comprehensive manuals have been developed, including an expansion of Lovaas's original manual (Lovaas 2002) and handbooks by Leaf and McEachin (1999), Maurice et al. (1996, 2001), and Harris and Weiss (1998). Guidebooks are also available that address specific teaching methods or skill areas, including the use of activity schedules to facilitate independent play and daily living skills (McClannahan and Krantz 1999), incidental teaching approaches such as pivotal response treatment (Koegel and Koegel 2006), strategies for reducing problem behavior (O'Neill et al. 1997), and methods for enhancing motivation (Delmolino and Harris 2004), social skills (Weiss and Harris 2001), conversation and language concepts (Freeman and Dake 1997), and augmentative communication (Bondy and Frost 2001).

Conclusions

In this chapter we have highlighted several key points that are of significance to practitioners:

1. ABA is the psychosocial intervention for ASDs that has generated the most extensive research. For this reason, some guidelines identify ABA as the treatment of choice for individuals with ASDs.
2. ABA is an applied science employed in diverse educational, occupational, and health settings. It emphasizes the study of functional relations between environmental events and behavior.

3. ABA programs should be supervised by certified behavior analysts or professionals with equivalent credentials (master's- or doctoral-level training in behavior analysis); these professionals should have 1 year or more of specialized training in ABA for individuals with ASDs.

4. The most favorable outcomes may be achieved when ABA is begun early (before age 4 years) and implemented intensively (20 hours or more per week for 2 or more years). Early, intensive ABA is designed to be comprehensive, addressing all areas of need. This intervention may enable many children with autism to make major developmental gains, such as increases in IQ and other standardized test scores, enhanced socioemotional functioning, and mainstreamed school placements.

5. Comprehensive programs such as ABA classrooms and residential settings also are available to older children and adults with ASDs. In addition, programs are available that focus on a more circumscribed set of skills and may involve training parents, teachers, or others to implement interventions. Research documents that both comprehensive and specific programs for older children and adults yield short-term benefits, although additional evidence on long-term effects is needed.

6. A variety of ABA intervention methods have been developed to help individuals with ASDs improve their skills in interacting with peers, playing and engaging in other leisure skills, performing self-help skills and occupational tasks, and regulating repetitive activities and other problem behaviors.

Numerous single-case studies document the effectiveness of many different ABA methods for teaching a variety of skills, and efforts continue to refine these methods. Outcome studies provide support for comprehensive ABA models, particularly EIBI. However, additional studies are needed to confirm these exciting findings. Outcome studies are also needed on other ABA models. In addition, more research is needed to evaluate ABA interventions with adolescents and adults with ASDs, as well as individuals of all ages with high-functioning autism or Asperger's disorder.

References

Autism Special Interest Group: Revised Guidelines for Consumers of Applied Behavior Analysis Services to Individuals with Autism and Related Disorders. September 15, 2004. Available at: http://www.behavior.org. Accessed April 18, 2007.

Bailey JS, Burch MR: Research Methods in Applied Behavior Analysis. Thousand Oaks, CA, Sage, 2002

Bailey JS, Burch MR: Ethics for Behavior Analysts. Mahwah, NJ, Erlbaum, 2005

Baron-Cohen S: Autism and symbolic play. Br J Dev Psychol 5:139–148, 1987

Barry TD, Klinger LG, Lee JM, et al: Examining the effectiveness of an outpatient clinic-based social skills group for high-functioning children with autism. J Autism Dev Disord 33:685–701, 2003

Behavior Analyst Certification Board: Behavior Analyst Certification Board Guidelines for Responsible Conduct for Behavior Analysts. August 2004. Available at: http://www.bacb.com/pages/conduct.html. Accessed April 18, 2007.

Bibby P, Eikeseth S, Martin NT, et al: Progress and outcomes for children with autism receiving parent-managed intensive interventions. Res Dev Disabil 23:81–104, 2002

Bijou SW, Ghezzi PM: The behavioral interference theory of autistic behavior in young children, in Autism: Behavior Analytic Perspectives. Edited by Ghezzi PM, Williams WL, Carr JE. Reno, NV, Reno Press, 1999, pp 33–43

Bodfish JW: Treating the core features of autism: are we there yet? Ment Retard Dev Disabil Res Rev 10:318–326, 2004

Bondy A, Frost L: The Picture Exchange Communication System. Behav Modif 25:725–744, 2001

Bundy AC, Lane SJ, Murray EA (eds): Sensory Integration: Theory and Practice, 2nd Edition. Philadelphia, PA, FA Davis, 2002

Carr EG, Durand VM: Reducing behavior problems through functional communication training. J Appl Behav Anal 18:111–126, 1985

Charlop-Christy MH, Le L, Freeman KA: A comparison of video modeling with in vivo modeling for teaching children with autism. J Autism Dev Disord 30:537–552, 2000

Cuvo AJ, May ME, Post TM: Effects of living room, Snoezelen room, and outdoor activities on stereotypic behavior and engagement by adults with profound mental retardation. Res Dev Disabil 22:183–204, 2001

Delmolino L, Harris SL: Incentives for Change: Motivating People With Autism Spectrum Disorders to Learn and Gain Independence. Bethesda, MD, Woodbine House, 2004

Durand VM, Carr EG: An analysis of maintenance following functional communication training. J Appl Behav Anal 25:777–794, 1992

Durand VM, Crimmins D: Identifying the variables maintaining self-injurious behavior. J Autism Dev Disord 18:99–117, 1988

Eason LJ, White MJ, Newsom C: Generalized reduction of self-stimulatory behaviors: an effect of teaching appropriate play to autistic children. Analysis and Intervention in Developmental Disabilities 2:157–169, 1982

Engelmann S, Becker WC, Carnine D, et al: The Direct Instruction Follow Through Model: design and outcomes. Education and Treatment of Children 11:303–317, 1988

Farmer-Dougan V: Increasing requests by adults with developmental disabilities using incidental teaching by peers. J Appl Behav Anal 27:533–544, 1994

Fisher WW, Lindauer S, Alterson C, et al: Assessment and treatment of destructive behavior maintained by stereotypic object manipulation. J Appl Behav Anal 31:513–527, 1998a

Fisher WW, Adelinis JD, Thompson RH, et al: Functional analysis and treatment of destructive behavior maintained by termination of "don't" (and symmetrical "do") requests. J Appl Behav Anal 31:339–356, 1998b

Freeman S, Dake L: Teach Me Language: A Language Manual for Children With Autism, Asperger's Syndrome, and Related Developmental Disorders. Langley, BC, Canada, SKF Books, 1997

Goldstein H: Communication intervention for children with autism: a review of treatment efficacy. J Autism Dev Disord 32:373–396, 2002

Handleman JS, Harris SL (eds): Preschool Education Programs for Children With Autism, 2nd Edition. Austin, TX, Pro-Ed, 2001

Haring TG, Kennedy CH, Adams MJ, et al: Teaching generalization of purchasing skills across community settings to autistic youth using videotape modeling. J Appl Behav Anal 20:89–96, 1987

Harris SL, Weiss MJ: Right From the Start: Behavioral Intervention for Young Children With Autism. Bethesda, MD, Woodbine House, 1998

Harris SL, Handleman JS, Alessandri M: Teaching youths with autism to offer assistance. J Appl Behav Anal 23:297–305, 1990

Holmes DL: Autism Through the Lifespan: The Eden Model. Bethesda, MD, Woodbine House, 1997

Horner RH, Carr EG, Strain PS, et al: Problem behavior interventions for young children with autism: a research synthesis. J Autism Dev Disord 32:423–446, 2002

Howard JS, Sparkman CR, Cohen HG, et al: A comparison of intensive behavior analytic and eclectic treatments for young children with autism. Res Dev Disabil 26:359–383, 2005

Ingersoll B, Schreibman L: Teaching reciprocal imitation skills to young children with autism using a naturalistic behavioral approach: effects on language, pretend play, and joint attention. J Autism Dev Disord 36:487–505, 2006

Iwata BA, Dorsey MF, Slifer KJ, et al: Toward a functional analysis of self-injury. J Appl Behav Anal 27:197–209, 1994

Iwata BA, Roscoe EM, Zarcone JR, et al: Environmental determinants of self-injurious behavior, in Self-injurious Behavior: Gene-Brain-Behavior Relationships. Edited by Schroeder SR, Oster-Granite ML, Thompson T. Washington, DC, American Psychological Association, 2002, pp 93–103

Jacobson JW, Foxx RM, Mulick JA (eds): Controversial Therapies for Developmental Disabilities. Mahwah, NJ, Erlbaum, 2005

Kamps DM, Leonard BR, Vernon S, et al: Teaching social skills to students with autism to increase peer interactions in an integrated first-grade classroom. J Appl Behav Anal 25:281–288, 1992

Kamps DM, Barbetta PM, Leonard BR, et al: Classwide peer tutoring: an integration strategy to improve reading skills and promote peer interactions among students with autism and general education peers. J Appl Behav Anal 27:49–61, 1994

Kennedy CH, Shukla S: Social interaction research for people with autism as a set of past, present, and emerging propositions. Behav Disord 21:21–36, 1995

Kennedy CH, Meyer KA, Knowles T, et al: Analyzing the multiple functions of stereotypical behavior for students with autism: implications for assessment and treatment. J Appl Behav Anal 33:559–571, 2000

Koegel LK, Koegel RL, Hurley C, et al: Improving social skills and disruptive behavior in children with autism through self-management. J Appl Behav Anal 26:341–353, 1992

Koegel RL, Koegel LK: Pivotal Response Treatments for Autism. Baltimore, MD, Paul H Brookes Publishing, 2006

Kok AJ, Kong TY, Bernard-Opitz V: A comparison of the effects of structured play and facilitated play approaches on preschoolers with autism: a case study. Autism 6:181–196, 2002

Krantz PJ, McClannahan LE: Teaching children with autism to initiate to peers: effects of a script-fading procedure. J Appl Behav Anal 26:121–132, 1993

Laushey KM, Heflin J: Enhancing social skills of kindergarten children with autism through the training of multiple peers as tutors. J Autism Dev Disord 30:183–193, 2000

Layton TL: Language training with autistic children using four different modes of presentation. J Commun Disord 21:333–350, 1988

Leaf R, McEachin J: A Work in Progress: Behavior Management Strategies and a Curriculum for Intensive Behavioral Treatment of Autism. New York, DRL Books, 1999

Lilienfeld SO: Scientifically unsupported and supported interventions for childhood psychopathology: a summary. Pediatrics 115:761–764, 2005

Lindberg JS, Iwata BA, Kahng SW: On the relation between object manipulation and stereotypic self-injurious behavior. J Appl Behav Anal 32:51–62, 1999

Lord C, Hopkins JM: The social behavior of autistic children with younger and same age nonhandicapped peers. J Autism Dev Disord 16:249–262, 1986

Lord C, Bristol-Power M, Cafiero JM, et al (eds): JADD special issue: NAS workshop papers. J Autism Dev Disord 32:349–508, 2002

Lovaas OI: Teaching Developmentally Disabled Children: The Me Book. Austin, TX, Pro-Ed, 1981

Lovaas OI: Behavioral treatment and normal educational and intellectual functioning in young autistic children. J Consult Clin Psychol 55:3–9, 1987

Lovaas OI: Teaching Individuals With Developmental Delays: Basic Intervention Techniques. Austin, TX, Pro-Ed, 2002

Lovaas OI, Smith T: A comprehensive behavioral theory of autistic children: paradigm for research and treatment. J Behav Ther Exp Psychiatry 20:17–29, 1989

Maine Administrators of Services for Children with Disabilities: Report of the MAD-SEC Autism Task Force. Manchester, ME, Maine Administrators of Services for Children with Disabilities, 2000

Matson JL, Vollmer TR: Questionnaire About Behavioral Function Manual. Baton Rouge, LA, Scientific Publishers, 1995

Matson JL, Benavidez, DA, Compton LS, et al: Behavioral treatment of autistic persons: a review of research from 1980 to the present. Res Dev Disabil 17:433–465, 1996

Maurice C, Green G, Luce SC: Behavioral Intervention for Young Children With Autism. Austin, TX, Pro-Ed, 1996

Maurice C, Green G, Foxx RM: Making a Difference: Behavioral Intervention for Autism. Austin, TX, Pro-Ed, 2001

McClannahan LE, Krantz PJ: Princeton Child Development Institute. Behavior and Social Issues 7:65–68, 1997

McClannahan LE, Krantz PJ: Activity Schedules for Children With Autism: Teaching Independent Behavior. Bethesda, MD, Woodbine House, 1999

McClannahan LE, MacDuff GS, Krantz PJ: Behavior analysis and intervention for adults with autism. Behav Modif 26:27–48, 2002

McClintock K, Hall S, Oliver C: Risk markers associated with challenging behaviours in people with intellectual disabilities: a meta-analytic study. J Intellect Disabil Res 47:405–416, 2003

McConnell SR: Interventions to facilitate social interaction for young children with autism: review of available research and recommendations for educational intervention and future research. J Autism Dev Disord 32:351–372, 2002

McEachin JJ, Smith T, Lovaas OI: Long-term outcome for children with autism who received early intensive behavioral treatment. Am J Ment Retard 97:359–372, 1993

McGee GG, Krantz PJ, Mason D, et al: A modified incidental-teaching procedure for autistic youth: acquisition and generalization of receptive object labels. J Appl Behav Anal 16:329–338, 1983

Miller N, Neuringer A: Reinforcing variability in adolescents with autism. J Appl Behav Anal 33:151–165, 2000

Mruzek DW, Cohen C, Smith T: Contingency contracting with students with autism spectrum disorders in a public school setting. J Dev Phys Disabil 19:103–114, 2007

Mudford OC, Cross BA, Breen S, et al: Auditory Integration Training: no behavioral benefits detected. Am J Ment Retard 105:119–129, 2000

Myles BS, Simpson RL, Ormsbee CK, et al: Integrating preschool children with autism with their normally developing peers: research findings and best practices recommendations. Focus Autism Other Devel Disabl 8:1–18, 1993

New York State Department of Health, Early Intervention Program: Autism/Pervasive Developmental Disorders: Assessment and Intervention for Young Children (Age 0–3 years) (DOH Publ No 4217). Albany, New York State Department of Health, 1999

Odom SL, McConnell SR, McEvoy MA, et al: Relative effects of interventions supporting the social competence of young children with disabilities. Topics in Early Childhood Special Education 19:75–91, 1999

O'Neill RE, Horner RH, Albin RW, et al: Functional Assessment and Program Development for Problem Behavior: A Practical Handbook, 2nd Edition. Pacific Grove, CA, Brooks/Cole, 1997

Patel MR, Carr JE, Kim C, et al: Functional analysis of aberrant behavior maintained by automatic reinforcement: assessments of specific sensory reinforcers. Res Dev Disabil 21:393–407, 2000

Pioggia G, Igliozzi R, Ferro M, et al: An android for enhancing social skills and emotion recognition in people with autism. IEEE Trans Neural Syst Rehabil Eng 13:507–515, 2005

Reese RM, Richman DM, Zarcone J, et al: Individualizing functional assessments for children with autism: the contribution of perseverative behavior and sensory disturbances to disruptive behavior. Focus Autism Other Devel Disabl 18:89–94, 2003

Rogers SJ, Bennetto L: Intersubjectivity in autism: the roles of imitation and executive function, in Autism Spectrum Disorders: A Transactional Developmental Perspective. Edited by Wetherby AM, Prizant BM. Baltimore, MD, Paul H Brookes Publishing, 2000, pp 79–107

Runco MA, Charlop MH, Schreibman L: The occurrence of autistic children's self-stimulation as a function of familiar versus unfamiliar stimulus conditions. J Autism Dev Disord 16:31–44, 1986

Sallows GO, Graupner TD: Intensive behavioral treatment for children with autism: four-year outcome and predictors. Am J Ment Retard 110:417–438, 2005

Sarokoff RA, Sturmey P: The effects of behavioral skills training on staff implementation of discrete-trial teaching. J Appl Behav Anal 37:535–538, 2004

Schopler E: Implementation of TEACCH philosophy, in Handbook of Autism and Pervasive Developmental Disorders, 2nd Edition. Edited by Cohen DJ, Volkmar FR. New York, Wiley, 1997, pp 767–795

Schreibman L, Koegel RL: Training for parents of children with autism: pivotal responses, generalization, and individualization of interventions, in Psychosocial Treatments for Child and Adolescent Disorders: Empirically Based Strategies for Clinical Practice, 2nd Edition. Edited by Hibbs ED, Jensen PS. Washington, DC, American Psychological Association, 2005, pp 605–631

Smith T: Outcome of early intervention for children with autism. Clinical Psychology: Research and Practice 6:33–49, 1999

Smith T: Discrete trial training in the treatment of autism. Focus Autism Other Devel Disabl 16:86–92, 2001

Smith T, Mruzek D, Mozingo D: Sensory integrative therapy, in Controversial Therapies for Developmental Disabilities. Edited by Jacobson JW, Foxx RM, Mulick JA. Mahwah, NJ, Erlbaum, 2005, pp 333–350

Smith T, McAdam D, Napolitano D: Autism and applied behavior analysis, in Autism Spectrum Disorders: Applied Behavior Analysis, Evidence, and Practice. Edited by Sturmey P, Fitzer A. Austin, TX, Pro-Ed, 2007, pp 1–29

Stahmer AC, Ingersoll B, Carter C: Behavioral approaches to promoting play. Autism 7:401–413, 2003

Strain PS, Cordisco LK: LEAP preschool, in Preschool Education Programs for Children With Autism, 2nd Edition. Edited by Harris SL, Handleman JS. Austin, TX, Pro-Ed, 1994, pp 225–244

Strain PS, Hoyson M: The need for longitudinal, intensive social skill intervention: LEAP follow-up outcomes for children with autism. Topics in Early Childhood Special Education 20:116–123, 2000

Sulzer-Azaroff B, Mayer GR: Behavior Analysis for Lasting Change. Fort Worth, TX, Holt, Rinehart, & Winston, 1991

Thiemann KS, Goldstein H: Effects of peer training and written text cueing on social communication of school-age children with pervasive developmental disorder. J Speech Hear Res 47:126–144, 2004

Weiss MJ, Harris SL: Teaching social skills to people with autism. Behav Modif 25:785–802, 2001

Whalen C, Schreibman L, Ingersoll B: The collateral effects of joint attention training on social initiations, positive affect, imitation, and spontaneous speech for young children with autism. J Autism Dev Disord 36:655–664, 2006

Wolf MM: Social validity: the case for subjective measurement or how applied behavior analysis is finding its heart. J Appl Behav Anal 11:203–214, 1978

Woods DW, Miltenberger RG: Are persons with nervous habit nervous? A preliminary examination of habit function in a nonreferred population. J Appl Behav Anal 29:259–261, 1996

Yoder PJ, Warren SF: Facilitating self-initiated proto-declaratives and proto-imperatives in prelinguistic children with developmental disabilities. Journal of Early Intervention 22:79–76, 1999

Young JM, Krantz PJ, McClannahan LE, et al: Generalized imitation and response-class formation in children with autism. J Appl Behav Anal 27:685–697, 1994

Zarcone JR, Lindauer SE, Morse PA, et al: Effects of risperidone on destructive behavior of persons with developmental disabilities: III. Functional analysis. Am J Ment Retard 109:310–321, 2004

The Developmental Individual-Difference, Relationship-Based (DIR/Floortime) Model Approach to Autism Spectrum Disorders

Stanley I. Greenspan, M.D.

Serena Wieder, Ph.D.

Most nonprogressive developmental and learning disorders, including autism spectrum disorders (ASDs), are nonspecific with regard to etiology and pathophysiology. Nonprogressive developmental disabilities are best characterized in terms of types and degrees of limitations in fundamental developmental areas of functioning such as auditory processing and engaging with others purposefully, as well as symptoms (e.g., echolalia). Yet, both historically and recently, we have focused on symptoms and very specific behaviors.

A functional developmental approach can change not only the way we think about developmental disabilities, including ASDs, but what is included in the research base to improve assessment and interventions. For example, research reviews on autism are often limited to assessment, intervention, or etiological studies on children with ASDs. However, instead, the research base should be defined by the relevant areas of developmental functioning, some of which are impaired in a variety of syndromes or problems. For example, almost all children with autism have severe motor planning and sequencing problems, as do lots of other children. Therefore, the general literature on motor planning and sequencing is relevant.

In the functional developmental approach, assessment and intervention must include all relevant areas of developmental functioning and deal with each child and family in terms of their unique profile. We have developed a model that identifies the relevant areas of functioning, helps with the construction of each child's functional developmental profile, and provides a developmental framework for the assessment and intervention process: the Developmental Individual-Difference, Relationship-Based (DIR) model, sometimes referred to as *Floortime*.

The DIR/Floortime Model

There are three components to the DIR/Floortime model: 1) functional emotional developmental level, 2) individual differences in sensory, modulation, processing, and motor planning, and 3) relationships and interactions.

Functional Emotional Developmental Level

The child's functional emotional developmental level (FEDL) examines how children integrate all their capacities (motor, cognitive, language, spatial, sensory) to carry out emotionally meaningful goals. The support for these FEDLs is reviewed elsewhere (Greenspan 1979, 1989, 1992, 1997b). These capacities include the ability to

1. Attend to multisensory affective experience and organize simultaneously a calm, regulated state (e.g., looking at, listening to, and following the movement of a caregiver).
2. Engage with and evidence affective preference and pleasure for a caregiver or caregivers (e.g., joyful smiles and affection with a stable caregiver).
3. Initiate and respond to two-way presymbolic gestural communication (e.g., back-and-forth use of smiles and sounds).

4. Organize chains of two-way social problem-solving communications (opening and closing many circles of communication in a row), maintain communication across space, integrate affective polarities, and synthesize an emerging prerepresentational organization of self and other (e.g., taking Dad by the hand to get a toy on the shelf). In this case, the child is aware of what he or she can and cannot do (self) to get the real toy he or she wants, and therefore seeks the help of someone else (other) and does so through gestures and actions before the child can represent his or her intent or idea in words or using figures.

5. Create and functionally use ideas as a basis for creative or imaginative thinking, giving meaning to symbols (e.g., pretend play, using words to meet needs, "Juice!").

6. Build bridges between ideas as a basis for logic, reality testing, thinking, and judgment (e.g., engage in debates, opinion-oriented conversations, and/or elaborate, planned pretend dramas).

Individual Differences in Sensory Modulation, Sensory Processing, and Motor Planning

Individual differences in sensory, modulation, processing, and motor planning are the result of genetic, prenatal, perinatal, and maturational variations and/or deficits and can be characterized in at least four ways:

1. Sensory modulation, including hypo- and hyperreactivity in each sensory modality, such as touch, sound, smell, vision, and movement in space.

2. Sensory processing in each sensory modality, including auditory processing and language and visuospatial processing. Processing includes the capacity to register, decode, and comprehend sequences and abstract patterns.

3. Sensory-affective processing in each modality (e.g., the ability to process and react to affect, including the capacity to connect "intent" or affect to motor planning and sequencing, language, and symbols). This processing capacity may be especially relevant in ASDs (Greenspan and Wieder 1997, 1998).

4. Motor planning and sequencing, including the capacity to sequence actions, behaviors, and symbols, including symbols in the form of thoughts, words, visual images, and spatial concepts.

Relationships and Interactions

Relationship and affective interaction patterns include developmentally appropriate, or inappropriate, interactive relationships with caregiver, parent, and family patterns. Interaction patterns between the child and caregivers and family members bring the child's biology into the larger developmental progression and can contribute to the negotiation of the child's functional developmental capacities. Developmentally appropriate interactions mobilize the child's intentions and affects and enable the child to broaden his or her range of experience at each level of development and to move from one functional developmental level to the next. In contrast, interactions that do not deal with the child's functional developmental level or individual differences can undermine progress. For example, a caregiver who is aloof may not be able to engage an infant who is underreactive and self-absorbed.

The DIR/Floortime Assessment

Implementation of an appropriate assessment of all the relevant functional areas requires a number of sessions with the child and family. These sessions must begin with discussions and observations.

The DIR/Floortime assessment process, which is described in detail elsewhere (Greenspan 1992; Greenspan and Wieder 1998), includes 1) two or more 45-minute clinical observations of child-caregiver and/or clinician-child interactions; 2) developmental history and review of current functioning; 3) review of family and caregiver functioning; 4) review of current programs and patterns of interaction; 5) consultation with speech pathologists, occupational and physical therapists, educators, and mental health colleagues, including the use of structured tests on an as-needed, rather than routine, basis; and 6) biomedical evaluation.

The Functional Developmental Profile

The DIR/Floortime assessment leads to an individualized functional profile that captures each child's unique developmental features and creates individually tailored intervention programs (i.e., tailoring the program to the child rather than fitting the child to a general program). The profile describes the child's functional developmental capacities and contributing biological processing differences and environmental interactive patterns, including the different interaction patterns available to the child at home, at school, with peers, and in other settings.

Subtypes of Autism Spectrum Disorders

Understanding children's developmental variations has enabled the formulation of subtypes for ASDs, which also may be described from a functional perspective as neurodevelopmental disorders of relating and communicating (NDRC), that can guide treatment and research. Table 9–1 and Figure 9–1 offer a summary and overview of the clinical subtypes of NDRC and related motor- and sensory-processing profile, respectively. (Please see the *Interdisciplinary Council on Developmental and Learning Disorders Diagnostic Manual for Infancy and Early Childhood Mental Health Disorders, Developmental Disorders, Regulatory-Sensory Processing Disorders, Language Disorders, and Learning Challenges [ICDL-DMIC]* [Interdisciplinary Council on Developmental and Learning Disorders 2005] for a more detailed description and discussion.[1])

Core Psychological Deficit in Autism and the Developmental Pathways to Joint Attention, Pattern Recognition, Theory of Mind, Language, and Thinking

The autism-specific developmental deficits that have been suggested include deficits in the following abilities:

1. Empathy and seeing the world from another person's perspective (theory of mind [Baron-Cohen 1994])

---

[1]This manual was put together by highly experienced clinicians and researchers from the fields of mental health, occupational therapy, speech and language pathology, education, and developmental optometry, who served on various task forces and provided the clinical expertise and consensus necessary to define the specific diagnostic classifications in the manual. Each task force met regularly for several years to review cases, view videotapes, and formulate and discuss definitions. The task force working on the NDRC also established reliability on the specific subtypes.

Table 9–1.   Overview of clinical subtypes of neurodevelopmental disorders of relating and communicating (NDRC) and related motor- and sensory-processing profile

Type I	Intermittent capacities for attending and relating; reciprocal interaction; and, with support, shared social problem solving and the initial use of meaningful ideas (i.e., with help, the child can relate and interact and even use a few words but not in a continuous and stable age-expected manner).
	Children with this pattern tend to show rapid progress in a comprehensive program that tailors meaningful emotional interactions to their unique motor- and sensory-processing profile.
Type II	Intermittent capacities for attention, relating, and a few back-and-forth reciprocal interactions, with only fleeting capacities for shared social problem solving and repeating some words.
	Children with this pattern tend to make steady, methodical progress.
Type III	Only fleeting capacities for attention and engagement. Occasionally a few back-and-forth reciprocal interactions with a great deal of support. Often no capacity for repeating words or using ideas, although may be able to repeat a few words in a memory-based (rather than meaningful) manner.
	Children with this pattern often make slow but steady progress, especially in the basics of relating with warmth and learning to engage in longer sequences of reciprocal interaction. Over long periods of time, often gradually master some words and phrases.
Type IV	Similar to Type III above but with a pattern of multiple regressions (loss of capacities). May also evidence a greater number of associated neurological challenges, such as seizures, marked hypotonia, etc.
	Children with this pattern often make very, very slow progress. The progress can be enhanced if the sources of the regressive tendencies can be identified.

2. Higher level abstract thinking, including making inferences (Minshew et al. 1997)

3. Shared attention, including social referencing and problem solving (Mundy et al. 1990)

4. Emotional reciprocity (Baranek 1999; Dawson and Galpert 1990)

5. Functional (pragmatic) language (Wetherby and Prizant 1993)

Neuropsychological models that have been proposed to account for the clinical features of autism further elaborate these autism-specific developmental deficits (Baron-Cohen 1989; Baron-Cohen et al. 1985; Bowler 1992; Dahlgren and Trillingsgaard 1996; Dawson et al. 1998; Frith 1989; Greenspan 2002; Klin et al. 1992; Ozonoff 1997; Pennington and Ozonoff 1996; Sperry 1985).

Our clinical work and research (Greenspan 2002; Greenspan and Shanker 2004, 2007), however, suggests that the deficits in abilities listed above stem from an earlier capacity that is compromised in children with ASDs (they are downstream phenomena). This earlier capacity is an infant's ability to connect emotions or intent to motor planning and sequencing and to sensations and, later, to early forms of symbolic expression of their intent or emotions, such as pretending to have a tea party or acting mad when playing, which later leads to more elaborate use of symbols to create ideas (Greenspan 1979, 1989, 1997b). We hypothesized that the biological differences associated with ASDs may express themselves through the derailing of this connection, leading to both the primary and secondary features of ASDs.

Sensory-Affect-Motor Connections

In healthy development, an infant connects the sensory system to the motor system through affect (e.g., seeing and turning to look at a caregiver's smiling face and wooing voice and not looking at a harsh voice). We have found that all sensation has both physical and affective qualities (Greenspan 1997a; Greenspan and Shanker 2004). The infinite variations in the affective aspect of sensation enable a person to use emotion to code, store, and retrieve information. The ability to create links between the physical and emotional qualities of sensation and motor behavior allows the growing infant to begin to perceive and organize patterns, such as seeing mother and reaching for her. These purposeful units grow into larger patterns, multiple back-and-forth problem-solving interactions. By the second year of life, these patterns lead to a sense of self as the purposeful agent and a sense of others, and ultimately enable a child to form and give meaning to symbols and develop higher levels of thinking.

We have formulated a number of stages through which the connection between sensation, affect, and motor behavior progresses (see Greenspan and Shanker 2004). This has allowed us to identify infants at risk for ASDs. Because the compromise to this connection is not all or nothing in children at risk for ASDs, early intervention that works with the child's affect and individual differences can foster improvement. Creating states of heightened

Overview of Motor and Sensory Processing Profile

Children with neurodevelopmental disorders of relating and communicating (NDRC) (which includes children with autism spectrum disorders) tend to evidence very different biologically based patterns of sensory reactivity, processing, and motor planning. These differences may have diagnostic and prognostic value, and therefore it may be helpful to describe them. The child's tendencies can be briefly summarized in the framework outlined below. (Note: Almost all the children with an NDRC diagnosis evidence language, sequencing, and visuospatial thinking challenges.)

The patterns listed in this figure are the ones that tend to differ among the children. To determine aspects of common patterns found in this population, parents are asked to complete this checklist. One may check all boxes that apply and, if sufficient clinical information is available, also use the box to indicate the degree to which that characteristic applies on a 1–3 scale (with 1 indicating minimum and 3 indicating the maximum degree).

Sensory Modulation

☐ Tends to be overresponsive to sensations, such as sound or touch (e.g., covers ears or gets dysregulated with lots of light touch)

☐ Tends to crave sensory experience (e.g., actively seeks touch, sound, and different movement patterns)

☐ Tends to be underresponsive to sensations (e.g., requires highly energized vocal or tactile support to be alert and attend)

Figure 9–1. Overview of Motor- and Sensory-Processing Profile

Motor Planning and Sequencing

☐ Relative strength in motor planning and sequencing (e.g., carries out many-step action patterns, such as negotiating obstacle courses or building complex block designs, etc.)

☐ Relative weakness in motor planning and sequencing (e.g., can barely carry out simple movements and may tend to simply bang blocks or do other one- to two-step action patterns)

Auditory Memory

☐ Relative strength in auditory memory (remembers or repeats long statements or materials from books, television, records, etc.)

☐ Relative weakness in auditory memory (difficulty remembering even simple sounds or words)

Visual Memory

☐ Relative strength in visual memory (tends to remembering what is seen, such as book covers, pictures, eventually words, etc.)

☐ Relative weakness in visual memory (difficulty remembering even simple pictures or objects)

Figure 9–1.   Overview of Motor- and Sensory-Processing Profile *(continued).*

pleasurable affect tailored to the child's unique motor- and sensory-processing profile helps to develop and strengthen the connection between sensation, affect, and motor action, which leads to more purposeful affective behavior, which in turn leads to reciprocal signaling, a sense of self, symbolic functioning, and higher level thinking skills. Relatively pleasurable and regulated emotional interaction helps a child to use all his or her senses, along with his or her motor and language abilities, together (for example, in looking, listening, and moving all at once while engaging in meaningful problem-solving–thinking interactions). These interactions, tailored to a child's individual processing differences, must occur in the context of a comprehensive, intensive intervention, as outlined in the DIR/Floortime intervention program later in this chapter.

Role of Affect Transformations and the Affect Diathesis Hypothesis in Pattern Recognition, Joint Attention, Intention Reading, Theory of Mind, and Higher Level Symbolic Thinking

As the infant negotiates the first four stages of affective transformation, he or she engages in progressively more complex patterns of affective signaling with caregivers (Greenspan and Shanker 2004). These long chains of coregulated affective gesturing enable the child to recognize various patterns involved in satisfying his or her emotional needs. The child learns, for example, how to solicit a caregiver's assistance to obtain some out-of-reach desired object and enter into finely tuned, back-and-forth interactions (through vocalizations and facial expressions) in a coregulated solution of the problem (for example, multiple joint-attention interactions). The child also learns what different gestures or facial expressions signify the connection between, on the one hand, certain kinds of facial expressions, tones of voice, or behavior and, on the other hand, an individual's mood or intentions and so on. This ability to read the patterns of others and, through recognition of one's own patterns, form a sense of self is the basis for what is called *intention reading* or *theory of mind*.

This ability is also essential if a child is to have and act on expectations—to know when to expect different kinds of responses from his or her caregiver or to know what love, anger, respect, shame, and so forth feel like. It is equally essential if the child is to know what others are thinking or feeling or to grasp their intentions. The ability to recognize the intentions of others does not come out of the blue. Rather, pattern recognition, intention reading, and joint attention emerge from and require mastery of all of the earlier stages of affective transformation. These capacities are downstream effects of the emotional capacities that have been developing in the first three stages of functional emotional development and reach a more complex configuration in the critical fourth stage of affective transformation (see Greenspan and Shanker 2007).

Understanding the complexity of this process has enabled the formulation of interventions that are tailored to the child's biological profile and vulnerabilities and increase the likelihood of his or her achieving some relative mastery of these critical early affective transformations and the subsequent abilities for joint attention, theory of mind, and higher levels of language and symbolic thinking (Greenspan and Wieder 1998).

The theory just outlined was tested on a representative population of more than 1,500 children whose parents were administered the Greenspan Social-Emotional Growth Chart (Greenspan 2004). Mastery of the early stages of affect transformation was found to be necessary for children to progress to the subsequent stages, and the first four stages were required for the capacities for symbol formation, pragmatic language, and higher level thinking (including theory-of-mind capacities such as empathy), and for social referencing and joint-attention capacities (such as reciprocal, shared social problem solving). (For a description of this study, see the new Bayley Scales Kit and manual at www.harcourtassessment.com and Bayley 2005).

This data set provides support for the DIR/Floortime model and opens the door to further research on what occurs in the central nervous system that is associated with compromises in these early emotional interactions.

The DIR/Floortime Intervention Program

The theory just summarized has enabled the formation of a comprehensive intervention program for infants, toddlers, and preschoolers with ASDs and other developmental challenges that involves helping them to reestablish the developmental sequence that went awry (with a special focus on helping them become more affectively connected and intentional). The program determines which of the functional emotional levels described earlier have been mastered fully, partially, or not at all. It also uses an understanding of children's individual differences in sensory modulation, processing, and motor planning to establish a relationship that creates interactive, affective opportunities to negotiate the partially mastered or unmastered functional emotional developmental process. Rather than focus only on isolated behaviors or skills, the DIR/Floortime approach focuses on these more essential functional emotional developmental processes and differences that underlie particular symptoms or behaviors. For example, rather than trying to teach a child who is perseveratively spinning the wheels on a car to play with something else or to play with the car appropriately, the therapist, in the DIR/Floortime approach, would use the child's interest and, warmly smiling, spin the wheel in the opposite direction to get reciprocal, affective interaction going.

The goal is to help the child construct the developmental foundations for healthy emotional, social, and intellectual functioning. The DIR/Floortime model provides a developmental framework for conceptualizing these foundations and pinpointing what is compromised in different children with ASDs. The DIR/Floortime model, however, is not an assessment tool or a discrete intervention. It helps to systematize many of the traditionally helpful assessments and interventions and to emphasize elements of a comprehensive approach that are often ignored or only dealt with superficially.

All the elements in the DIR/Floortime model have a long tradition, including speech and language therapy, occupational therapy, special and early childhood education, and Floortime-type interactions with parents (which is consistent with the developmentally appropriate practice guidelines of the National Association for the Education of Young Children [NAEYC]) [Bredekamp and Copple 1997] and pragmatic speech therapy practices, both of which attempt to foster preverbal and symbolic communication and thinking). The DIR/Floortime model, however, contributes to these traditional practices by further defining the child's developmental level, individual processing differences, and the need for certain types of affective interactions in terms of a comprehensive program in which all the elements can work together toward common goals.

In this model, the therapeutic program must begin as soon as possible so that the children and their parents are reengaged in emotional interactions that use their emerging but not fully developed capacities for communication (often initially with gestures rather than words).

The DIR/Floortime intervention is fundamentally different from behavioral therapy, skill building, play therapy, or psychotherapy. The primary goal of this intervention is to enable children to form a sense of themselves as intentional, interactive individuals; to develop cognitive, language, and social capacities from this basic sense of intentionality; and to progress through the six DIR/Floortime FEDLs. Floortime is the most important component of a DIR/Floortime comprehensive program and refers to unstructured "play" sessions in which the child is in the lead and initiates the ideas, and the adult both follows and challenges the child to support spontaneous, purposeful, and flowing interactions at both presymbolic and symbolic levels. In addition, a comprehensive DIR/Floortime intervention includes the additional interactive activities and therapies described below. These components are always developmentally appropriate and are selected and balanced to fit the profile of the child and the family, and together constitute a complete and full-time approach that addresses the individual and changing goals of the child and family. Elements of a comprehensive program often include the following:

- Home-based, developmentally appropriate interactions and practices (Floortime).
- Spontaneous, Floortime interactions (following the child's lead), in which the focus is initially on joint attention, engagement, and problem-solving interaction to establish a continuous flow. The therapist and child then move on to creative pretend play that supports mastering the full range of emotional and cognitive abilities and prepares the child for higher levels of abstract thinking. As the child gets older, more reality-based conversations and reflective "talktime" become the later forms of Floortime (20–30 minutes, eight or more times a day; as children improve they can usually engage in longer sessions).
- Semistructured, affect-based problem solving, such as dealing with real-life situations in which the child encounters problems through relevant daily experiences where he or she must interact with the parent to solve problems (e.g., finding his or her favorite crackers, which are in a ziplock bag; finding the tub empty when asked if ready for a bath; searching for Dad, who is calling from somewhere in the house; negotiating with a sibling for a toy;

or working on tasks together to support reasoning, planning, and sequencing), all requiring back-and-forth problem-solving discussions. Some children also benefit from semistructured problem solving found in the affect-based language curriculum (Greenspan and Lewis 2002) (20 or more minutes, four to eight times a day).

- Spatial, motor, and sensory activities (15–30 minutes or longer, four times a day):
  - Running and changing direction, jumping, spinning, swinging, deep tactile pressure.
  - Perceptual motor challenges, including looking and doing games.
  - Visuospatial processing and motor-planning games, including treasure hunts and obstacle courses.
  - The activities above can become integrated with the pretend play of Floortime.
- Speech therapy, typically three or more times a week.[2]
- Sensory integration– and sensory motor–based occupational therapy and/or physical therapy, typically two or more times a week.[2]
- Play dates with older or younger peers who are natural play partners and will pursue and interact with the child or respond to the adult's coaching and mediation. The number of play dates a week should match the age of the child (i.e., a 3-year-old should have three play dates a week). Later, these can expand to small groups and semistructured activities with other children in clubs and music, art, drama, and sports activities.
- Family consultation and counseling to help parents design and implement their comprehensive programs, support family functioning, and provide advocacy where needed.

---

[2]Frequency of specific therapies will vary depending on the child's needs, the implementation of the home program, and the services obtained in an education setting. For example, some children at the start will benefit from more intensive speech and language and oral motor therapy, but later this may be decreased as the child has more opportunities for conversations and symbol language. Similarly, occupational and sensory motor therapies will vary depending on individual needs, activities organized at home, and participation in sports and may later change to visuospatial cognitive therapy.

- Educational program, daily, with parent collaboration.

  - For children who can interact and imitate gestures and/or words and engage in preverbal problem solving, either an integrated inclusion program or a regular preschool program with an aide.

  - For children not yet able to engage in preverbal problem solving or imitation, a special education program in which the major focus is on engagement, preverbal purposeful gestural interaction, preverbal problem solving (a continuous flow of back-and-forth communication), and learning to imitate actions, sounds, and words. As children prepare for academic learning, some may require individualized instruction or tutoring in reading, mathematics, and visual thinking, as well as specific learning techniques, such as Lindamood-Bell Learning Processes (see www.lblp.com). The other considerations involve smaller class size and facilitative environments that do not overwhelm the child.

- Biomedical interventions, including consideration of medication, to enhance motor planning and sequencing, self-regulation, concentration, and/or auditory processing and language.

- A consideration of 1) nutrition and diet and 2) technologies geared to improve processing abilities, including auditory processing, visuospatial processing, sensory modulation, and motor planning.

Most children with ASDs require most if not all of these components for a comprehensive program because each component addresses a major area requiring further development, and each provides countless opportunities for successful spontaneous and semistructured interactions that have been derailed. It is a dynamic program and, depending on the individual profile of the children and family, there will be variations in this program at various stages of progress, although Floortime and, later, reflective talk time remain constant. In some cases, therapies and other program components can be modified if a strong home program guided by the therapist is implemented. In addition, specific techniques or tools may be indicated such as augmentative communication, assistive technology, and activities to support imitative and ritualized learning, such as social games, drama, and sports. As the child progresses, various activities will become part of the child's social activities, such as clubs, sports, music, and drama. A comprehensive program is quite full-time during the early years when intensive intervention is very important, but then it transitions into more typical child activities as the child progresses.

Comments on the Therapeutic Process

The DIR/Floortime therapeutic process is described in detail elsewhere (Greenspan 1992; Greenspan and Wieder 1998). Only a few essential features will be described here. Children with ASDs often lack the most basic foundation for interpersonal experiences (e.g., they are often not interactive in the purposeful way that typically developing 8-month-olds are) Therefore, the earliest therapeutic goals are to mobilize shared attention, engagement, and intentional back-and-forth signaling. Interactive experiences enable them to abstract a sense of self and form higher level cognitive and social capacities.

As focus and engagement are fostered, attention must be paid to the children's profile of individual processing differences (regulatory profile), as described earlier. For example, if they are overreactive to sound, talking to them in a loud voice may lead them to become more aimless and withdrawn. If they are overreactive to sights, bright lights and even very animated facial expressions may be overwhelming to them. On the other hand, if they are underreactive to sensations of sound and visuospatial input, talking in a strong voice and using animated facial expressions in a well-lighted room may help them attend. Similarly, in terms of their receptive language skills, if they are already at the point where they can decode a complex rhythm, making interesting sounds in complex patterns may be helpful. On the other hand, if they can only decode very simple two-sequence rhythms, simpler rhythms will be better.

One may find that children remain relatively better focused in motion, such as when they are being swung. Certain movement rhythms may be more effective than others.

It is especially difficult to foster a sense of intimacy. As children are encouraged to attend and engage, it is critically important to take advantage of their own natural interests. It is most helpful to follow their lead and look for opportunities for that visceral sense of pleasure and intimacy that leads them to *want* to relate to the human world. Intimacy is further supported as children are helped to form simple, and then more complex, gestural communications.

A major challenge is children's tendency to perseverate. One child may only open and close a door. Another may only bang blocks together. The key is to transform the perseveration into an interaction. We use the children's intense motivation to their advantage to get gestural circles of communication opened and closed. For example, we get stuck in a door or our hands caught between some blocks. We are gentle and playful as they try to get us out of their way (as in a cat and mouse game). As gestural interactions occur, behavior becomes purposeful and affective. We modulate their feelings of annoyance and help soothe and comfort as well, although often children find our playful obstruction amusing.

As children become more purposeful, we have found that they can imitate gestures and sounds more readily and can copy feeding a doll or kissing a bear. With continuing challenges to be intentional, they copy complex patterns and imitate sounds and words, often gradually beginning to use words and pretend on their own. Another challenge, as one moves toward more representational or symbolic elaboration, is to help children differentiate their experiences. They need to learn cause-and-effect communication at the level of ideas and to make connections between various representations or ideas.

Caregivers become the representation for reality. The ability of clinicians or parents to enter the symbolic world of children becomes the critical vehicle for fostering emotional differentiation and higher levels of abstract and logical thinking.

Relating to children when they are feeling strong affects is critical. They are connecting words to underlying affects that give them purpose and meaning. When children are motivated, for example, in trying to negotiate to get a certain kind of food or to go outside, there is often an opportunity to open and close many symbolic circles. The child who tries to open the door to go outside and is angry that he or she cannot may, in the midst of feeling annoyed, open and close 20 circles of communication if the adult soothingly tries to find out what the child wants to do outside.

Children with pervasive developmental disabilities find it especially difficult to shift from concrete to abstract modes of thinking because they do not easily generalize from a specific experience to other similar experiences. There is a temptation to teach them answers and repeat the same question by scripting the dialogue. However, they can learn to abstract and generalize only through active, emotionally meaningful experiences. Long conversations with debates are most helpful because it helps the child express his or her own opinions (e.g., "I like juice because it tastes good") rather than memorized elaborations of facts (e.g., "The juice is orange").

As the child progresses through the six functional emotional milestones, the therapeutic program works on mobilizing all six levels at the same time in each and every interaction. The therapeutic program often evolves to a point in which the child and family are involved in three types of activities: 1) spontaneous, creative interactions (Floortime); 2) semistructured, problem-solving interactions to learn new skills, concepts, and master academic work (e.g., creating problems to solve, like negotiating for cookies or mastering spatial concepts such as "behind" and "next to" by discovering where the favorite toy is located); and 3) motor, sensory, and spatial play to strengthen fundamental processing skills.

Selected Research on the DIR/Floortime Model and Outcome Studies

In the following section, we briefly review selected studies on the DIR/Floortime approach.

Review of 200 Cases of Children With Autism Spectrum Disorders

In this study (Greenspan and Wieder 1997), we looked systematically at the cases of 200 children, whom we had seen for consultation or treatment over an 8-year period. The children had varying presenting impairments (see Table 9–2), all diagnosed on the autistic spectrum by two or three other evaluation teams.

The children were treated with methods based on the developmental model described earlier. In reviewing the original diagnoses of these children, and their subsequent progress over 2–8 years after the start of intervention, we divided the children into groups as indicated in Table 9–3.

The first group—those with good-to-outstanding outcome—did better than any current prognosis for children with ASDs would have predicted. After 2 or more years of intervention, these children became warm and interactive, relating joyfully with appropriate, reciprocal preverbal gestures; could engage in lengthy, well-organized, and purposeful social problem solving and share attention on various social, cognitive, or motor-based tasks; used sym-

Table 9–2. Presenting conditions in 200 cases of children with autism spectrum disorders

Functional developmental component	Description of functional developmental component	Percent patients with mild to severe impairment
Presenting functional, emotional, developmental level	Partially engaged and purposeful, with limited use of symbols (ideas)	24
	Partially engaged, with limited complex problem-solving interactive sequences (half of this group evidenced only simple purposeful behavior)	40
	Partially engaged, with only fleeting purposeful behavior	31
	No affective engagement	5
Sensory modulation	Overreactive to sensation	19
	Underreactive to sensation (with 11% craving sensation)	39
	Mixed reactivity to sensation	36
	Not classified	6
Motor-planning dysfunction	Mild to moderate motor-planning dysfunction	52
	Severe motor-planning dysfunction	48
Low muscle tone	Motor-planning dysfunction with significant degree of low muscle tone	17
Visuospatial processing dysfunction	Relative strength (e.g., can find toys, good sense of direction)	22
	Moderate impairment	36
	Moderate to severe impairment	42
Auditory processing and language	Mild to moderate impairment, with intermittent abilities to imitate sounds and words or use selected words	45
	Moderate to severe impairment, with no ability to imitate or use words	55

Table 9–3.   Floortime intervention outcomes

Good to outstanding	58%
Medium	25%
Ongoing difficulties	17%

bols and words creatively and logically, based on their intent and desires, rather than using rote sequences; and progressed to high levels of thinking, including making inferences and experiencing empathy. Some children in this group developed precocious academic abilities two or three grade levels above their ages.

These children all mastered basic capacities such as reality testing, impulse control, organization of thoughts and emotions, differentiated sense of self, and ability to experience a range of emotions, thoughts, and concerns. Finally, they no longer showed symptoms such as self-absorption, avoidance, self-stimulation, or perseveration. As rated on the Childhood Autism Rating Scale (CARS; Schopler et al. 1988), they shifted into the nonautistic range, although some still exhibited auditory or visuospatial difficulties (which were improving), and most had some degree of fine or gross motor-planning challenges.

The second, or medium, group made slower and more gradual progress but still made significant gains in their ability to relate and communicate with gestures, entering into long sequences of purposeful interaction but not necessarily a continuous flow. They could share attention and engage in problem solving. They developed some degree of language and could talk in phrases; many could answer "why" questions. However, they still had significant problems developing their symbolic capacities. They, too, became very warm and loving; in fact, the first thing that changed was their relatedness and ability to show affection. But they had less sophisticated or abstract thinking skills. Some of these children had more involved neurological challenges to begin with. As with the first group, the children in this group no longer exhibited self-absorption, avoidance, self-stimulation, or perseveration.

The third group—those with ongoing difficulties who had the most complicated neurological pictures, including other neurological disorders such as seizure disorders—made very slow progress. Although most eventually learned how to communicate with gestures or simple words and phrases or both, they continued to have difficulties with attention and with sequences of gesturing, and still evidenced self-absorption, avoidance, self-stimulation, and persever-ation. However, many were making progress in their ability to relate warmly to others, and their problematic behaviors decreased. Of this last group, eight children were wavering or losing abilities.

Because all the children in this study were brought to us by their families, who were motivated to work with this approach, this was not a representative population of children with ASDs. However, it is reasonable to assume based on our observations that a subgroup of children with ASDs can make enormous progress. Only future clinical trial studies will determine what percentage of children is in this subgroup.

We observed that children who made progress tended to improve in a cer-tain sequence. First, within several months, they began showing more emotion and pleasure in relating to others. Contrary to the stereotypes of autism, they seemed eager for emotional contact; the problem was that they had trouble fig-uring out how to achieve it. They seemed grateful when their parents helped them express their desire for interaction. After parents learned to draw them out by being playfully obstructive, even children who had been very avoidant and self-absorbed began seeking out their parents for relatedness and taking the initiative.

Overall, most of the children, including many in the third group, initially showed improvement in the range and depth of their engagement and expres-sion of emotions, particularly pleasure. Once engaged, many then moved from simple to complex emotional and motor gestures, which in turn led to the emer-gence of functional symbolic capacities. Presymbolic communication always preceded creative symbolic elaboration and the expressive use of language. Many children went through a transitional stage of using scripted words and then became increasingly creative with their gestural interactions. Children who remained rigid in their gestural interactions often remained stereotyped in their use of language. Flexibility in nonverbal interactions led to the spon-taneous and creative use of language.

Once they became more symbolic, many of the children could not stop talking, as if they were excited to use their new abilities. Their ideas were at first jumbled and occasionally illogical and scripted; over time, however, over half of the children could use their symbols creatively and logically. Most of the children learned to express their own ideas much more quickly than they learned to understand the ideas of others. Eventually, if their caretakers and therapists focused on rapid, two-way, symbolic communication, challenging the children to process incoming information in long, back-and-forth exchanges, children learned to comprehend the ideas of others and express abstract "why" ideas.

The children in the good-to-outstanding outcome group who became creative and logical then became able to hold spontaneous, affect-driven, two-way symbolic communication. This allowed them to differentiate their internal worlds and develop logical thinking, impulse control, and an organized sense of self. For many, this was a two-step process. First, they learned to hold "islands" of logical dialogue. Over time, they learned to integrate and expand these islands, and a cohesive sense of self and capacity for logic emerged, along with their ability for functional logical exchanges, two-way thinking, problem solving, and working with others. In consequence, their academic abilities also improved, as did their peer relationships, although in the latter case a great deal of practice was required. With appropriate dynamic and secure academic environments, many of the children in the first group developed average to superior academic skills; however, those in overly structured academic settings tended to remain more rigid, concrete, and rote.

This pattern of progress occurred in the context of a comprehensive DIR/Floortime intervention, as described earlier.

Detailed Study of 20 Good-to-Outstanding Outcome Group Patients

As part of the above study, we also studied in detail 20 of the children in the good-to-outstanding group who had made the most progress, using videotape analysis and the Vineland Adaptive Behavior Scales (Sparrow et al. 1984) to compare them with children with no challenges at all who were functioning both emotionally and intellectually at or above age level. We also compared these two groups with a group of children who continued to have chronic problems in relating and communicating.

The 20 children we studied ranged in age from 5 to 10 years old, had all started intervention between age 2 and 4 years, and had received between 2 and 8 years of intervention or follow-up consultation, or both. At the time of outcome, all were attending regular schools, enjoyed relationships with friends, and participated in community activities. Many had been assessed for cognitive abilities using standardized tests and were functioning in the superior range.

As measured by the Functional Emotional Assessment Scale (FEAS; Greenspan et al. 2001), children who never had challenges and the 20 children from the DIR/Floortime subgroup originally diagnosed with ASDs were indistinguishable. The FEAS is a reliable, validated clinical rating scale that can be applied to videotaped interactions between infants or children and caregivers to measure emotional, social, and intellectual functioning. The Vineland Adaptive Behavior Scales address adaptive behavior in the domains of communication, daily living, and socialization.

On the Vineland scales, all the children scored higher than age level in the communication domain, with 60% scoring 1–2 years higher than age level. In the socialization domain, 90% of the children received scores 2–3 years ahead of age level, which is particularly notable given that children with ASDs typically continue to evidence significant social impairments even when there is some progress in language and cognition. Scores for daily living improved less in comparison with the other two domains. Because of motor-planning difficulties that affect daily living, self-care skills are often more challenging for this population.

Finally, the adaptive behavior composite scores, which average the three domains, were all above age level except in one child, who had significant motor difficulties. None of the children presented maladaptive behavior patterns. Overall, the longer the child was in treatment and the older he or she was, the higher the child's scores relative to his or her age, suggesting that children continued to function progressively better as they grew older.

For the FEAS ratings, each child in each of the groups was videotaped while interacting with a caregiver for 15 minutes or more. A reliable judge blind to the identity of the children used FEAS to rate the children on the DIR/Floortime FEDLs (Greenspan et al. 2001). As stated previously, the intervention group was indistinguishable from the normal healthy control group. Both groups were significantly different from the group with continuing difficulties. Table 9–4 shows the scoring breakdown for each of the groups, with 76 representing the top of the scale.

The findings in the FEAS clinical ratings are especially important because they can be used to reliably rate the subtle, high-level personality functions (e.g., quality of intimacy, emotional expressiveness and reciprocity, creativity and imagination, and abstract, flexible thinking, as well as problem solving and reality testing) that are expected to be relatively permanently impaired in children with ASDs, even those who make considerable progress in their lan-

Table 9–4.   Functional Emotional Assessment Scale (FEAS) outcomes

	N	Mean FEAS	Range
DIR/Floortime intervention group	20	74.8	70–76
Normal comparison group	14	74.9	65–76
Continuing significant difficulties	2	23.7	10–40

guage and cognitive abilities. The fact that the intervention group was comparable with a peer group without developmental disorders suggests, at a minimum, that children initially given an autism spectrum diagnosis can develop sustainable patterns of healthy emotional, social, and adaptive behavior.

Long-Term Follow-Up Study

Subsequent to the study just described, we performed a 10- to 15-year follow-up study of 16 children who were in the good-to-outstanding outcome group of the original 200 subjects (Wieder and Greenspan 2005). In this study we attempted to determine whether a subgroup of children initially diagnosed with ASDs could, with an optimal developmentally based program, go beyond expectations for high-functioning ASDs and learn to be interactive, empathetic, creative, and reflective thinkers, and to sustain these gains into adolescence.

At the time of the study, these children (all males) were between the ages of 12 and 17 years. This follow-up study was comprehensive, addressing the full range of emotional, social, and sensory-processing variables in addition to traditional cognitive and academic outcomes. The study showed that this group had developed high levels of empathy and were often more empathetic than their peers. Some became very talented in music and writing, including poetry. Most were outstanding students, excelling in many academic areas; others were average students; a few struggled academically with learning disabilities because of executive functioning and sequencing problems. As a group, they showed the expected range of mental health problems, which often depended on family circumstances (a few were anxious or depressed as adolescents). Importantly, however, they coped with the stresses of puberty and family concerns while maintaining their core gains in relating, communicating, and reflective thinking and making further progress as well. For this subgroup of children, the core deficits and symptoms of ASDs were no longer observed 10–15 years after they initially presented.

For this study we conducted parent interviews and asked parents to complete a Functional Emotional Developmental Questionnaire (FEDQ) through which they could rate the children's development in the various domains described previously. We also rated our impressions of the children independently, using videotapes made by parents, our direct interviews with the children, or audiotapes recorded via telephone. We also collected school reports and obtained IQ tests when available (most parents indicated there was no need to have their children tested for IQ). Finally, to provide an objective assessment, we administered the Achenbach Child Behavior Checklist scales (Achenbach 1991), which rates competence and clinical syndromes.

Short-Term Changes

In addition, we conducted a study looking at short-term changes in children with ASDs who received DIR/Floortime consultation (Greenspan and Breinbauer 2005). We looked at 10 cases in detail for this pilot study.

This study showed positive changes in emotional and social functioning after "coaching" in the second half of the first session as well as 1 and 2 years later, suggesting that the DIR/Floortime approach works on the very processes it purports to address and helps to explain the mechanisms through which children with ASDs can change and learn to master the building blocks of relating, communicating, and thinking. The study also shows the value of coaching caregivers in bringing out the child's highest levels to help ascertain the child's range, which is necessary for organizing an appropriate intervention program. We will soon replicate this pilot effort with a larger sample.

Other Research Support for the DIR/Floortime Model

As we have described, children with ASDs typically have challenges at two levels: 1) compromises in the basic foundations of relating, communicating, and thinking; and 2) symptoms such as repetitive behavior, self-stimulation, and self-absorption. Modern developmental, relationship-based approaches for children with ASDs and other disorders of relating and communicating—such as the DIR/Floortime model—attempt to help children master both levels at the same time. In contrast, older approaches—such as behavioral ones, including the widely used Applied Behavior Analysis (ABA) discrete trial approach—tend to focus on changing surface behaviors and symptoms without attention to underlying individual differences or the missing basic foundations of relating and thinking. Although early reports on behavioral approaches suggested positive educational gains for children with ASDs, later, more definitive studies have shown only modest educational gains and little to no emotional or social gains for highly structured behavioral approaches (McEachin et al. 1993; Shea 2004; Smith 2001; Smith et al. 2000).

The National Academy of Sciences (NAS), in its report *Educating Children With Autism* (National Research Council 2001), stated that there is research support for a number of approaches, including DIR/Floortime and behavioral interventions, but that there are no proven "relationships between any particular intervention and children's progress" (p. 5) and "no adequate comparisons of different comprehensive treatments" (p. 8). The report concluded that effective interventions vary depending on an individual child's and family's needs.

The NAS analysis further indicated that behavioral interventions are moving toward naturalistic, spontaneous types of learning situations that follow the child's interests and note that "studies have reported that naturalistic approaches are more effective than traditional discrete trial at leading to generalization of language gains to natural contexts" (Koegel et al. 1998; McGee et al. 1985).

In the chapter "Evaluating Effective Interventions for Children with Autism and Related Disorders: Widening the View and Changing the Perspective," Elizabeth Tsakiris, M.Ed. (Tsakiris 2000), reviews the research support for each of the different component parts of the DIR/Floortime model. This review shows that a great deal of research supports the importance of the different elements that constitute the DIR/Floortime model, including relationships and emotional/social interactions in facilitating emotional and cognitive development. There is also a great deal of support for interventions that work with auditory processing and language functioning. There is significant support (but less than for the two areas listed above) for interventions that focus on motor planning and sequencing, executive functioning, sensory modulation, and visuospatial processing.

In a study (Simpson et al. 2003) on the new Bayley Scales of Infant and Toddler Development (Bayley 2005), which includes the Greenspan Social-Emotional Growth Chart, a parent questionnaire on the DIR/Floortime FEDLs was field-tested on a representative sample of 1,500 infants and young children and found to discriminate between children with problems and disorders and those without. The study also validated the age predictions of the DIR/

Floortime FEDLs. (See the Psychological Corporation, Harcourt Assessment Web site at www.harcourtassessment.com for more information and to obtain a manual with the data.) Furthermore, in a recent national survey of over 15,000 families, the federal government's National Center for Health Statistics used questions on the DIR/Floortime FEDLs and found that it identified 30% more infants and children at risk (most of whom were not receiving services) than prior health surveys (Simpson et al. 2003). This was the first time emotional variables were used in this national health survey.

In the Michigan PLAY Project, Rick Solomon, M.D., has analyzed the results of a community-based application of the DIR/Floortime model. He found significant gains for a group of children with ASDs in social, cognitive, and language functioning, and demonstrated that the DIR/Floortime model can be applied to a large community with public funding at low cost (Solomon et al. 2007).

In addition, other developmental relationship-based approaches are showing promising results. For example, Gerald Mahoney, Ph.D., and Frida Perales, M.Ed., of the Mandel School of Applied Social Sciences at Case Western Reserve University have conducted a number of studies on developmental relationship-based approaches (Mahoney and Perales 2005). The work of Sally Rogers, Ph.D., and colleagues (the Denver model) (Rogers and DiLalla 1991; Rogers et al. 2000) is another example.

Summary

In this chapter we presented a brief overview of the DIR/Floortime model and discussed its implications for assessment, intervention, and understanding the developmental pathways leading to ASDs. We also presented an overview of selected studies that support the DIR/Floortime model. For further information, see Greenspan and Wieder 1998, 2006; Interdisciplinary Council on Developmental and Learning Disorders 2005; and Tsakiris 2000; as well as the www.icdl.com and www.Floortime.org Web sites.

References

Achenbach TM: Integrative Guide to the 1991 CBCL/4–18, YSR, and TRF Profiles. Burlington, VT, University of Vermont, Department of Psychiatry, 1991

Baranek GT: Autism during infancy: a retrospective video analysis of sensory-motor and social behaviors at 9–12 months of age. J Autism Dev Disord 29:213–224, 1999

Baron-Cohen S: The theory of mind hypothesis of autism: a reply to Boucher. Br J Disord Commun 24:199–200, 1989

Baron-Cohen S: Mindblindness: An Essay on Autism and Theories of Mind. Cambridge, MA, MIT Press, 1994

Baron-Cohen S, Leslie AM, Frith U: Does the autistic child have a "theory of mind"? Cognition 21:37–46, 1985

Bayley N: Bayley Scales of Infant and Toddler Development, 3rd Edition. Bulverde, TX, Psychological Corporation, 2005

Bowler DM: "Theory of mind" in Asperger's syndrome. J Child Psychol Psychiatry 33:877–893, 1992

Bredekamp S, Copple C: Developmentally Appropriate Practices in Early Childhood Programs. Washington, DC, National Association for the Education of Young Children, 1997

Dahlgren SO, Trillingsgaard A: Theory of mind in non-retarded children with autism and Asperger's syndrome: a research note. J Child Psychol Psychiatry 37:759–763, 1996

Dawson G, Galpert I: Mother's use of imitative play for facilitating social responsiveness and toy play in young autistic children. Dev Psychopathol 2:151–162, 1990

Dawson G, Meltzoff A, Osterling J, et al: Neuropsychological correlates of early symptoms of autism. Child Dev 69:1276–1285, 1998

Frith U: Autism: Explaining the Enigma. London, Blackwell, 1989

Greenspan SI: Intelligence and adaptation: an integration of psychoanalytic and Piagetian developmental psychology. Psychol Issues 12:1–408, 1979

Greenspan SI: The Development of the Ego: Implications for Personality Theory, Psychopathology, and the Psychotherapeutic Process. New York, International Universities Press, 1989

Greenspan SI: Infancy and Early Childhood: The Practice of Clinical Assessment and Intervention With Emotional and Developmental Challenges. Madison, CT, International Universities Press, 1992

Greenspan SI: Developmentally Based Psychotherapy. Madison, CT, International Universities Press, 1997a

Greenspan SI: The Growth of the Mind and the Endangered Origins of Intelligence. Reading, MA, Addison Wesley Longman, 1997b

Greenspan SI: The affect diathesis hypothesis: the role of emotions in the core deficit in autism and the development of intelligence and social skills. Journal of Developmental and Learning Disorders 5:1–45, 2002

Greenspan SI: Greenspan Social-Emotional Growth Chart. San Antonio, TX, Psychological Corporation, 2004

Greenspan SI, Breinbauer C: Short-term changes in emotional, social and intellectual functioning in children with ASD with the DIR-Floortime approach. January 30, 2005. Available at: http://www.icdl.com.

Greenspan SI, Lewis D: The Affect-Based Language Curriculum: An Intensive Program for Families, Therapists and Teachers. Bethesda, MD, Interdisciplinary Council on Developmental and Learning Disorders, 2002

Greenspan SI, Shanker S: The First Idea: How Symbols, Language and Intelligence Evolved From Our Primate Ancestors to Modern Humans. Reading, MA, Perseus Books, 2004

Greenspan SI, Shanker S: The developmental pathways leading to pattern recognition, joint attention, language and cognition. New Ideas in Psychology 2(2):128–142, 2007

Greenspan SI, Wieder S: Developmental patterns and outcomes in infants and children with disorders in relating and communicating: a chart review of 200 cases of children with autistic spectrum diagnoses. Journal of Developmental and Learning Disorders 1:87–141, 1997

Greenspan SI, Wieder S: The Child With Special Needs: Encouraging Intellectual and Emotional Growth. Reading, MA, Perseus Books, 1998

Greenspan SI, Wieder S: Engaging Autism: The Floortime Approach to Helping Children Relate, Communicate, and Think. Cambridge, MA, DaCapo Press/Perseus Books, 2006

Greenspan SI, DeGangi GA, Wieder S: The Functional Emotional Assessment Scale (FEAS) for Infancy and Early Childhood: Clinical and Research Applications. Bethesda, MD, Interdisciplinary Council on Developmental and Learning Disorders, 2001

Interdisciplinary Council on Developmental and Learning Disorders Diagnostic Manual for Infancy and Early Childhood Mental Health Disorders Workgroup: Interdisciplinary Council on Developmental and Learning Disorders Diagnostic Manual for Infancy and Early Childhood Mental Health Disorders, Developmental Disorders, Regulatory-Sensory Processing Disorders, Language Disorders, and Learning Challenges (ICDL-DMIC). Bethesda, MD, Interdisciplinary Council on Developmental and Learning Disorders, 2005

Klin A, Volkmar FR, Sparrow S: Autistic social dysfunction: some limitations of the theory of mind hypothesis. J Child Psychol Psychiatry 33:861–876, 1992

Koegel JK, Camarata SM, Valdez-Menchaca M, et al: Setting generalization of question-asking by children with autism. Am J Ment Retard 102:346–357, 1998

Mahoney G, Perales F: Relationship-focused early intervention with children with pervasive developmental disorders and other disabilities: a comparative study. J Dev Behav Pediatr 26:77–85, 2005

McEachin JJ, Smith T, Lovaas OI: Long-term outcome for children with autism who received early intensive behavioral treatment. Am J Ment Retard 97:359–372, 1993

McGee GC, Krantz PJ, McClannahan LE: The facilitative effects of incidental teaching on preposition use by autistic children. J Appl Behav Anal 18:17–31, 1985

Minshew NJ, Goldstein D, Siegel DJ: Neuropsychologic functioning in autism: profile of a complex information processing disorder. J Int Neuropsychol Soc 3:303–316, 1997

Mundy P, Sigman M, Kasari C: A longitudinal study of joint attention and language development in autistic children. J Autism Dev Disord 20:115–128, 1990

National Research Council: Educating Children With Autism. Committee on Educational Interventions for Children With Autism. Edited by Lord C, McGee JP. Division of Behavioral and Social Sciences and Education. Washington, DC, National Academy Press, 2001

Ozonoff S: Causal mechanisms of autism: unifying perspectives from an information-processing framework, in Handbook of Autism and Pervasive Developmental Disorders, 2nd Edition. Edited by Cohen D, Volkmar F. New York, Wiley, 1997, pp 868–879

Pennington J, Ozonoff S: Executive functions and developmental psychopathology. J Child Psychol Psychiatry 37:51–87, 1996

Rogers S, DiLalla D: A comparative study of the effects of a developmentally based instructional model on young children with autism and young children with other disorders of behavior and development. Topics in Early Childhood Special Education 11:29–47, 1991

Rogers SJ, Hall T, Osaki D, et al: The Denver model: a comprehensive, integrated educational approach to young children with autism and their families, in Preschool Education Programs for Children With Autism, 2nd Edition. Edited by Handleman JS, Harris SL. Austin, TX, Pro-Ed, 2000, pp 95–133

Schopler E, Reichler RJ, Renner BR: The Childhood Autism Rating Scale (CARS). Los Angeles, CA, Western Psychological Services, 1988

Shea V: A perspective on the research literature related to early intensive behavioral intervention (Lovaas) for young children with autism. Autism 8:349–367, 2004

Simpson GA, Colpe L, Greenspan SI: Measuring functional developmental delay in infants and young children: prevalence rates from the NHIS-D. Paediatr Perinat Epidemiol 17:68–80, 2003

Smith T: Discrete trial ABA approaches. Paper presented at the annual meeting of the Interdisciplinary Council on Developmental and Learning Disorders. Tysons Corner, VA, November 2001

Smith T, Groen AD, Wynn JW: Randomized trial of intensive early intervention for children with pervasive developmental disorder. Am J Ment Retard 105:269–285, 2000

Solomon R, Necheles JW, Ferch C, et al: Evaluation of a training program for young children with autism: the Michigan P.L.A.Y. Project for home consultation model. Autism 11(3):205–224, 2007

Sparrow S, Balla DA, Cicchetti D: Vineland Adaptive Behavior Scales. Circle Pines, MN, American Guidance Service, 1984

Sperry RW: Consciousness, personal identity, and the divided brain, in The Dual Brain. Edited by Benson F, Zaidel E. New York, Guilford, 1985, pp 11–27

Tsakiris E: Evaluating effective interventions for children with autism and related disorders: widening the view and changing the perspective, in Interdisciplinary Council on Developmental and Learning Disorders' Clinical Practice Guidelines: Redefining the Standards of Care for Infants, Children, and Families With Special Needs. Interdisciplinary Council on Developmental and Learning Disorders Clinical Practice Guidelines Workgroup. Bethesda, MD, Interdisciplinary Council on Developmental and Learning Disorders, 2000, pp 725–819

Wetherby AM, Prizant BM: Profiling communication and symbolic abilities in young children. J Childhood Comm Disord 15:23–32, 1993

Wieder S, Greenspan SI: Can children with core deficits become empathetic, creative, and reflective? A ten- to fifteen-year follow-up of a subgroup of children with autism spectrum disorders (ASD) who received a comprehensive Developmental, Individual-Difference, Relationship-based (DIR) Approach, Journal of Developmental and Learning Disorders 9:39–61, 2005

10

Educational Approaches for Autism—TEACCH

Lee Marcus, Ph.D.

Eric Schopler, Ph.D.

In this chapter we discuss an approach to education based on the experience, principles, and practices of the Treatment and Education of Autistic and Related Communication-Handicapped Children (TEACCH) program in North Carolina (Mesibov et al. 2005). Following the presentation of an overview and background of TEACCH, we review the fundamental empirical principles and values that form the basis of the program, then describe in a developmen-

In Memoriam: Dr. Schopler passed away on July 7, 2006, after a long and distinguished career as one of the pioneers and leaders in the field of autism. Having received many other awards, in 2006 he was presented the Lifetime Achievement Award by the International Meeting for Autism Research and the Gold Medal Award for Life Achievement in the Application of Psychology by the American Psychological Association.

Acknowledgment: The authors want to thank Brenda Denzler, Ph.D., for her help with this manuscript. Not only did she provide thoughtful edits, but, more impressively, she took on the publisher's elaborate, daunting electronic formatting requirements. Without her dedicated help, we would have faced endless delays to complete this manuscript.

tal framework how these are utilized across the age spectrum. The concluding section focuses on the empirical basis for TEACCH methods and the evidence for their effectiveness.

Background and Structure of TEACCH

TEACCH had its origins in the late 1960s as a National Institute of Mental Health (NIMH)–funded research project that demonstrated that children with autism could be best helped by using their parents as cotherapists (Schopler and Reichler 1971). Parents are now commonly accepted as potential teachers, advocates, and support agents for their autistic children (Marcus et al. 2005), but in the past they were viewed as being the cause of their children's problems and in need of psychotherapy. In addition to dispelling that myth, Schopler and Reichler used the project to develop the diagnostic and assessment tools (Schopler et al. 1988, 2005) and many of the intervention strategies that continue to be used at TEACCH and in other programs worldwide (Schopler 2000). As the research project was concluding in 1971, parents and professionals who had been involved in it convinced the North Carolina state legislature not just to maintain the program but to expand it to include 3 statewide regional diagnostic and treatment centers and 11 public school classrooms (see Schopler 1986). These classrooms were among the first in the United States to be designed for students with autism. When national laws were passed mandating access to a free and appropriate public education for the disabled, additional TEACCH-affiliated clinics and classrooms were established. Currently there are over 300 autism-specific classrooms in North Carolina whose teaching and support staff can receive training and consultation from one of the now 9 regional TEACCH centers.

TEACCH is a unique organization in that it is a division in the Department of Psychiatry at the University of North Carolina School of Medicine, with its mission of teaching, clinical service, and research, as well as being a mandated state agency with a mission of high-quality service to persons with autism, their families, and other professionals. This combination of being both a significant part of a major university and a state agency has enabled TEACCH to integrate the scientific and empirical aspects with the practical aspects of understanding and helping individuals with autism and their support systems. Table 10–1 provides an overview of TEACCH principles, values, and program components.

Table 10–1. Overview of TEACCH program concepts and strategies

Principles	Core values	Methods	Structured teaching components
Empirical bases for clinical practice	Understand and appreciate people with autism spectrum disorders	Assessment	Physical structure
Improved adaptation	Professionals function as generalists, not specialists	Direct intervention: structured teaching and working with parents	Individual daily schedule
Parent–professional collaboration	Spirit of cooperation and collaboration	Consultation	Work system
Role of assessment	Understand and appreciate people with autism spectrum disorders	Training	Visual structure
Structured teaching	Understand and appreciate people with autism spectrum disorders	Research	Routines
Skill enhancement	Understand and appreciate people with autism spectrum disorders	Collaboration with other state agencies	Visual structure
Community involvement	Spirit of cooperation and collaboration	Collaboration with other state agencies	All components
Holistic orientation	Professionals as generalists		

Note. TEACCH = Treatment and Education of Autistic and Related Communication-Handicapped Children.

Core Principles and Values

Although the TEACCH program has evolved in its methods and techniques, its basic principles, derived from years of empirical research, have remained constant over the years (Schopler 1997):

1. *Importance of empirical bases for clinical practice.* Incorporating scientifically derived evidence into decisions about basic practices and methods is important and increasingly discussed in psychology and medicine (Rogers 1998; Schopler et al. 2001). This principle has guided the clinical and educational methods used by TEACCH from its inception. In addition to building our intervention programs on sound research-based methods, TEACCH has always critically evaluated the myriad treatment approaches and etiological explanations that have peppered the field for a half century or more. Whether it is megavitamins, psychopharmacology, inclusion, diets, sensory integration therapy, or facilitated communication, TEACCH has carefully and systematically reviewed the existing literature (or lack thereof) and advised families and others about the potential value or harmfulness of these therapies (Schopler et al. 2001). Our commitment to these principles guides both our clinical practice and research (Mesibov et al. 2005).

2. *Commitment to improved adaptation.* As the biological basis of autism became more widely established (Schopler and Mesibov 1987), it became evident that a meaningful treatment program for most people on the autism spectrum would need to be long term. Accordingly, rather than expecting a cure, our treatment focuses on improved adaptation, which also tends to be any parent's goal for their own child. Optimum adaptation can be achieved in two ways: by teaching the individual new or improved skills or, when skill acquisition is blocked by either short-term or long-term developmental delay, by modifying the environment to accommodate the deficit. Both new skills and environmental accommodation will produce improved adaptation.

3. *Parent–professional collaboration.* The belief that parents of children with autism should be viewed as partners in their relationships with professionals is now commonly accepted (Dunlap 1999; Harris 1998; Marcus et al. 2005; Seligman and Darling 1997; Singer and Powers 1993). However, in the 1960s parents were seen as the primary cause of autism. Our early em-

pirical studies in the Child Research Project that preceded TEACCH demonstrated that parents had been misinterpreted and misunderstood (Schopler and Loftin 1969a, 1969b; Schopler et al. 2001). Since then, parents and TEACCH professionals have worked collaboratively at every step, starting with the initial diagnostic evaluation (Marcus and Stone 1993), through home teaching, counseling, and support sessions (Schopler 1995; Schopler et al. 1984), to helping to establish public school classrooms, group homes, supported employment, and other services. The development and growth of this partnership led to the establishment and expansion of TEACCH and to the formation of the Autism Society of North Carolina.

4. *Role of assessment.* The role of assessment, both formal and informal, is to help plan a specific program of education (individualized education program [IEP]) and treatment. Formal assessment systematically identifies the features people share to be grouped in the autism spectrum, whereas informal assessment identifies the ways in which each person varies in his or her learning patterns within the formal diagnosis. Diagnostic instruments such as the Revised Child Autism Rating Scale (CARS; Schopler et al. 1988) and the Autism Diagnostic Observation Schedule (Lord et al. 2002) can help with diagnosis, but the developmental-behavioral-educational scale for children, the Psychoeducational Profile, 3rd Edition (PEP-3; Schopler et al. 2005), and the functional assessment scale for adolescents and adults, the TEACCH Transition Assessment Profile (TTAP; Mesibov et al. 2007) were developed at TEACCH to identify and measure specific learning needs. These formal assessment instruments, along with informal assessment methods that teachers and others are encouraged to use, have been helpful in designing IEPs, home programs, transitional activities, and strategies, as well as intervention methods in supported employment settings.

5. *Structured teaching.* The importance of learning and perceptual problems in autism was identified in early studies by Schopler (1964, 1965, 1966) and Reichler and Schopler (1971). One of the early studies of the Child Research Project demonstrated that children with these kinds of difficulties did better when in a structured situation than in an unstructured one (Schopler et al. 1971). Since then, this finding has been supported repeatedly across programs and settings (e.g., Dawson and Osterling 1997; National Research Council 2001; Rutter and Bartak 1973) and become an axiom in the field. Within TEACCH, the idea of structure, with emphasis

on the use of visual structures (Schopler 1994; Schopler et al. 1995), has been developed and fine-tuned to become a cornerstone of our program.

6. *Skill enhancement.* The most effective treatment approach is to give priority to recognizing the skills of the person with autism and to acknowledge and accept his or her deficits. This important principle parallels a major finding from behavioral treatment that the most effective results are achieved from frequent use of positive reinforcement or rewards. This holds true not only for children's skill acquisition but also for parents' and teachers' use of consultation and for professional staff development (Schopler and Loftin 1969a, 1969b).

7. *Community involvement.* As of now, autism still has lifelong effects in most cases. In the early years of TEACCH, both parents and staff recognized that most persons with autism and their families would require some special help throughout the autistic person's lifespan (Mesibov 1983). Such continuing services are most cost-effective when coordinated with consistency in teaching strategy and support systems as needed throughout the life cycle.

8. *Holistic orientation.* TEACCH-based programs have often been started in reaction to parental complaints about professionals' misunderstanding. This was most noticeable when parents' unconscious wishes and attitudes were seen as the primary cause of the symptoms of autism. However, parental complaints that their child was misunderstood frequently also referred to professionals from various disciplines who viewed the child narrowly within the focus of their specialized field of study. Relying on their specialized training, professionals often would be interested in the specific behavior problem, speech deficit, perceptual-motor impairment, or new pharmaceutical agent—but they did not see the whole child within the context of a unique family. That is why a holistic orientation at TEACCH has shaped our treatment approach and our training of teachers and professionals, becoming a core value of our program.

In a recent book on the TEACCH program, Mesibov et al. (2005) reported the results of a survey on the core values of TEACCH. Program therapists and staff, outside professionals, client families, and people with autism reported three main values. First, *TEACCH understands and appreciates people with autism spectrum disorders,* seeing the condition not only as a challenge but as an integral part of who each client is. Such respect greatly facilitates the assessment and intervention process. Second, *TEACCH professionals function as generalists, not specialists.* This stance aids their ability to understand and deal with autism from multiple perspectives as well as to appreciate the multiple roles parents must play in working with their children. Parents cannot be specialists; they have to know about language, motor, and cognitive development from infancy through adulthood, and they have to be able to communicate effectively about these topics. Professionals need to be equally well versed across these many dimensions. Finally, *TEACCH fosters a spirit of cooperation and collaboration* with families, clients, colleagues within TEACCH, and outside professionals. Whether the task is helping parents teach their child the first steps in communication, mentoring a new staff member, or consulting with a classroom teacher about a serious behavior problem, TEACCH staff approach these working relationships with mutual respect and a commitment to sharing expertise.

Applications of TEACCH Methods and Strategies

There are four main components of TEACCH's treatment methodology that are based on the values and principles just described: *assessment, direct intervention, consultation,* and *training.* These components are used with clients of any age and across ability levels (including those with high-functioning autism and Asperger's disorder)—from the preschool and elementary years through adolescence and adulthood.

Assessment

As noted earlier in this chapter, individualized assessment has always been an integral part of the TEACCH program. The rationale for the first version of the Psychoeducational Profile (PEP) included the need for an assessment tool that could reliably measure developmental skills at a time when most professionals believed that autistic children were "untestable," and the need to find a systematic method for individualizing an educational program to meet the needs of children whose learning patterns varied although they showed the common criteria defining autism (Schopler and Reichler 1979). The PEP demonstrated that a test that reduced language demands and could be flexibly administered resulted in more accurate developmental information and could help in program planning. By the late 1980s more children were being identified at the preschool age, so the PEP was revised (becoming the PEP-R) to better assess children under age 3 years. Most recently, the PEP-3 revision (Schopler et al. 2005) has brought the test further in line with current concepts of cognitive functioning and psychometric properties. The strengths of the PEP include its ability to be used with the entire range of preschool- and elementary school–aged children with autism regardless of the severity of their autism, its integration of the behavioral and the developmental domains, and its value for educational and home programming. In our work with teachers, we demonstrate how the basic features of the formal PEP assessment instrument can be translated into informal assessment methods in the classroom, and we urge them to use these methods to help with day-to-day decision making regarding curriculum and behavior management issues. Specifically, we emphasize the concept of emerging skills and the importance of noting the child's interests and learning style, spotting possibly interfering autism characteristics, and recognizing parent priorities as they pertain to various curriculum areas.

As the student moves out of childhood and preadolescence and into the teenage years, assessment shifts from the developmental to the functional as the curriculum emphasis changes. The assessment process remains critical, but the focus and location of assessment moves from the classroom to in-school settings such as the office or cafeteria and to actual life space areas in the community such as work sites. Even for those students who can continue on an academic track, there is a need to assess functionally communication, social, and work behavior skills. The Adolescent and Adult Psychoeducational Profile (AAPEP) (Mesibov et al. 1988) was designed to provide a functional assessment for adolescents and adults with autism and mental retardation. It recently has been revised to serve more explicitly as a tool to help with transition planning, becoming the TTAP (Mesibov et al. 2007). An important feature of the AAPEP/TTAP is that it enables a direct and consistent evaluation of a person's skills in a number of functional domains, across home, school, and work settings. In addition to the formal assessment instrument that constituted the older AAPEP, the newer TTAP also includes an informal measure for older adolescents and adults who are candidates for supported employment services. This instrument, which has been developed and fine-tuned for nearly two decades through our TEACCH supported employment program, evaluates work skills and behaviors that are needed in actual work settings (Keel et al. 1997).

The information gathered with these two assessment instruments is used to help with job placement decisions and determining strategies for on-the-job instructional programs. For high-functioning individuals, traditional psychological and achievement tests may also be used to clarify cognitive patterns and strengths and weaknesses. These are supplemented by tasks from neuropsychological tests and measures of social understanding and expression, theory of mind, and central coherence. Observations and results from all of these measures help pinpoint subtle social and communication problems, and specific thinking and learning issues such as literalness, difficulties with perspective taking, and cognitive inflexibility that may need to be specially addressed in a job setting.

A very important aspect of assessment is gathering and sharing information from and with parents. At the preschool level, the initial assessment process is usually geared to determining a diagnosis and answering questions about its implications (Marcus and Stone 1993). This time is also used to introduce the parents to our philosophy, approach, and commitment to ongoing support. Because we provide direct follow-up (see subsection "Consultation and Training" later in this chapter), the initial evaluation serves as a relationship-building experience that does not end. Seeking and using parents' observations and opinions is integral to the assessment process as well as to making treatment decisions, such as appropriate school placement, need for medication, and future residential and vocational placements.

Direct Intervention

TEACCH does not just provide diagnostic services; our mission includes the provision of direct treatment and intervention services as well. There are several components to the TEACCH intervention model, most of which are used at all developmental stages, although tailored, of course, to the specific needs of different age and ability groupings. These components include 1) individualized assessment; 2) use of structured teaching methods (Schopler et al. 1995); 3) particular focus on the curriculum areas of social, communication, independence, coping, and adaptive behavior skills; 4) incorporation of specific techniques that may be adapted to a given situation such as use of the Picture Exchange Communication System (PECS; Frost and Bondy 1994), social stories (Gray 1998), incidental teaching (McGee et al. 1994), and joint-attention training (Mundy and Crowson 1997), among others; 5) use of constructs from developmental psychology where appropriate; and 6) close working partnership with parents to address their concerns, integrate their perspective, and help with generalization of skills between school or work settings and home. Two of the most important of these components are structured teaching and working with parents.

Structured Teaching

The rationale behind the use of structured teaching is that it provides a stable, predictable environment in which the person with autism can be more productive, learn to become more independent, and feel more in control of his or her surroundings, thus becoming calmer and more able to behave appropriately. Structured teaching embodies a set of strategies that enable the person with autism, regardless of age or ability level, to focus his or her attention on what is relevant, to be organized, to understand the abstract through concrete representations, to generalize learning and responses, and to understand what is being communicated by the teacher, parent, or other helper. Within the structured teaching environment, the individual with autism can better cope with and compensate for social, communication, and learning problems that in an unstructured, unpredictable, and confusing environment can become overwhelming.

There are three specific components to the structured teaching approach, all of which emphasize the visual modality: *physical structure, the individual daily schedule,* and *work systems.* The use of visual structure is critical, as it governs how information is organized and presented to help the child be as successful and as independent as possible (Schopler et al. 1995). This is done using a variety of visual cues, such as templates, step-by-step instructions, highlighting and labeling, and other types of cuing (Eckenrode et al. 2003). Physical structure pertains to how the environment is set up through the visual organization of furniture and through the establishment of boundaries to help the student (or worker) understand the intended use of the space, as well as to reduce unnecessary and distracting or unpleasant sensory stimulation. The individual daily schedule provides information about where the individual should be and the sequence of events that will be happening there. What makes it individualized are the type of cue that is used (i.e., object, picture, or written words, depending on the abilities of the individual), the length of time it covers, how the schedule gets manipulated (i.e., whether cards listing a task are moved to a "finished" folder or a checklist is marked), where it is located, what cue gets the student to the schedule, and so on. For instance, one student might have a picture schedule with three activities on it, whereas another might have a written schedule for the entire day. The work system serves as a kind of how-to-do list that answers four questions about the task to be completed: *What work? How much work? How do I know when I am finished?* and *What comes next?* A work system is different from the schedule (a what-and-when-to-do list), which mainly gets the person to where the next activity will occur, in that it informs the student about what he or she will be doing during the activity period. For example, for a preschooler having a one-on-one session with his or her teacher, the work system might be a set of three bins in which there is one activity per bin. The teacher presents and teaches the activity from each bin in a left-to-right fashion (from the child's point of view), with the completed work deposited into a large container. When all the activities in a work system are completed, the person might be rewarded with a favorite activity. In this case, the preschool child might get to play for a limited time with a favorite toy (i.e., What comes next?).

These three structured teaching components can be implemented in all age groups, for all developmental levels. For example, in the home of a preschooler, a parent can designate and set up areas for play, teaching time, and snack time. For a preverbal child, the parent can use a row of objects to indicate the order in which activities will occur, such as a cup for mealtime followed by a ball for play time. For a preschooler who has emerging language and an understanding of pictures, a photo or line drawing schedule of two or three activities in sequence can be posted in a convenient area. Students in elementary school classrooms, whether self-contained or included, can also be provided with these elements of a structured program. Because no two children are exactly the same, a good classroom should reflect a diversity of schedules, work systems, and visually structured tasks.

Structure is intended to be portable. That is, it can be used in a wide variety of settings. For the comfort and independence of people with autism, all of their normal, daily environments should be physically organized with a schedule and a work system. For example, a hygiene list (work system) in the bathroom that uses pictures or words to indicate the personal care tasks that need to be done (if necessary, showing all the steps involved in each task) enables the student to carry out independently all of his or her grooming needs. By the same token, students transitioning to work sites or adults in supported employment or other work venues benefit enormously from clearly defined spatial environments, schedules, work checklists, and other aspects of a structured setting. For the high school student placed in either a volunteer or paid job, the routines taught and practiced in the classroom can and should be replicated and adapted to the nonclassroom, community setting. For example, for the student who can read, a written work system that lists a series of classroom tasks or chores is now transformed into a written job list in a setting such as a library (e.g., 1) shelve one row of books, 2) vacuum carpet, and then 3) take a break). Virtually any work site lends itself to this type of organization and structured approach. The success of TEACCH's supported employment program is largely a result of the creative use of each of these components of structured teaching in a wide range of employment environments and with clients having a wide range of functional levels and structural needs.

Working With Parents

Parents of children with autism face a number of special stressors, such as understanding their child's complex condition, dealing with difficult behavior at home and in public situations, figuring out what is willful behavior and what is a learning deficit, confusion over their child's uneven and atypical development, and sorting through myriad unproven but highly touted fads and therapies (Marcus et al. 2005). Therefore, intervention goals, approaches, and techniques need to be selected not only in light of the unique characteristics of autism, the individual child's needs, and the treatment program's professional capabilities, but also with respect to the family's needs and priorities. Since its inception, the TEACCH program has been dedicated to meeting this complex set of challenges.

Work with parents at TEACCH begins with the diagnostic and assessment processes, which are tailored to the age and approximate developmental level of the individual child. The staff carefully gathers information from the parents, listens to their concerns and perspectives, and then sensitively but candidly shares the findings, answering all questions about the implications of the diagnosis. At that point, the serious work begins. The foundation of our relationship with parents and the central premise of our program is the parents-as-cotherapists model that served as the impetus for the original NIMH grant

(Schopler and Reichler 1971). This holistic and interactive model is based on the concept that parents are the first and best authorities on their children's behaviors and abilities, and can and should be able to teach and guide their autistic child at home with support and direction from professional staff. This support consists of the formulation of individualized teaching programs, use of a playroom/observation room to observe how therapists work with their child, and being coached in how to do the same teaching activities, then carrying out those activities at home and coming back later to demonstrate them in the clinic. In addition, the model provides opportunities for parents to discuss any home- or community-based issues of concern. A key factor in this model is close communication between the staff therapists to ensure that the goals being worked on with the client are consistent with the needs expressed by the parents.

The parent-as-cotherapist model is as effective in working with teens and adults as it is with younger children. Many families whose older child is finally diagnosed with autism require as much attention and support as those with an 18-month-old, although the focus and approach differ. Although issues of privacy and confidentiality preclude the use of parent observation of the therapist's direct work with the client, still, the focus is on collaboration, sharing information, and dealing with issues of mutual concern to both parent and client.

There are four types of parent–professional role relationships that emerge from this extended parent–therapist interaction (Schopler et al. 1984). First, parents may relate to professionals as trainees who want to learn about home teaching programs, behavior management, and related issues. Second, parents often serve as trainers of professionals, with emphasis on sharing information with staff and broadening the professionals' understanding of autism and how families cope. Third, parents and professionals often provide mutual emotional support, utilizing techniques such as ongoing discussions, parent counseling, and support groups. Fourth, parents and professionals work together to develop advocacy skills as a means of promoting improved public and private services and addressing other social action issues. Not all of these relationships emerge in every case, and TEACCH staff therapists and parents usually shift among these different roles. In all cases, however, the goal is to attempt to strengthen the parent-child relationship and to help families cope effectively with this chronic disorder.

Over the years, as an adjunct to its regular functions, the TEACCH program has sponsored support groups for mothers, for parents of adolescents, for fathers, and for parents and siblings of adults with autism (Marcus et al. 1995). All groups use open enrollment, are confidential, and share in common a format where specific topics and issues are discussed with a TEACCH professional as facilitator. They serve a number of important purposes: 1) to provide information that is practical and meaningful; 2) to provide an opportunity for giving and receiving valuable mutual support; 3) to help parents realize that they are not "alone," which has a powerful positive effect on families' coping ability; 4) to serve as a springboard for social action that can lead to the development of services; and 5) to empower participants, many of whom eventually learn leadership skills that translate into important roles in their community. An additional positive side effect has been that many of the parents have developed enduring friendships through the group.

In the past several years, we have capitalized on the power of the "parents together" idea behind the parent groups by initiating and expanding a parent mentor program at TEACCH (Palmer and Marcus 1998). This program matches experienced, TEACCH-trained parents with parents of newly identified or diagnosed children or adults with autism. With support and guidance from TEACCH, as necessary, the role of the parent mentor is to provide support to families of children with autism by listening and understanding, providing information about resources in the community, and providing information about autism and related topics. Mentors are chosen with several criteria in mind: parents who have a child with autism, have been through the TEACCH program, are coping well, are involved in the community, and are comfortable speaking with others about their child. Many of the mentors in our program have reported that they benefited as much from what they received as from what they were able to give to the new families.

Consultation and Training

In line with the principle of community involvement, the TEACCH program has spent considerable effort in developing consultation and training services. As the numbers of individuals in need of specialized autism-based services has virtually exploded, there has been an equivalent need for providers of quality services. TEACCH has been in the forefront of training service providers from a wide variety of disciplines, programs, and agencies since the early 1970s, when we were among the first to develop a model for training public school personnel to teach children with autism in the classroom in order to comply with new federal legislation. Over the years, TEACCH has developed an extensive set of training opportunities, including specialized seminars, workshops, inservices, conferences, and intensive hands-on training programs (Mesibov et al. 2005) that attract thousands of participants each year from around the world.

The 5-day, hands-on, structured teaching training program perhaps best illustrates TEACCH's commitment to preparing professionals for direct work with children or adults with autism. The training can be geared to age groups ranging from preschoolers to adults, and to settings ranging from the classroom to residential environments. It includes basic lectures on key topics, such as assessment, the philosophy and protocols of structured teaching, and communication and social skills. Participants are assigned to groups of five and spend a portion of each day observing and interacting with one of five autistic student trainers in a model classroom that is set up for training purposes and staffed by experienced TEACCH staff. These personnel both demonstrate how to work with the student trainers and supervise the workshop participants as they complete their assigned activities. Each day there is a different theme (e.g., communication), with activities provided to illustrate critical teaching points. At the end of the day, the participants and TEACCH staff gather in small and large groups to discuss what they learned and the implications for their work. This multimodal approach uses a combination of didactic, experiential, interactive, and peer-to-peer learning to teach the concepts, principles, and practices that have defined the TEACCH program for nearly four decades.

As important as training is, of equal importance is follow-up consultation with staff therapists, who provide consultation services to teachers and other professionals either on individual cases or in regard to general programmatic questions. Case consultation involves responding to learning and/or behavioral questions about a child or adult who has been previously evaluated or treated at TEACCH, and it requires the therapist who is most familiar with the client going on site to observe the client, meet with the teacher, and make recommendations for addressing the issue(s). Program consultation involves a collaborative relationship between TEACCH and another program such as a classroom or group home that is designed to serve several persons with autism. The consultation covers a wide range of issues, such as how the physical environment is organized, how schedules are deployed, the nature of the curriculum, behavior management, relationships within the school, and other systems issues.

We have discussed the research-based principles and the application of those principles in the TEACCH program. In the next section, we review the empirical evaluation of treatment programs for individuals on the autism spectrum.

Treatment Effectiveness

In reviewing evidence for the effectiveness of the TEACCH model, two types of information should be considered: 1) the empirical bases for the basic principles and practices of the program, and 2) documentation of the positive impact of different components of the model on learning and behavior of the child and improved functioning of the family.

The scientific bases for TEACCH methods include findings from the neuropsychological literature regarding intact and impaired cognitive skills (e.g., Dawson 1996; Hermelin and O'Connor 1970; Ozonoff 1998), which can be helped with structured teaching strategies. For example, deficits in executive functioning such as poor planning, organizational, and sequencing skills can be addressed through the use of daily schedules, work systems, and visual structuring of activities. Research has highlighted the problems individuals with autism have with expressive communication, in particular, spontaneous, directed, and intentional communication. The TEACCH approach emphasizes teaching the spontaneity of communication, not the reliance on prompting and rote language development (Watson et al. 1989). The scientific literature also highlights the importance and value of visual supports for individuals with autism (e.g., Bryan and Gast 2000; Pierce and Schreibman 1994), supports that are integrated into TEACCH interventions.

The diagnostic and assessment instruments developed by TEACCH have been widely used in both research and clinical practice. The instruments were initially developed and later revised on the basis of current empirically based concepts and knowledge of the nature of autism. For example, the PEP has been revised twice to reflect changes in the understanding of the early developmental markers of autism. The CARS is being revised to address the need for an empirically validated tool for identifying high-functioning individuals with autism.

Both early and recent formal research and later informal evidence support TEACCH effectiveness (e.g., Mesibov 1997; Schopler 1997, Schopler and Mesibov 2000). The earlier, more formal research included studies demonstrating the nature of the sensory processes characterizing autism (Schopler 1964, 1965, 1966, 1971; Reichler and Schopler 1971); the need for structured rather than unstructured environments (Mesibov et al. 2005; Rutter and Bartak 1973; Schopler et al. 1971); a further refinement of the structured environment concept with an emphasis on visual structure (Mesibov et al. 1994; Schopler et al. 1995); evidence that parents of autistic children were misunderstood (Marcus et al. 1978; Schopler 1971; Schopler and Loftin 1969a, 1969b; Schopler and Mesibov 1984; Schopler and Reichler 1971, 1972); support for the effectiveness of structured teaching in the home (Ozonoff and Cathcart 1998); and the generalization of learning from the clinical setting into the home (Short 1984). More informal evidence of the program's effectiveness has included multiple national and state recognitions, peer acceptance, the number of grants received, and replication in countries on every continent (Schopler and Mesibov 2000).

Although there have been a limited number of studies documenting the effectiveness of the visually based strategies associated with and practiced at TEACCH (e.g., Ozonoff and Cathcart 1998; Persson 2000), a recent study on the effects of the work system on students' independent functioning is a good illustration of how this central component of structured teaching can be scientifically assessed (Hume and Odom 2006). The study examined the effects of an individual work system on the independent work and play of two children and one adult with autism, using a single subject as its own control design. A single-subject withdrawal of treatment design with replications across the three participants was used to assess the on-task behavior and work completion skills of the subjects in classroom and employment settings as a result of the intervention. Observational data indicated that all subjects showed positive increases in on-task behavior, increases in the number of tasks completed or play materials utilized, and reduction in teacher prompts. Results were maintained through a 1-month follow up, and teachers expressed satisfaction and noted the social importance of the participant outcomes. This well-designed and well-executed study yielded results consistent across subjects. The subjects were moderately to severely impaired—a group often unresponsive or minimally responsive to a specific intervention such as this. Of added importance was the use of the work system in natural settings of play and workplace, addressing the issue of generalization of learning.

One of the challenges of assessing the effectiveness of the TEACCH involves the enormous complexity and diversity of the program, and its many levels and layers. It can be argued that one measure of its effectiveness is the efforts to replicate many of its components, embodied in part in the structured teaching model, by programs and professionals across the United States and in many countries across the world. For example, TEACCH and Japan have developed and sustained a close working relationship since 1982, with professionals from Japan receiving training at TEACCH centers and returning to their country to implement what they have learned. Classrooms and centers in Japan have replicated all facets of the TEACCH program. To one degree or another, similar experiences have occurred elsewhere in Europe, Scandinavia, Latin America, and the Middle East. The widespread influence of the TEACCH philosophy and methods of assessment and intervention is an indicator of its effectiveness.

The ongoing support of the program by the North Carolina legislature is another informal measure of effectiveness. This support, in part, also reflects the appreciation and value parents have attached to the program. A study in the early 1980s (Schopler et al. 1981) analyzed questionnaires from 348 families who had participated in the program. With consistent enthusiasm, parents reported that interventions with TEACCH were positive, productive, and extremely helpful. One specific illustration of a positive outcome was the high percentage of adolescents and adults living in the community in contrast to other studies at the time, which indicated much higher percentages of older individuals living in institutions. The support of parents mirrors one of the core components of the TEACCH program: the emphasis on parents as partners.

Another relevant informal measure of effectiveness has been peer recognition with respect to awards give to the program and TEACCH faculty. Starting in 1972, with the Gold Award given to the program by the American Psychiatric Association, the number of honors bestowed on TEACCH and its leaders has been impressive. In 2005 alone, the TEACCH founder, its director, one of its clinical directors, and a teaching faculty member were awarded high honors from the University of North Carolina for excellence in teaching, community service, and leadership. In 2006, Dr. Schopler received the Gold Medal Award for Life Achievement in the Application of Psychology from the American Psychological Association and the Lifetime Achievement Award from the International Meeting for Autism Research.

The combination of evidence from these three critical sources—scientific foundations underlying TEACCH principles and methods, empirical support for specific components of the program, and informal measures—provides an accumulation of compelling documentation for the success of the program over a 40-year period.

Conclusions

The educational approach of the TEACCH model is based on solid, empirical, experimental data buttressed by decades of clinical validation. Both our research and our application of the research are based on cognitive and behavioral concepts applied in a developmental context. The outcomes derived from all of this research and its application are summarized in the principles and concepts outlined in this chapter. From our long experience with both research on and treatment of autism, we feel that multiple approaches and designs, rather than reliance on a single methodology such as a randomized controlled trial, are required for evaluating effective treatment outcomes. Our commitment to the understanding of autism through a highly individualized approach necessitates a comparable perspective when doing careful assessment of psychosocial interventions.

More research is needed in evaluating the various components of the structured teaching methodology of TEACCH, including how the visual presentation of tasks and activities helps learning, how varying the types and other aspects of schedules can improve independence, and how and to what extent the use of this approach reduces behavior problems. Because the TEACCH model is robust and relevant for the entire age spectrum and levels of severity, including patients with high-functioning autism/Asperger's disorder, studying how modifications are made for varying groups and which aspects of structure are effective would also be useful.

References

Bryan L, Gast D: Teaching on-task and on-schedule behaviors to high functioning children with autism via picture activity schedules. J Autism Dev Disord 30:553–567, 2000

Dawson G: Brief report: Neuropsychology of autism: a report on the state of the science. J Autism Dev Disord 26:179–184, 1996

Dawson G, Osterling J: Early intervention in autism: effectiveness and common elements of current approaches, in The Effectiveness of Early Intervention: Second Generation Research. Edited by Guralnick MJ. Baltimore, MD, Paul H Brookes Publishing, 1997, pp 307–326

Dunlap G: Consensus, engagement, and family involvement for young children with autism. J Assoc Pers Sev Handicaps 24:222–225, 1999

Eckenrode L, Fennell P, Hearsey K: Tasks Galore. Raleigh, NC, Tasks Galore, 2003

Frost LA, Bondy AS: The Picture Exchange Communication System Training Manual. Cherry Hill, NJ, Pyramid Educational Consultants, 1994

Gray C: Social stories and comic strip conversations with students with Asperger syndrome and high functioning autism, in Asperger Syndrome or High-Functioning Autism? Edited by Schopler E, Mesibov GB, Kunce LJ. New York, Plenum, 1998, pp 167–198

Harris SL: Behavioral and educational approaches to the PDDs, in Autism and Pervasive Developmental Disorders. Edited by Volkmar FR. New York, Cambridge University Press, 1998, pp 195–208

Hermelin B, O'Connor N: Psychological Experiments With Autistic Children. London, Pergamon, 1970

Hume K, Odom S: Effects of an individual work system on the independent functioning of students with autism. J Autism Dev Disord 2006 Oct 27 [Epub ahead of print]

Keel JH, Mesibov GB, Woods A: TEACCH supported employment programs. J Autism Dev Disord 27:3–9, 1997

Lord C, Rutter M, Dilavore PC, et al: Autism Diagnostic Observation Schedule. Los Angeles, CA, Western Psychological Services, 2002

Marcus LM, Stone WL: Assessment of the young autistic child, in Preschool Issues in Autism and Related Developmental Handicaps. Edited by Schopler E, Van Bourgondien ME, Bristol M. New York, Plenum, 1993, pp 149–173

Marcus L, Lansing M, Andrews C, et al: Improvement of teaching effectiveness in parents of autistic children. J Am Acad Child Psychiatry 17:625–639, 1978

Marcus L, Wertheimer A, Clement S, et al: Support groups for parents of autistic children from preschool to adulthood. Paper presented at the National Conference on Autism of the Autism Society of America, Greensboro, NC, July 1995

Marcus LM, Kunce L, Schopler E: Working with families, in Handbook of Autism and Pervasive Developmental Disorders, Vol 2: Assessment, Interventions, Policy, 3rd Edition. Edited by Volkmar F, Paul R, Klin A, et al. Hoboken, NJ, Wiley, 2005, pp 1055–1086

McGee G, Daly T, Jacobs HA: The Walden Preschool, in Preschool Education Programs for Children With Autism. Edited by Harris S, Handleman, JS. Austin, TX, Pro-Ed, 1994, pp 127–162

Mesibov GB: Current perspectives and issues in autism and adolescence, in Autism in Adolescents and Adults. Edited by Schopler E, Mesibov GB. New York, Plenum, 1983, pp 37–53

Mesibov GB: Formal and informal measures of the effectiveness of the TEACCH program. Autism 1:25–35, 1997

Mesibov GB, Schopler E, Schaffer B, et al: Adolescent and Adult Psychoeducaitonal Profile. Austin, TX, Pro-Ed, 1988

Mesibov GB, Schopler E, Hearsey K: Structured teaching, in Behavioral Issues in Autism. Edited by Schopler E, Mesibov GB. New York, Plenum, 1994, pp 195–207

Mesibov GB, Shea V, Schopler E: The TEACCH approach to Autism Spectrum Disorders. New York, Kluwer Academic/Plenum, 2005

Mesibov GB, Thomas J, Chapman M, et al: Adolescent and Adult Psychoeducational Profile (AAPEP): Revised TEACCH Transition Assessment Profile (TTAP). Austin, TX, Pro-Ed, 2007

Mundy P, Crowson M: Joint attention and early social communication: implications for research on intervention with autism. J Autism Dev Disord 27:653–676, 1997

National Research Council, Committee on Educational Interventions for Children With Autism: Educating Children With Autism. Edited by Lord C, McGee JP. Washington, DC, National Academy Press, 2001

Ozonoff S: Assessment and remediation of executive dysfunction in autism and Asperger syndrome, in Asperger Syndrome or High-Functioning Autism? Edited by Schopler E, Mesibov GB, Kunce LJ. New York, Plenum, 1998, pp 327–348

Ozonoff S, Cathcart K: Effectiveness of a home program intervention for young children with autism. J Autism Dev Disord 28:25–32, 1998

Palmer A, Marcus L: Developing a parent mentoring program for families with children with autism. Paper presented at the 10th Annual Leo M. Croghan Conference, Raleigh, NC, December 1998

Persson B: Brief report: A longitudinal study of quality of life and independence among adult men with autism. J Autism Dev Disord 30:61–66, 2000

Pierce K, Schreibman L: Teaching daily living skills to children with autism in unsupervised settings through pictorial self-management. J Appl Behav Anal 27:471–481, 1994

Reichler RJ, Schopler E: Observations on the nature of human relatedness. J Autism Child Schizophr 1:283–296, 1971

Rogers SJ: Empirically supported comprehensive treatments for young children with autism. J Clin Child Psychol 27:168–179, 1998

Rutter M, Bartak L: Special education treatment of autistic children: a comparative study—2. Follow-up findings and implications for services. J Child Psychiatry 14:241–270, 1973

Schopler E: On the relationship between early tactile experiences and the treatment of an autistic and a schizophrenic child. Am J Orthopsychiatry 34:339–340, 1964

Schopler E: Early infantile autism and receptor processes. Arch Gen Psychiatry 13:327–335, 1965

Schopler E: Visual versus tactual receptor preference in normal and schizophrenic children. J Abnorm Psychol 71:108–114, 1966

Schopler E: Parents of psychotic children as scapegoats. Journal of Contemporary Psychology 4:17–22, 1971

Schopler E: Relationship between university research and state policy: division TEACCH—Treatment and Education of Autistic and related Communication handicapped CHildren. Pop Gov 51:23–32, 1986

Schopler E: Neurobiologic correlates in the classification and study of autism, in Atypical Cognitive Deficits in Developmental Disorders: Implication for Brain Function. Edited by Broman S, Grafman J. Hillsdale, NJ, Erlbaum, 1994, pp 87–100

Schopler E: Parent Survival Manual: A Guide to Crisis Resolution in Autism and Related Developmental Disorders. New York, Plenum, 1995

Schopler E: Implementation of TEACCH philosophy, in Handbook of Autism and Pervasive Developmental Disorders, 2nd Edition. Edited by Cohen DJ, Volkmar FR. New York, Wiley, 1997, pp 767–795

Schopler E (ed): Special issue: International priorities for developing autism services via the TEACCH model. Int J Ment Health 29:3–184, 2000

Schopler E, Loftin J: Thinking disorders in parents of psychotic children. J Abnorm Psychol 74:281–287, 1969a

Schopler E, Loftin J: Thought disorders in parents of psychotic children: A function of test anxiety. Arch Gen Psychiatry 20:174–181, 1969b [also in Chess S, Thomas A (eds): Annual Progress in Child Psychiatry and Child Development. New York, Brunner/Mazel, 1970, pp 472–486]

Schopler E, Mesibov GB: Professional attitudes toward parents: a forty-year progress report, in The Effects of Autism on the Family. Edited by Schopler E, Mesibov GB. New York, Plenum, 1984, pp 3–17

Schopler E, Mesibov GB (eds): Neurobiological Issues in Autism. New York, Plenum, 1987

Schopler E, Mesibov GB: Cross cultural priorities in developing autism services. Int J Ment Health 293–21, 2000

Schopler E, Reichler RJ: Parents as cotherapists in the treatment of psychotic children. J Autism Child Schizophr 1:87–102, 1971

Schopler E, Reichler RJ: How well do parents understand their own psychotic child? J Autism Child Schizophr 2:387–400, 1972

Schopler E, Reichler RJ: Individualized Assessment and Treatment for Developmental Disabled Children, Vol I: Psychoeducational Profile. Baltimore, MD, University Park Press, 1979

Schopler E, Brehm S, Kinsbourne M, et al: Effect of treatment structure on development in autistic children. Arch Gen Psychiatry 24:415–421, 1971

Schopler E, Mesibov GB, DeVellis R, et al: Treatment outcome for autistic children and their families, in Frontiers of Knowledge in Mental Retardation, Vol 1: Social, Educational, and Behavioral Aspects. Baltimore, MD, University Park, 1981, pp 293–301

Schopler E, Mesibov GB, Shigley RH, et al: Helping autistic children through their parents: the TEACCH model, in The Effects of Autism on the Family. Edited by Schopler E, Mesibov GB. New York, Plenum, 1984, pp 65–81

Schopler E, Reichler RJ, Renner BR: The Childhood Autism Rating Scale (CARS), Revised. Los Angeles, CA, Western Psychological Services, 1988

Schopler E, Mesibov GB, Hearsey K: Structured teaching in the TEACCH system, in Learning and Cognition in Autism. Edited by Schopler E, Mesibov GB. New York, Plenum, 1995, pp 243–268

Schopler E, Yirmiya N, Shulman C, et al: The Research Basis for Autism Intervention. New York, Kluwer Academic/Plenum, 2001

Schopler E, Lansing MD, Reichler RJ, et al: The Psychoeducational Profile, 3rd Edition. Austin, TX, Pro-Ed, 2005

Seligman M, Darling RB: Ordinary Families, Special Children: A Systems Approach to Childhood Disability. New York, Guilford, 1997

Short A: Short-term treatment outcomes using parents as co-therapists with their own autistic children. Journal of Child Psychiatry, Psychology, and Allied Disciplines 25:443–458, 1984

Singer GHS, Powers LE: Contributing to resilience in families: an overview, in Families, Disability, and Empowerment: Active Coping Skills and Strategies for Family Interventions. Edited by Singer GHS, Powers LE. Baltimore, MD, Paul H Brookes Publishing, 1993, pp 1–25

Watson L, Lord C, Schaffer B, et al: Teaching Spontaneous Communication to Autistic and Developmentally Handicapped Children. Austin, TX, Pro-Ed, 1989

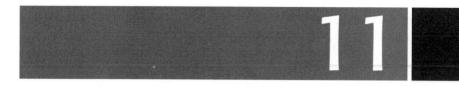

Peer Relationships of Children With Autism

Challenges and Interventions

Connie Kasari, Ph.D.

Erin Rotheram-Fuller, Ph.D.

Positive peer relationships are a critical ingredient for healthy development across the lifespan. Peer relationships provide an invaluable context for refining interpersonal skills and developing a sense of self in relation to others. Out of these peer relationships, friendships often develop, and the value of friendships has been noted in many studies. For example, the presence of even a single friend can buffer an individual from the negative effects of stressful life events, including anxiety and depressive symptoms (Furman 1989). Friends can also promote the development of social competence, self-esteem, and problem solving (Nelson and Aboud 1985).

This work was supported by National Institutes of Health Grant NIH MH068172 to Dr. Kasari and the Center for Autism Research and Treatment at UCLA.

235

Whereas some children may have brief periods of difficulty with peers, others find peer relationships a constant challenge. Children with autism are one group of children who report difficulties with peer relationships across ages and ability levels. Wing (1988) classified children with autism into categories of "passive," "aloof," and "interactive but odd." Those children classified as aloof, for example, appeared to lack even the most basic social motivation. Although there was a stronger social motivation among those children with autism who would be considered interactive but odd, the children still lacked the considerable skill needed to build positive social relationships. Indeed, for children with autism, the social world can bring major challenges, which if not properly addressed can lead to social rejection and victimization. The purpose of this chapter is to describe the significant social challenges children with autism face and to explore the treatment research aimed at improving their social situation.

Peer Interaction Challenges for Children With Autism

Studies have shown that children with autism initiate interactions less often with peers, are less proximal and engaged with peers, show more nonsocial behaviors, and score below expected levels on teacher ratings and standardized measures of social behavior (Koegel et al. 2001; McConnell 2002). Compared with typical children, even high-functioning children with autism report having poorer peer relationships, including having fewer friends and less satisfying companionship with their friends (Bauminger and Kasari 2000). Not surprisingly, children with autism also report more loneliness at school compared with typical children (Bauminger and Kasari 2000).

The difficulty these children have in developing and maintaining positive peer relationships and friendships continues well into adulthood. Howlin et al. (2004) determined that of 68 children with autism who were followed up as adults, 56% of them reported no friends or acquaintances. Similarly, Orsmond et al. (2004) asked 235 parents about the peer relationships of their adolescent and adult children with autism. Again, nearly half reported no peer relations at all. Moreover, school inclusion with typical age mates was not associated with having peer relationships. Thus, an individual's participation in an inclusive setting did not result in a greater chance of having a friend.

The difficulty children with autism show in interactions with peers is likely a result of a number of factors, including experience with peers and the lack of social skills and social understanding. There is some evidence that all three contribute to peer difficulties and are reflected in peer interaction studies of children with autism.

Experience With Peers

Children with autism have less experience with peers than typically developing children. The reason for this lack of experience, however, is complicated. Certainly caregivers make extraordinary attempts to provide their children with opportunities for social interactions (Chamberlain et al. 2006). They also identify experience with typical peers as a major motivating factor in having their children in inclusive school settings (Kasari et al. 1999). Despite these efforts, when children with autism are observed in the presence of other children, studies indicate they make fewer attempts to engage with other children and are less responsive to others' bids for social interaction (Sigman and Ruskin 1999). Thus, the children appear to distance themselves from interactions and not take advantage of the social opportunities surrounding them.

Kanner (1943) suggested that children with autism have a "powerful desire for aloneness" (p. 249). Yet, when asked about this desire, high-functioning children with autism reported feeling lonely at school, thus countering the notion that they prefer aloneness (Bauminger and Kasari 2000). Children with autism have also shown awareness of their own social rejection when it occurs, causing them both behavioral and emotional distress (Bullock 1988; Ochs et al. 2001). It is probably more likely that instead of wanting to be alone, children with autism are simply not able to make the most of their experiences with peers because of a lack of social skill and understanding.

Social Skills and Social Understanding

Effective social interactions require a certain level of social skill and social understanding. In particular, the development of friendships requires a set of sophisticated interpersonal skills, such as the ability to offer fun companionship, express feelings of affection, and help when needed (Asher et al. 1998). But friendship also requires an ability to attune oneself with another, to understand what the other is thinking and feeling, and a basic understanding of oneself as a person distinct from the other. This knowledge that self and other are separate and unique individuals with distinct reference points may not be immediately evident to children with autism (Hobson 1990). Children with autism who lack an understanding of persons as subjects assume initially that others have access to their same thoughts and perceptions. Friendships can provide a context for developing that sense of self in relation to others and acquiring new social skills. However, for children with autism, friendships can be fraught with difficulties, risks of communication failure, rejection, and even victimization.

Communication difficulties are particularly significant for children with autism. Whereas young children with autism may need to develop basic communication skills with peers (for example, greeting other children or responding to another child's bid for interaction), older and higher functioning children with autism must learn complex rules of communicating with others. The difficulties these high-functioning children face are incredibly complex. They must figure out the social nuances of interaction, such as when someone is joking or serious. It is critical to interpret both nonverbal as well as verbal language. Unfortunately, children with autism frequently fail to use language appropriately in social interactions and consequently may be misunderstood by their peers. Part of the issue may be a result of difficulty in taking the perspective of others. Understanding nonliteral language, whether humor, irony, or teasing, requires an understanding of another person's perspective as well as the social context in which the language takes place (Heerey et al. 2005; Lyons and Fitzgerald 2004; Martin and McDonald 2004). For example, Martin and McDonald (2004) found that young adults with Asperger's syndrome were less likely than control subjects to use the social context for interpreting the conversational meaning of ironic jokes. Although they seemed to have an understanding of the cognitive basis of humor, particularly around topics they were interested in, they lacked understanding of the intent of humor—that is, to share enjoyment with others.

Children with autism also have difficulty with the social perceptions of their own peer relationships. Thus, often there is a difference between how children with autism see themselves and how others see them. Children with autism may see themselves as more socially involved than their peers or their parents report. For example, in a social network study, the friendship nominations of children with autism were less likely to be reciprocated than were typical peers (Chamberlain et al. 2006). The children with autism identified more peers as friends than the same peers identified them as friends. Moreover, parents concede that many of the "friends" they identify for their children with autism are more desired friends than actual relationships (Bauminger and Kasari 2000).

Peer Relations, Social Acceptance, and Inclusion

Inclusion of children with autism in general education classrooms is an increasing practice. Despite the peer interaction difficulties of children with autism, parents increasingly prefer mainstreaming and/or inclusion of their children (Kasari et al. 1999). Professionals also advocate inclusion, with the belief that placement of children with autism in general educational settings increases their involvement in the mainstream of society by improving both the children's social behavior repertoires and society's acceptance and appreciation of people with differences (Guralnick 1990; Villa and Thousand 1995).

The evidence that inclusion actually benefits the social interactions of these children is less clear. For example, Sigman and Ruskin (1999) found that children with autism were more socially engaged at school if they had access to typical children on the playground. Similarly, Bauminger et al. (2003) found that high-functioning children with autism were more likely to engage with a typical peer on the playground than with children with special needs. Some parents report their child's inclusive experience as being characterized by peer acceptance and even being able to form meaningful friendships with their non-disabled classmates (Ryndak et al. 1995; Staub et al. 1994). There are also reports indicating that children with autism show improvements in both their number of social initiations and their ability to generalize social skills that they learn while in this context (Carr and Darcy 1990; Strain 1984). Mainstreamed classrooms may offer an ideal context to use typical peers as social models, encouraging the maintenance and generalization of skills from interventions that are often not achieved when using an adult as the interventionist (Carr and Darcy 1990; Roeyers 1996; Shearer et al. 1996).

In contrast, other studies demonstrate that inclusion may be insufficient to truly integrate children with autism into the social networks of their typical peers (Burack et al. 1997; Chamberlain 2001) and may even be to their social detriment (MacMillan et al. 1996; Ochs et al. 2001; Sale and Carey 1995). Children's social abilities affect whether they are accepted and included by others.

Thus, peers are more likely to reject children with autism on the basis of their social behavior and respond to them less favorably, even when they are given an explanation for their differences. For example, Swaim and Morgan (2001) showed third- and sixth-graders two video clips of a typical 12-year-old boy, who in one clip acted normally and in the other acted autistic. For some children viewing the clip, the boy was given a label of autism, and for other children he was not. Children rated the boy in the video acting autistic less favorably regardless of whether they had a label for his behavior. Indeed, an explanation for his behavior did not seem to affect their opinions of the boy.

The quality of interaction also affects children's level of social inclusion. Strain (1984) compared how typical children behaved toward their peers in a mainstream preschool and found a qualitative difference in their relationships. Toward nondisabled peers, typical children tended to address compliments, play suggestions, and sharing. However, toward children with disabilities, typical children tended to show more physical help and conflict management. Typical children also preferred to select other typical children as playmates, and if they did select a child with a disability, it was usually a chronologically older child who was, therefore, closer in developmental age. Therefore, even with increased interactions with peers the interactions of children with autism still lack the reciprocal quality associated with true friendships.

In other studies investigating social acceptance and using social network methodology, children with autism were found to be less socially connected to other children in their class. In studies using the Cairns method of social network analysis (Cairns and Cairns 1994), children were asked, "Who hangs out with whom?" From this information, the researchers developed classroom network maps showing all of the connections between children in the class. In one study with second- and third-graders, children with autism were most often socially attached to a group of children by a connection to only one child in the group, or were members of a small group that was set apart from the most prominent groupings in the class (Chamberlain et al. 2006). Children with autism were also less accepted by their classmates. Fewer children named them as a friend, and children identified by the children with autism as friends less often reciprocated that friendship. While most of the children with autism were boys, they were more likely to have peer connections with girls. This tendency is significantly different from typical children at this age, who most often have same-gender friendships. It may be that girls were more likely than boys to take on a caregiving role among their classmates and therefore were more likely to associate with the children with autism.

Over time, peer relationships of children with autism often become more difficult. In a subsequent study of peer social networks, third- to fifth-graders were significantly less included in their class social networks than were kindergarten through second-graders (Rotheram-Fuller 2005). Still, these young children did not report more loneliness than their typical classmates (in contrast to the increased loneliness reported by adolescents with autism [Bauminger and Kasari 2000]). These studies suggest that children with high-functioning autism at younger ages are less able to recognize the relative weakness of their social relationships, resulting in a kind of "ignorant bliss." Parents of the children with autism similarly reported that their children seemed "oblivious" to social involvement cues. Unlike typical peers, whose peripheral and isolated social network involvement was associated with more loneliness, children with autism showed less sensitivity to their own lack of involvement (Chamberlain et al. 2006). Another indication of typical children's awareness of their own social status was in their nominations of peers as friends. Typical children were likely to nominate approximately as many children as friends as nominated them in return. Children with autism, on the other hand, were more likely to nominate a much larger number of friends than they received nominations (Rotheram-Fuller 2005).

An impressive database is accumulating on children's perceptions of their own social situation; observations of their social behavior in their natural environments, such as school playgrounds; and opinions of their social behavior from others, including peers, teachers, and parents. However, studies have rarely linked children's perceptions with their actual behaviors. Future studies are needed that combine perceptions and observations to inform interventions for particular subsets of children with autism.

Peer Interventions and Autism

Given the poor peer relationships of children with autism, and some data suggesting that inclusion alone is not enough to improve these relationships, targeted peer interventions are necessary (Myles et al. 1993). Since the mid-1980s, a number of interventions have been tried with children with autism. These interventions fall into two general classes of peer intervention. The first—

the *target-child* approach—targets the social skills of the child with autism. The second—the *peer-mediated* approach—focuses on teaching typical children how to engage the child with autism. Both have met with some success but have not been subjected to direct comparison using rigorous research designs in the child's natural environment (see Table 11–1). Indeed, three recent reviews of this literature suggest that most peer intervention work has been conducted with preschool-age children with autism in specialized settings, is behavioral in nature, and is single subject in design (Goldstein 2002; McConnell 2002; Rogers 2000). Few researchers have replicated an intervention approach across multiple studies, and thus only a handful of children may have received any one type of intervention. Given this state of the science, we currently cannot recommend to practitioners (teachers and parents) one particular approach over another for specific children.

Within these classes of peer-related interventions, several different therapeutic approaches have been tried, and the skill that is the target of intervention has varied. For young children, behavioral approaches dominate, with a focus on increasing peer initiations and responses. For older and higher functioning children, cognitive-behavioral approaches often have focused on emotional understanding and responsiveness.

Target-Child Interventions

McConnell (2002) reviewed the peer intervention literature and concluded that social skills programs specifically targeting social and communication skills can increase the frequency and quality of children with autism's social communication behaviors with peers. For example, Odom and Strain (1986) employed a child-centered prompting and reinforcement program and found that children with autism increased their number of social initiations toward peers, obtained more social initiations from peers, and increased their mean length of interaction with peers. Using similar prompting and reinforcement procedures by adults, other researchers have also reported increases in children with autism's social initiations with peers and overall amount of interaction (Belchic and Harris 1994; Davis et al. 1994; Zanolli and Daggett 1998).

Some common techniques used in working directly with the child with autism have included self-management (Koegel et al. 1992; Shearer et al. 1996; Strain et al. 1994), pivotal response training (Pierce and Schreibman 1995, 1997; Stahmer 1995), differential reinforcement of appropriate behavior (Kodak et al. 2003; Reed et al. 2005), discrete trial training (Grindle and Remington 2002; Miranda-Linne and Melin 1992; Prizant and Wetherby 1998; Taubman et al. 2001), reciprocal imitation training (Field et al. 2001; Ingersoll et al. 2003), in vivo modeling (Charlop et al. 1983; Charlop-Christy et al. 2000; Egel et al. 1981; Gena et al. 2005; Tryon and Keane 1986), and video modeling (Charlop and Milstein 1989; Charlop-Christy et al. 2000; Gena et al. 2005; LeBlanc et al. 2003; Nikopoulos and Keenan 2004). Each technique has met with varying degrees of success, but all have shown at least limited effectiveness in improving some aspects of social relationships (Stahmer et al. 2003). Specific situations and populations with which each technique is most effective have not been explored, and such work is necessary to truly address the specific needs of each child with autism.

One issue with target-child approaches has concerned generalization of skills to new settings or new partners. Skills learned with interventionists or specific peers must be then translated into interactions with new peers in different settings. Self-monitoring techniques have shown generalization to others in nontreatment settings, even among children as young as preschool age (Koegel et al. 1992; Shearer et al. 1996; Strain et al. 1994). However, combining intervention methods such as direct teaching of appropriate social and communication behaviors using prompting and reinforcement strategies along with self-monitoring techniques for generalization may offer the best potential to increase appropriate peer-interactive behavior in children with autism.

One method of target-child intervention that is gaining in popularity is video feedback. A study used a computer-based, virtual environment to tap the ability of adolescents with autism to navigate a "virtual café" (Parsons et al. 2004). Results showed that the adolescents with autism successfully completed a number of tasks in the virtual environment and that they were able to interpret the environment as a representation of reality. Despite this understanding, more adolescents with autism bumped into people in this virtual environment, suggesting they had less understanding of the social appropriateness of personal space. This study was not a treatment study but used a method that may be useful in future social skills interventions.

Some studies have used video modeling as a method of teaching social skills to children with autism. Two types of video modeling have been used: the *self-as-model method* and the *other-as-model method*. Using the self-as-model method, children can be videotaped and then shown their own behaviors as a

Table 11–1.   Comparison of social skills intervention types for children with autism

Intervention type	Advantages	Disadvantages
Inclusion	Increases proximity to typical peers. Can improve the frequency of interactions. Can improve peers' understanding of disabilities.	Can increase loneliness for children with autism. Does not necessarily include children with autism fully into the classroom social networks. Social inclusion is more difficult with increasing grades. Peers rate children with autism less favorably than typical peers.
Target-child interventions	Have shown limited improvements in social skills. Multiple methods available and tested with limited success: • Self-management • Pivotal response training • Differential reinforcement of appropriate behavior • Discrete trial instruction • Reciprocal imitation training • In vivo modeling • Video modeling	Generalization of skills is limited. Methods have not been systematically compared. It is unclear if there are specific interventions that might differentially benefit subsets of children.

Table 11–1.   Comparison of social skills intervention types for children with autism *(continued)*

Intervention type	Advantages	Disadvantages
Peer-mediated interventions	Have shown limited improvements in social and communication skills. Largest, best developed group of social interaction interventions for children with autism. Potential to teach skills to both children with autism and their peers. Can train multiple individuals around the child for increased generalization. Multiple methods tested with limited success. • Peer tutors • Modeling • Social skills groups • Pivotal response training • Priming	Methods have not been systematically compared. Maintenance of improvements may be limited. Generalization has been inconsistent across studies. Most studies have looked at preschool-age children and may not be representative of the experiences of older children with autism.
Combined interventions	Can involve multiple individuals in the child's life for better generalization and maintenance of skills Can improve skills above using either type of intervention alone Can improve skills of multiple individuals in the child's life (i.e., parents, teachers, peers)	Methods have not been systematically compared It is unclear which types of interventions might be most effective with specific subsets of children

reinforcement of what is desired. Generally, researchers use only positive behaviors exhibited by the child to reinforce those actions. In contrast, the other-as-model method teaches children to observe and emulate the behavior of others.

Video modeling has been shown to be effective in teaching a wide variety of skills, including conversational speech (Charlop and Milstein 1989; Sherer et al. 2001), perspective taking (LeBlanc et al. 2003), verbal responding (Buggey et al. 1999), social initiations (Nikopoulos and Keenan 2004), and play skills (Nikopoulos and Keenan 2004) relating to social interactions. Video modeling has also been compared with in vivo modeling and has been shown to be as good as (Gena et al. 2005), as well as more cost-effective and efficient as using live models (Charlop and Milstein 1989; Charlop-Christy et al. 2000). There have been concerns about the ability of children to generalize skills learned from video modeling (LeBlanc et al. 2003); however, there has been some evidence of generalization to other adults and topics (Charlop and Milstein 1989; Charlop-Christy et al. 2000). This technique offers a promising and efficient treatment alternative to improve children's social competence.

Given results from the social network studies described previously, it appears that some approaches may be more successful with children at different ages. Given peers' reluctance to assist their disabled peers in the older elementary school grades (third through fifth grade) (Rotheram-Fuller 2005), using the target-child approach with children with autism in this age group may assist children with autism in addressing their own behaviors so they can be more accepted. More information is needed, however, to systematically compare interventions with different ages of children to identify which might be the most effective at each level.

Peer-Mediated Interventions

A number of studies have also found that using typical peers as tutors can increase the social and communication skills of targeted children with autism. Some of the most common peer-mediated interventions include using peer tutors (Kamps et al. 1997; McGee et al. 1992), modeling (Dewey et al. 1988; Laushey and Heflin 2000; Shafer et al. 1984), social skills groups (Kamps et al. 1992), pivotal response training (Pierce and Schreibman 1997), and priming (Zanolli et al. 1996). Each of these interventions has shown effectiveness targeting specific social skills, but these approaches also have not been compared systematically.

Kamps et al. (1997) used peer networks as a cooperative learning strategy for language and social skills in three 6- to 7-year-old children with autism. Five typical first-graders with high social status were matched with the children with autism and trained to use an augmentative communication system. The intervention resulted in increased peer interaction and acceptance. Similarly, teaching typical peers how to use pivotal response techniques, Pierce and Schreibman (1997) found increases in language and social skills for three children with autism, including increases in nontargeted joint-attention skills. Peer-mediated network interventions have been effective at increasing social initiations, both to and from students with autism, particularly when the peers self-monitor their initiations and meet regularly with an adult facilitator (Haring and Breen 1992; Sainato et al. 1992). However, if prompts were removed without training in self-monitoring, nondisabled peers showed reductions in their initiations to students with autism (Odom and Watts 1991).

As with target-child approaches, generalization of skills to new peers for both typical children and children with autism has been inconsistent with peer-mediated approaches. Pierce and Schreibman (1997) demonstrated that pivotal response training generalized to other people, situations, and materials, whereas Kamps et al. (1997) found generalization of skills using a cooperative learning strategy for only two out of three children studied. In a study by Laushey and Heflin (2000), social interactions in an inclusive school setting were successfully improved when a typical child and a child with autism were paired as "buddies"; however, only one of the two children with autism studied was able to generalize his learned skills to a new classroom. Even in a study combining target-child and peer-mediated methods there are problems with generalization and sustainability. Kohler et al. (1995) taught peers and target children simultaneously through a group-reinforcement intervention. During active treatment phases of the study, children were responsive to the reinforcement and provided supportive prompts to peers in the group, as instructed. However, when reinforcement was removed, prompts correspondingly decreased. Longer term interventions with natural community reinforcers included may be needed to maintain gains in social improvements.

Even with these noted limitations, McConnell (2002) suggests that peer-mediated procedures are the largest and best-developed group of social interaction interventions for children with autism. Odom and Strain (1986) reviewed three different peer-mediated treatment approaches: proximity alone (in which peers are told to simply play with the autistic peer), prompt/reinforcement (in which peers prompt and reinforce the autistic child for desired social behavior), and peer initiation (in which peers are instructed to make social overtures) interventions. All three types of interventions resulted in increased social behaviors by the child with autism. Although Odom and Strain (1986) suggest that prompt/reinforcement and peer-initiation methods are more powerful than proximity alone, no effect sizes were reported because of the small number of participants evaluated using single-subject designs and the fact that none of the treatments were compared experimentally in the same study.

Combined Interventions

Although peer-mediated approaches appear to increase the social behaviors of children with autism, it is not clear whether these approaches are superior to a target-child approach or whether they may need to be used in combination for maximum efficacy. Both approaches reportedly improve social initiations, social responding, and increased amounts of interaction, especially when used in combination with self-monitoring to improve generalization and maintenance of effects. Yet questions remain as to the sustainability of any intervention method and whether we need to develop new combinations of longer term interventions to maintain gains in social improvements.

Some studies have incorporated more than one modality of treatment and have shown promising results. In a study by Bauminger (2002), 15 high-functioning children with autism were provided cognitive-behavioral therapy incorporating their teacher, parent, and peers as interventionists, for 3 hours a week over 7 months. This intensive intervention led to improvements in social functioning and understanding in several areas. Children improved in their problem-solving skills, understanding of complex emotions, and expression of emotions. They also had increased interactions with peers, with improved eye contact and the ability to share experiences and interest in their peers. Teachers rated the children overall as having improved social skills as the result of treatment.

Another study by Solomon et al. (2004) used a 20-week social adjustment curriculum for 18 children with autism and a psychoeducational program for the parents. Improvements were noted in children's facial expression recognition and problem solving. Mothers in this intervention reported lower depression ratings and fewer problem behaviors in their children as a result of treatment.

The previously described programs involved several members of the child's immediate environment. Such an approach may prove to increase maintenance of these skills over the longer term. Moreover, there is general recognition that not all treatments work equally well for all children. In determining who benefits most from what type of treatment, it is important to examine predictors of treatment outcome. Likewise, we need to better understand the effect of specific treatments on related areas of social and academic performance.

Predictors and Correlates of Treatment Response

Most treatment studies have not examined the role that pretreatment characteristics play in predicting treatment response. In part, this is a result of the preponderance of single-subject designs that do not allow for such analyses. However, Solomon et al. (2004) found that their social skills intervention was most successful for older and lower functioning children with autism, suggesting a unique response to the intervention by this subgroup. Parents of these children reported greater improvement in depression scores compared with parents of higher functioning and younger children.

Although not treatment studies, a number of studies have examined the correlates of peer interactions of children with autism. For example, a number of studies have found that children who have higher mental and language ages are more socially engaged than children with lower mental and language ages (Sigman and Ruskin 1999; Stone and Caro-Martinez 1990). Thus, developmental age may be an important moderator of treatment response.

Finally, the presence of a coexisting psychological disorder may interfere uniquely with the child with autism's ability to engage with peers. For example, anxiety disorder is a common comorbid condition for children with autism. As many as 35%–85% of children with autism may also suffer from significant social anxiety (Green et al. 2000; Kim et al. 2000; Muris et al. 1998). For many children with autism, a coexisting anxiety disorder may reduce significantly the effects of a social skills treatment. Thus, even if children demonstrate improved social skills under controlled conditions (e.g., social skills groups), persistent anxiety may prevent the effective use of these newly acquired skills in real-world situations. Although it is possible that some existing social skills programs are effective in reducing anxiety, the extent to which anxiety is addressed or measured in social skills programs for children with autism is unknown.

Outcomes of Peer Interventions

Although a number of studies have demonstrated efficacy of a particular intervention for increasing specific measures of peer interactions, rarely have these effects been extended to related areas of overall peer acceptance, social networks, and friendships. These social outcomes are important to consider because they reflect larger and more qualitative aspects of peer interactions. Thus, improving peer interactions for children with autism may also increase the number or quality of their friendships, or their social acceptance among their classmates. Moreover, improving peer interactions may also have a positive effect on later adaptive behavior (McGovern and Sigman 2005).

Conclusions

Children with autism have specific and pervasive challenges with peer relationships. These children demonstrate less engagement, poorer skill, and less understanding in social situations with others. Yet children with autism show desire for relationships with peers and particularly for friendships.

These peer interaction problems have prompted a number of interventions for children with autism at all ages and ability levels. Most studies focus on the preschool age and are focused on either the target child with autism or typical peers who are taught to engage the target child. Nearly all studies note the immediate effects of intervention, but generalization and maintenance of skills have been more elusive. Indeed, there are currently no accepted, well-established, and efficacious treatments for social skills of children with autism (Rogers 2000).

A goal of future research studies should be to isolate, through use of scientifically rigorous research designs, the active ingredients of interventions (Kasari 2002). For example, comparing peer-mediated models with target-child models may yield information on which treatment is most efficacious for children with autism. Moreover, few studies have examined the moderators of treatment success or examined outcomes that extend beyond the immediate effects of the intervention. Because a particular treatment cannot be expected to benefit all children with autism, it will be important to determine the best fit between a particular child and treatment approach in future studies.

Finally, there are a number of clinical implications of current research studies. One issue has been the consistent problem in generalization of social skills programs. Children with autism likely need many levels of support to learn and to implement effective social behaviors. It may be that the targeted social programs that have been the focus of most research are inadequate for helping children with autism develop lifelong satisfying peer relationships because they are too narrow and too short term. Teaching skills to both the child with autism as well as those in their natural context such as family or friends can be an important key to generalizing skills in the absence of interventionists. This structural approach may also be critical to provide families with guidance and support in navigating their child's developmental needs and transitions.

Comprehensive social inclusion programs show considerable potential, particularly for children at the middle and high school ages, for whom there is far less intervention research. A clinical program that is trying to think outside the box at the high school age is the Spectrum Program, which is located on a regular high school campus (London 2007). Children with high-functioning autism or Asperger's syndrome at this high school are supported in their social development by two academic periods that focus on their ability to develop narratives, to understand nonliteral language, and to improve executive functions in planning and implementing social interactions. The goal of this activity-based program is to move away from teaching discrete or scripted behaviors by enhancing children's ability to project, to problem solve, and to improvise—the skills necessary to living life as it unfolds daily. Indeed, it may take an intensive and comprehensive effort to successfully affect and improve the social inclusion of individuals with autism.

References

Asher S, Parker J, Walker A: Distinguishing friendship from acceptance: implications for intervention and assessment, in The Company They Keep: Friendship in Childhood and Adolescence. Edited by Bukowski WM, Newomb AF, Hartup WW. New York, Cambridge University Press, 1998, pp 366–405

Bauminger N: The facilitation of social-emotional understanding and social interaction in high-functioning children with autism: intervention outcomes. J Autism Dev Disord 32:283–298, 2002

Bauminger N, Kasari C: Loneliness and friendships in high-functioning children with autism. Child Dev 71:447–456, 2000

Bauminger N, Shulman C, Agam G: Peer interaction and loneliness in high-functioning children with autism. J Autism Dev Disord 33:489–507, 2003

Belchic JK, Harris SL: The use of multiple peer exemplars to enhance the generalization of play skills to the siblings of children with autism. Child and Family Behavior Therapy 16:1–25, 1994

Buggey T, Toombs K, Gardener P, et al: Training responding behaviors in students with autism: using videotaped self-modeling. Journal of Positive Behavioral Interventions 1:205–214, 1999

Bullock CC: Interpretive lines of action of mentally retarded children in mainstreamed play settings. Studies in Symbolic Interaction: A Research Annual 9:145–174, 1988

Burack JA, Root R, Zigler E: Inclusive education for students with autism: reviewing ideological, empirical, and community considerations, in Handbook of Autism and Pervasive Developmental Disorders, 2nd Edition. Edited by Cohen DJ, Volkmar F. New York, Wiley, 1997, pp 796–807

Cairns RB, Cairns BD: Lifelines and Risks: Pathways of Youth in Our Time. New York, Cambridge University Press, 1994

Carr EG, Darcy M: Setting generality of peer modeling in children with autism. J Autism Dev Disord 20:45–59, 1990

Chamberlain B: Isolation or involvement? The social networks of children with autism included in regular classrooms. Dissertation Abstracts International Section A: Humanities and Social Sciences 62:2680, 2001

Chamberlain B, Kasari C, Rotheram-Fuller E: Involvement or isolation? The social networks of children with autism in regular classrooms. J Autism Dev Disord 37:230–242, 2006

Charlop MH, Milstein JP: Teaching autistic children conversational speech using video modeling. J Appl Behav Anal 22:275–285, 1989

Charlop MH, Schreibman L, Tryon AS: Learning through observation: the effects of peer modeling on acquisition and generalization in autistic children. J Abnorm Child Psychol 11:355–366, 1983

Charlop-Christy MH, Le L, Freeman KA: A comparison of video modeling with in vivo modeling for teaching children with autism. J Autism Dev Disord 30:537–552, 2000

Davis C, Brady M, Hamilton R, et al: Effects of high-probability requests on the social interactions of young children with severe disabilities. J Appl Behav Anal 27:619–637, 1994

Dewey D, Lord C, Magill J: Qualitative assessment of the effect of play materials in dyadic peer interactions of children with autism. Can J Psychol 42:242–260, 1988

Egel EL, Richman GS, Koegel RL: Normal peer models and autistic children's learning. J Appl Behav Anal 14:3–12, 1981

Field T, Field T, Sanders C, et al. Children with autism display more social behaviors after repeated imitation sessions. Autism 5:317–323, 2001

Furman W: The development of children's social networks, in Children's Social Networks and Social Supports. Edited by Belle D. New York, Wiley, 1989, pp 151–172

Gena A, Couloura S, Kymissis E: Modifying the affective behavior of preschoolers with autism using in-vivo or video modeling and reinforcement contingencies. J Autism Dev Disord 35:1–12, 2005

Goldstein H: Communication intervention for children with autism: a review of treatment efficacy. J Autism Dev Disord 32:373–396, 2002

Green J, Gilchrist A, Burton D, et al: Social and psychiatric functioning in adolescents with Asperger syndrome compared with conduct disorder. J Autism Dev Disord 30:279–293, 2000

Grindle CF, Remington B: Discrete-trial training for autistic children when reward is delayed: a comparison of conditioned cue value and response marking. J Appl Behav Anal 35:187–190, 2002

Guralnick MJ: Major accomplishments and future directions in early childhood mainstreaming. Topics in Early Childhood Special Education 10:1–17, 1990

Haring T, Breen C: A peer mediated social network intervention to enhance the social integration of persons with moderate and severe disabilities. J Appl Behav Anal 25:319–333, 1992

Heerey EA, Capps LM, Keltner D, et al: Understanding teasing: lessons from children with autism. J Abnorm Child Psychol 33:55–68, 2005

Hobson P: On the origins of self and the case of autism. Dev Psychopathol 2:163–181, 1990

Howlin P, Goode S, Hutton J, et al: Adult outcome for children with autism. J Child Psychol Psychiatry 45:212–229, 2004

Ingersoll B, Schreibman L, Tran QH: Effect of sensory feedback on immediate object imitation in children with autism. J Autism Dev Disord 33:673–683, 2003

Kamps DM, Leonard BR, Vernon S, et al: Teaching social skills to students with autism to increase peer interactions in an integrated first-grade classroom. J Appl Behav Anal 25:281–288, 1992

Kamps DM, Potucek J, Lopez A, et al: The use of peer networks across multiple settings to improve social interaction for students with autism. Journal of Behavioral Education 7:335–357, 1997

Kanner L: Autistic disturbances of affective contact. Nerv Child 2:217–250, 1943

Kasari C: Assessing change in early intervention programs for children with autism. J Autism Dev Disord 32:447–461, 2002

Kasari C, Freeman S, Bauminger N, et al: Parental perceptions of inclusion: effects of autism and Down syndrome. J Autism Dev Disord 29:297–305, 1999

Kim JA, Szatmari P, Bryson S, et al: The prevalence of anxiety and mood problems among children with autism and Asperger syndrome. Autism 4:117–132, 2000

Kodak T, Miltenberger RG, Romaniuk C: The effects of differential negative reinforcement of other behavior and noncontingent escape on compliance. J Appl Behav Anal 36:379–382, 2003

Koegel LK, Koegel RL, Hurley C, et al: Improving social skills and disruptive behavior in children with autism through self-management. J Appl Behav Anal 25:341–353, 1992

Koegel LK, Koegel RL, Frea WD, et al: Identifying early intervention targets for children with autism in inclusive school settings. Behav Modif 25:745–761, 2001

Kohler FW, Strain PS, Hoyson M, et al: Using a group-oriented contingency to increase social interactions between children with autism and their peers: a preliminary analysis of corollary supportive behaviors. Behav Modif 19:10–32, 1995

Laushey KM, Heflin LJ: Enhancing social skills of kindergarten children with autism through training of multiple peers as tutors. J Autism Dev Disord 30:183–193, 2000

LeBlanc LA, Coates AM, Daneshvar S, et al: Using video modeling and reinforcement to teach perspective-taking skills to children with autism. J Appl Behav Anal 36:253–257, 2003

London N: Spectrum Program at New Roads School, Available at: http://www.newroads.org. Accessed April 20, 2007.

Lyons V, Fitzgerald M: Humor in autism and Asperger's syndrome. J Autism Dev Disord 34:521–531, 2004

MacMillan DL, Gresham FM, Forness SR: Full inclusion: an empirical perspective. Behavioral Disorders 21:145–159, 1996

Martin I, McDonald S: An exploration of causes of non-literal language problems in individuals with Asperger's syndrome. J Autism Dev Disord 34:311–328, 2004

McConnell SR: Interventions to facilitate social interaction for young children with autism: review of available research and recommendations for educational intervention and future research. J Autism Dev Disord 32:351–372, 2002

McGee GG, Almeida MC, Sulzer-Azaroff B, et al: Promoting reciprocal interactions via peer incidental teaching. J Appl Behav Anal 25:117–126, 1992

McGovern CW, Sigman M: Continuity and change from early childhood to adolescence in autism. J Child Psychol Psychiatry 46:401–408, 2005

Miranda-Linne F, Melin L: Acquisition, generalization, and spontaneous use of color adjectives: a comparison of incidental teaching and traditional discrete-trial procedures for children with autism. Res Dev Disabil 13:191–210, 1992

Muris P, Steerneman P, Merckelback H, et al: Comorbid anxiety symptoms in children with pervasive developmental disorders. J Anxiety Disord 12:387–393, 1998

Myles BS, Simpson R, Ormsbee C, et al: Integrating preschool children with autism with their normally developing peers: research findings and best practices recommendations. Focus on Autistic Behavior 8:1–18, 1993

Nelson J, Aboud FE: The resolution of social conflict between friends. Child Dev 56:1009–1017, 1985

Nikopoulos CK, Keenan M: Effects of video modeling on social initiations by children with autism. J Appl Behav Anal 37:93–96, 2004

Ochs E, Kremer-Sadlik T, Solomon O, et al: Inclusion as a social practice: views of children with autism. Soc Dev 10:399–419, 2001

Odom SL, Strain PS: A comparison of peer-initiation and teacher-antecedent interventions for promoting reciprocal social interaction of autistic preschoolers. J Appl Behav Anal 19:59–71, 1986

Odom SL, Watts E: Reducing teacher prompts in peer-mediated interventions for young children with autism. J Spec Educ 25:26–43, 1991

Orsmond GI, Krauss MW, Seltzer MM: Peer relationships and social and recreational activities among adolescents and adults with autism. J Autism Dev Disord 34:245–256, 2004

Parsons S, Mitchell P, Leonard A: Do adolescents with autistic spectrum disorders adhere to social conventions in virtual environments? Autism 9:95–117, 2004

Pierce K, Schreibman L: Increasing complex social behaviors in children with autism: effects of peer-implemented pivotal response training. J Appl Behav Anal 28:285–295, 1995

Pierce K, Schreibman L: Multiple peer use of pivotal response training social behaviors of classmates with autism: results from trained and untrained peers. J Appl Behav Anal 30:157–160, 1997

Prizant BM, Wetherby AM: Understanding the continuum of discrete-trial traditional behavioral to social-pragmatic developmental approaches in communication enhancement for young children with autism/PDD. Semin Speech Lang 19:329–352, 1998

Reed GK, Ringdahl JE, Wacker DP, et al: The effects of fixed-time and contingent schedules of negative reinforcement on compliance and aberrant behavior. Res Dev Disabil 26:281–295, 2005

Roeyers H: The influence of nonhandicapped peers on the social interactions of children with a pervasive developmental disorder. J Autism Dev Disord 26:303–320, 1996

Rogers S: Interventions that facilitate socialization in children. J Autism Dev Disord 30:399–409, 2000

Rotheram-Fuller E: Age-related changes in the social inclusion of children with autism in general education classroom. Dissertation Abstracts International 66:2493, 2005

Ryndak DL, Downing JE, Jacqueline LR, et al: Parents' perceptions after inclusion of their children with moderate or severe disabilities. J Assoc Pers Sev Handicaps 20:147–157, 1995

Sainato DM, Goldstein H, Strain PS: Effects of self-evaluation on preschool children's use of social interaction strategies with their classmates with autism. J Appl Behav Anal 25:127–141, 1992

Sale P, Carey DM: The sociometric status of students with disabilities in a full-inclusion school. Except Child 62:6–19, 1995

Shafer MS, Egel AL, Neef NA: Training mildly handicapped peers to facilitate changes in the social interaction skills of autistic children. J Appl Behav Anal 17:461–476, 1984

Shearer DD, Kohler F, Buchan K, et al: Promoting independent interactions between preschoolers with autism and their nondisabiled peers: an analysis of self-monitoring. Early Educ Dev 7:205–220, 1996

Sherer M, Pierce KL, Paredes S, et al: Enhancing conversation skills in children with autism via video technology: which is better, "self" or "other" as a model? Behav Modif 25:140–158, 2001

Sigman M, Ruskin E: Continuity and change in the social competence of children with autism, Down syndrome, and developmental delays. Monogr Soc Res Child Dev 64:1–114, 1999

Solomon M, Goodlin-Jones BL, Anders TF: A social adjustment enhancement intervention for high functioning autism, Asperger's syndrome, and pervasive developmental disorder NOS. J Autism Dev Disord 34:649–668, 2004

Stahmer A: Teaching symbolic play skills to children with autism using pivotal response training. J Autism Dev Disord 25:123–141, 1995

Stahmer AC, Ingersoll B, Carter C: Behavioral approaches to promoting play. Autism 7:401–413, 2003

Staub D, Schwartz IS, Galluci C, et al: Four portraits of friendship at an inclusive school. J Assoc Pers Sev Handicaps 19:314–325, 1994

Stone WL, Caro-Martinez LM: Naturalistic observations of spontaneous communication in autistic children. J Autism Dev Disord 20:437–453, 1990

Strain PS: Social behavior patterns of nonhandicapped and developmentally disabled friend pairs in mainstream preschools. Analysis and Intervention in Developmental Disabilities 4:15–28, 1984

Strain P, Kohler F, Storey K, et al: Teaching preschoolers with autism to self-monitor their social interactions: an analysis of results in home and school settings. Journal of Emotional and Behavioral Disorder 2:78–88, 1994

Swaim KF, Morgan SB: Children's attitudes and behavioral intentions toward a peer with autistic behaviors: does a brief educational intervention have an effect? J Autism Dev Disord 31:195–205, 2001

Taubman M, Brierley S, Wishner J, et al: The effectiveness of a group discrete trial instructional approach for preschoolers with developmental disabilities. Res Dev Disabil 22:205–219, 2001

Tryon AS, Keane SP: Promoting imitative play through generalized observational learning in autisticlike children. J Abnorm Child Psychol 14:537–549, 1986

Villa R, Thousand J: Creating an Inclusive School. Alexandria, VA, Association for Supervision and Curriculum Development, 1995

Wing L: The continuum of autistic characteristics, in Diagnosis and Assessment in Autism. Edited by Schopler E, Mesibov GB. New York, Plenum, 1988, pp 91–110

Zanolli K, Daggett J: The effects of reinforcement rate on the spontaneous social initiations of socially withdrawn preschoolers. J Appl Behav Anal 31:117–125, 1998

Zanolli K, Daggett J, Adams T: Teaching preschool age autistic children to make spontaneous initiations to peers using priming. J Autism Dev Disord 26:407–422, 1996

12

Complementary and Alternative Therapies for Autism

Michelle Zimmer, M.D.

Cynthia A. Molloy, M.D., M.S.

Complementary and alternative medicine (CAM) refers to medications, herbs, supplements, or nonbiological treatments such as massage therapy used outside the accepted practices of Western medicine to treat symptoms or medical conditions (American Academy of Pediatrics 2001). Recent estimates suggest that 33%–50% of children with autism spectrum disorders (ASDs) are using some form of CAM (Levy and Hyman 2003; Nickel 1996). Healthcare providers for these children are increasingly being asked to prescribe or give advice regarding these treatments.

The availability of information regarding CAM use in ASDs is astounding. A Google search using the search terms "autism" and "alternative medicine" yielded more than 600,000 sites. Most parents seeking information on this topic have difficulty sorting out solid medical advice from pseudoscience on the Internet.

Helping Parents Make Informed Choices About CAM Treatments

Healthcare providers need to balance support for parents' decisions regarding their child's treatment with solid advice based on best medical practice. Therefore it is important to use the principles of evidence-based medicine to evaluate any potential CAM therapy being considered for use. *Evidence-based medicine* refers to the practice of evaluating the strength of scientific evidence behind any proposed medical treatment. Many CAM therapies have no scientific evidence behind them, or use anecdotal reports or case series as evidence of efficacy.

Of great concern is the fact that some autism CAM Web sites actively discourage parents from considering evidence-based medicine in their decision-making process, citing that these types of studies are only necessary for potentially harmful treatments, not natural treatments. It is important for physicians to inform families that the distinction between natural and manufactured pharmaceuticals is not so clear. Many effective medications come from natural plant sources (i.e., tamoxifen for breast cancer) and *all* pharmaceuticals, natural or not, have potential side effects.

Healthcare practitioners need to communicate with families about how medical treatments are evaluated scientifically. In particular, they should understand the concept of placebo effects. A randomized, placebo-controlled clinical trial of secretin is an excellent example of such an effect. Parents' expectancy for this treatment was so high that over 30% of children receiving saline solution placebo were reported by parents to have significant improvement in their symptoms. Even more surprising was the fact that after the study was unblinded and families were told that their child received placebo, there was still intense interest in pursuing the treatment (A. Sandler 2005). This study illustrates issues related to mind–body connection and placebo effects. Parents should be aware of the possibility of the placebo effect coming into play with any treatment they choose to pursue for their child.

It is also important for the healthcare provider to build a partnership with families that allows for open discussion of any type of treatment the family would like to pursue. It is well known that families frequently do not disclose CAM use to their child's healthcare provider. It is also true that many families who suspect an autism spectrum diagnosis in their child have implemented one or more alternative treatments while they are waiting for an appointment with a specialist to confirm the diagnosis (Levy et al. 2003). Families, in fact, are often resentful of the fact that their healthcare provider does not provide them with information about alternative treatments when such information is so readily available from other sources such as the Internet. This leads to a disconnect between families and medical professionals, who are seen as uncaring, rigid, or not open to more "progressive" therapies and treatments.

The healthcare provider might open the door to discussions about CAM by actively asking the question during the course of the medical history. Example questions might include, Is your child taking any medications? Have you considered, or is your child currently taking, any vitamins, supplements, or herbs, or is he on any special diet restrictions? Receiving the responses nonjudgmentally is a good way to open the door to these types of discussions. It is important to make parents aware of alternative therapies early on in the diagnosis. One might provide families with a list of resources to parent support groups and reliable Web sites, book chapters, and review articles that feature balanced discussions of CAM. This can build trust in the provider-patient relationship and lead to a discussion of how to critically evaluate these treatments.

How Do I Find Reliable Information About CAM Therapies?

Healthcare providers frequently do not ask families about their use of CAM therapies because of lack of knowledge regarding how to advise families about the use of these therapies. Therefore, the healthcare provider needs to have resources available to help sift through this information. There are many good Web sites and books available to search for information regarding CAM treatments. AltMedDex is an excellent resource available through the Internet through Thomson Micromedex (AltMedDex 2007) and many medical center intranet sites (AltMedDex intranet database, version 5.1. Thomson Micromedex). AltMedDex lists peer-reviewed publications, treatment indications, and known side effects for many herbs and supplements used in alternative medical practice. The National Library of Medicine has developed a specific CAM Web search engine that will automatically link providers to the CAM subset of PubMed (http://nccam.nih.gov/camonpubmed). The National Center for Complementary and Alternative Medicine (http://nccam.nih.gov) provides information on herbs and supplements and other alternative treatments as well as

National Institutes of Health–funded studies of CAM therapies. It also provides several useful patient education handouts.

Should I Agree to Monitor Alternative Therapies for My Patients/Families?

Many healthcare practitioners are not willing to prescribe CAM treatments directly because they are outside the realm of standard medical practice. However, practitioners can agree to help the family become informed consumers and make smart choices about how to evaluate the effectiveness of the treatment. Practitioners can teach families to conduct their own "*N* of 1" experiment. In this model, the family sets a time period for the treatment under "study." Usually it is recommended to evaluate one treatment at a time. Practitioners can help families choose target symptoms to monitor improvements and can provide standardized behavior rating forms to assess target symptoms. These measures should be administered before starting the treatment and then at regular time intervals. Ideally, it is important to get opinions from objective raters such as teachers or therapists who do not have the same expectancy as the parents for improvement from the treatment. Additional support can be provided by scheduling regular follow-up visits to monitor progress. It is also important for the practitioner to document contents of the CAM discussion in the medical record to make it clear what services are being provided to the family.

Should Laboratory Testing Be Ordered?

Many alternative medicine practitioners offer parents a wide range of laboratory testing, the interpretation of which is difficult and not validated. Most of these tests are of dubious value and have no proven relationship to the etiology of autism. Furthermore, many of these tests do not have published norms for children with or without autism.

The healthcare provider needs to explain to families why lab testing is not offered and discuss the concept of chance associations, and the importance of having reference norms and knowing how to interpret a test result. If parents insist on lab testing, it is best to offer support, such as a list of resources to CAM autism clinical trials going on at medical centers as well as alternative medicine practitioners in the community. The healthcare provider may offer handouts such as those developed by the National Center for Complementary and Alternative Medicine that offer families advice about how to evaluate and choose an alternative practitioner (http://nccam.nih.gov/health). The provider may also explain that visits to alternative medicine practitioners usually are not covered by medical insurance. A follow-up visit to discuss recommendations of alternative practitioners and lab results may be useful.

Specific CAM Therapies

Table 12–1 summarizes the CAM therapies described in this section.

Therapies Aimed at Gastrointestinal Function

Evidence of Gastrointestinal Dysfunction in Autism Spectrum Disorders

Several studies have reported an increase in gastrointestinal (GI) symptoms among children with ASDs. In 1998, Wakefield et al. reported GI symptoms associated with the onset of autistic regression in a series of 12 children. They concluded that the timing was consistent with administration of the measles, mumps, and rubella vaccine and implicated this vaccine as a causative agent of autistic regression (Wakefield et al. 1998). Subsequently, the validity of this data has come under scrutiny. The article was retracted from *JAMA*, with a letter published by the Wakefield collaborators retracting the conclusions drawn from the study. Wakefield had failed to disclose a significant conflict of interest with families who had come to him interested in filing lawsuits against vaccine companies for causing their child's autism. Other studies have reported an increased prevalence of GI symptoms among this population (Molloy and Manning-Courtney 2003). However, in their nested case–control study, Black et al. (2002) found that GI symptoms occurred in only 9% of children with autism—a rate similar to that seen with control subjects.

Numerous hypotheses have been generated about the possible relationship between the GI tract and symptoms of autism. D'Eufemia et al. (1996) reported increased intestinal permeability in 43% of patients with autism, leading to a resurgence of the "leaky gut" hypothesis. In this hypothesis, opioid peptides formed from the breakdown of milk and wheat products are absorbed across a "leaky" GI tract in patients with ASDs (Cade et al. 2000; Reichelt et al. 1991; Shattock et al. 1990). These opioid peptides cause symptoms of autism, including hyporesponsiveness to pain, social withdrawal, and under- or over-

Table 12–1.   Specific complementary and alternative medicine therapies for the treatment of patients with autism spectrum disorders

Name of treatment	Research evidence in autism	Possible side effects
Secretin	14 clinical trials, including several randomized, double-blind, placebo-controlled trials, producing negative results	Abdominal cramps, abdominal discomfort, bradycardia, hypotension, diaphoresis, flushing, diarrhea, nausea, vomiting, headache, lightheadedness; allergic reaction possible
Gluten-/casein-free (GFCF) diet	Unblinded pre-/postevaluation of milk elimination diet; autistic behaviors improvement in five of seven autistic behaviors (Lucarelli et al. 1995) Single-blind, randomized trial of GFCF diet; improvements in attention, social and emotional functioning, communication, and cognition (Knivsberg et al. 2002) Double-blind, randomized trial of GFCF diet; no improvements in group data; small subset of individuals showed improvement in language and behavior (Elder et al. 2006)	Nutritional deficiencies possible (calcium, protein)
Digestive enzymes	None	Not known
Probiotics	None	Flatulence, constipation, skin rash, itching, urticaria; bacteremia has been reported with use in short gut syndrome
Antibiotics	Pre-/postevaluation of vancomycin in autistic children; improvements in chronic diarrhea and autistic symptoms in 8 of 11 children (R.H. Sandler et al. 2000)	Drug-induced erythroderma, nausea, vomiting, neutropenia, anaphylaxis (rare), ototoxicity (rare), nephrotoxicity (rare)
Antifungals	None	Nausea and vomiting; potential for hepatotoxicity with chronic use of oral antifungal agents

Table 12–1. Specific complementary and alternative medicine therapies for the treatment of patients with autism spectrum disorders *(continued)*

Name of treatment	Research evidence in autism	Possible side effects
Intravenous immunoglobulin	Improvement in symptoms suggested in two case series (Gupta et al. 1996; Plioplys 1998); in one case, no improvement over 6 months (DelGiudice-Asch et al. 1999)	Flushing, hypotension, chills, fever, headache, low back pain, nausea, chest tightness, acute renal failure (rare), aseptic meningitis (rare), neutropenia, elevation in serum creatinine, anaphylaxis (rare)
Dimethylglycine	Negative results in the two placebo-controlled clinical trials conducted (Bolman and Richmond 1999; Kern et al. 2001)	Not known
Amino acids	None	Not known
Chelation	None	Hematological, renal, and liver toxicity possible; death has occurred with intravenous use
Omega-3 fatty acids/ fish oil	Small, randomized, double-blind, placebo-controlled trial suggested trends toward improvement in hyperactivity (Amminger et al. 2007)	Belching, fishy odor, skin rash, abdominal distention, diarrhea, nosebleed, easy bruising
Glutathione	None	Not known
Vitamin B_6/ magnesium (Mg)	Improvement shown in several open-label single-blind studies (Barthelemy et al. 1980; Jonas et al. 1984; Martineau et al. 1985; Rimland et al. 1978), but negative findings in two randomized, double-blind, placebo-controlled trials (Findling et al. 1997; Tolbert et al. 1993)	B_6: photosensitivity, nausea, vomiting, abdominal pain, peripheral neuropathy Mg: cardiovascular effects possible with high doses, excessive sweating, flushing, nausea and vomiting, muscle weakness, prolonged bleeding time, decreased tendon reflex, central nervous system depression, respiratory tract paralysis

Table 12–1. Specific complementary and alternative medicine therapies for the treatment of patients with autism spectrum disorders (*continued*)

Name of treatment	Research evidence in autism	Possible side effects
Vitamin B$_{12}$	None	Pain at injection site, headache, diarrhea
L-Carnosine	Improvement on Gilliam Autism Rating Scale and Peabody Picture Vocabulary Test in one randomized, placebo-controlled trial (Chez et al. 2002)	Not known
Vitamin C	Reduction of symptoms in one double-blind, crossover trial in institutionalized children with autism	None in reasonable doses; diarrhea, iron overload, nephrolithiasis have been reported in large doses
Tryptophan	Dietary depletion of tryptophan exacerbated autistic symptoms (McDougle et al. 1993)	Eosinophilia myalgia syndrome, nausea, headache, lightheadedness, drowsiness
Melatonin	None specifically in autism; has been shown to improve sleep latency in children with neurodevelopmental disabilities (Phillips and Appleton 2004)	Minimal toxicity reported
St. John's wort	None	Gastrointestinal upset, diarrhea, nausea, anorexia, dry mouth, constipation, edema, frequent urination, anorgasmia, mania, hypomania, anxiety, schizophrenia relapse, photosensitivity, pruritus, exanthema, restlessness, fatigue, headache, paresthesia
S-adenosyl-methionine	None	Headache, nausea, dizziness, fatigue, urinary frequency, itching, abdominal pain, diarrhea, anxiety, mania

Table 12–1. Specific complementary and alternative medicine therapies for the treatment of patients with autism spectrum disorders (*continued*)

Name of treatment	Research evidence in autism	Possible side effects
Naltrexone	Reduction in hyperactivity and stereotyped and compulsive behaviors in open-label studies (Campbell et al. 1993; Herman et al. 1989; Panksepp and Lensing 1991); only marginal benefits seen in randomized, double-blind, placebo-controlled trials (Cazzullo et al. 1999; Feldman et al. 1999; Kolmen et al. 1997; Willemsen-Swinkels et al. 1996)	Abdominal pain, constipation, nausea, headache, anxiety, liver damage

response to environmental stimuli. In a follow-up study to his original report of GI symptoms in children with autism, Wakefield all but implicated measles vaccine as a potential factor in the etiology of autism. Wakefield performed endoscopies on 55 children with ASDs and 37 developmentally normal control subjects. He found an increased rate of ileal-lymphoid-nodular hyperplasia among the group with autism. This finding was taken as evidence for gut inflammation from viral disease and implied that measles virus from vaccination could be a potential etiological factor (Wakefield et al. 1998). Hypotheses from other investigators explaining the gut–brain interaction in autism have included overgrowth of neurotoxic bacteria (R.H. Sandler et al. 2000), dysfunction of secretin or its receptors (Horvath and Perman 2002; Horvath et al. 1999), and dysfunction of serotonin or its receptors (Fiorica-Howells et al. 2000).

Gastrointestinal Treatments

Secretin. Secretin is a 27–amino acid hormone released from S cells within the proximal duodenum in response to gastric acid secretion ("Secretin" 2006). In 1998, infusion of purified porcine secretin was reported to improve symptoms in three children with autism (Horvath et al. 1998). After the initial report of efficacy, an explosion of interest in secretin as a treatment for ASDs ensued. Many children with autism received secretin before more formalized research studies were developed. Now, secretin is probably the most well studied treatment for autism, with at least 14 well-designed, randomized, placebo-controlled trials conducted. The Cochrane Developmental, Psychosocial and Learning Problems Group performed a meta-analysis on these studies, which included more than 500 children, and concluded that no difference existed between placebo and intervention groups (Williams et al. 2005). Interestingly, in some of these studies, improvements were seen in both treatment and control groups, suggesting a strong placebo effect associated with receiving the intravenous injections (A. Sandler 2005). Potential side effects include abdominal cramps, abdominal discomfort bradycardia (mild), diaphoresis, flushing, diarrhea, nausea, vomiting, headache, lightheadedness, and hypotension. Caution should be used in administration in those with a history of allergy, asthma, atopic disease, inflammatory bowel disease, or concomitant use of anticholinergic medication ("Secretin" 2006). Given its lack of efficacy in well-designed treatment studies, the high cost of these treatments, and the potential side effects, secretin is not recommended for treatment of subjects with ASDs.

Gluten-/casein-free diet. A recent survey suggests that up to 15% of children with ASDs adhere to gluten-/casein-free (GFCF) diets (Levy and Hyman 2003). There are some preliminary data to suggest that elimination of gluten and casein from the diet of autistic children may reduce symptoms. Lucarelli and colleagues first published a study in 1995 suggesting the potential efficacy of a milk elimination diet in treating autistic symptoms (Lucarelli et al. 1995). This group was studying the possible link between allergy and autism and found that 36 children with autism who had eliminated milk products from their diet for 8 weeks had significantly fewer autistic behaviors in five of seven categories on a standardized observational assessment of autistic symptoms (Lucarelli et al. 1995). This study has significant limitations, including lack of a control group, unblinded raters, failure to control for other psychosocial interventions such as behavior therapy, and lack of information regarding use of other medications. Similarly, Knivsberg et al. (2002) conducted a small, randomized, single-blind clinical trial of gluten and casein elimination in 10 school-age children with autism. The diet intervention group showed significant improvements in a composite score that included verbal and nonverbal communication, behavior in learning situations, sharing of emotions, anxiety, rigidity, and peculiarity. However, no improvements in linguistic, cognitive, and motor abilities were noted. This study was limited by small sample size and the lack of control for other interventions such as use of medications or behavior therapy. Critics of the study suggest that increased attention and household structure needed to comply with the diet combined with the use of more traditional therapies such as behavior modification were not accounted for in the study and could be responsible for the positive result.

More recently, Elder et al. (2006) reported results of a small double-blind trial of GFCF diet. Language and videotaped behavioral interactions were coded. Change in autistic symptoms was measured with the childhood Autism Rating Scale. Overall, the authors found no group differences in any measure. However, they reported that individual children did show gains in language and behavior, and called for larger, blinded randomized controlled clinical trials.

Additionally, a literature search found no published studies assessing the safety of a GFCF diet. This is of great concern because many autistic children already have limited diets based on their sensory aversion to certain types and textures of foods. Elimination of milk products potentially runs the risk of inadequate intake of protein, calcium, and other essential vitamins in the diet, and there is preliminary evidence that a GFCF diet is associated with a decrease in bone density (Brudnak et al. 2002; Hediger et al. 2005). This is an area that has not yet been fully investigated.

Several studies of GFCF diets are ongoing in the United States, and data may soon be available to answer the question of whether this treatment has any therapeutic value. Families utilizing the diet should seek counsel from a nutritionist to ensure that they are providing adequately for their child's nutritional needs.

Digestive enzymes.   The theory behind the use of digestive enzymes is closely related to the leaky gut theory. Digestive enzymes are purported to break down food products into small "nontoxic" particles. Only one open-label trial of digestive enzymes combined with probiotics is reported in the literature (Brudnak et al. 2002). In the study, 46 children with ASDs were enrolled and received EnZymAid plus probiotics for 12 weeks. Only 22 remained in the study for the entire period. Those who remained in the study reported some behavioral improvements. Outcome measures were unblinded. There is currently not enough data to comment on the potential efficacy of this treatment for ASDs.

Probiotics.   Probiotics are products containing microflora in amounts sufficient to alter intestinal flora with the purpose of sustained health benefits. Recently, these products have been shown to be of value in treating atopic disease in children who have a family history of atopy (Kalliomaki et al. 2001), and antibiotic-associated diarrhea (Cremonini et al. 2002; D'Souza et al. 2002; Szajewska and Mrukowicz 2001; Van Niel et al. 2002). There is some evidence of their potential efficacy on other chronic GI– and allergy-mediated conditions. The only report of probiotic use in ASDs was in combination with the use of digestive enzymes (see previous subsection), with behavioral improvements reported. Recently several case reports of bacteremia with use of probiotics in children with short gut syndrome have been published (De Groote et al. 2005; Kunz et al. 2004). Other known side effects include flatulence, constipation, skin rash, itching, and urticaria ("Probiotics" 2007).

Therapies Targeting the Immune System

Evidence of Impaired Immunity in Autism Spectrum Disorders

There is mounting evidence that children with ASDs differ from normally developing control subjects on several measures of immune function. Although the evidence supports an association between the immune system and ASDs, no consistent pattern of dysfunction has been identified. Abnormalities in peripheral cytokines (Croonenberghs et al. 2002; Gupta et al. 1998; Jyonouchi et al.

2001), autoantibodies to neuronal elements (Connolly et al. 1999), cell-mediated (T_H1) response, and allergic (T_H2) immune response (Gupta et al. 1996) have been reported. Children diagnosed with ASDs are more likely to have a family history of autoimmune disease (Comi et al. 1999; Sweeten et al. 2003).

Immune Treatments

Antibiotics. Only one study of antibiotic use in autism has been published to date (R. H. Sandler et al. 2000). This study hypothesized that autistic symptoms were exacerbated by repeated use of antibiotics, leading to gut bacterial overgrowth and colonization by "neurotoxic" bacteria. These neurotoxic bacteria "cause" the autistic regression. On the basis of this hypothesis, the researchers gave oral vancomycin to 11 children with a recent diagnosis of autism, regression, and antibiotic use within 2 months of symptoms followed by the onset of diarrhea. Psychologists blinded to the study coded videotapes and reported improvements in autistic symptoms in 8 children studied. The improvements waned after the treatment was withdrawn. The authors did not purport this as a useful treatment but cited this as potential evidence of a gut–brain interaction in some individuals with autism.

Antifungals. Antifungals have been proposed as a treatment for colonic yeast overgrowth for individuals with autism. Some alternative practitioners propose that toxic yeast metabolites are absorbed through an inflamed intestinal wall and cause symptoms of autism (Pangborn 2002). Colonic yeast overgrowth in autistic individuals has not been documented in peer-reviewed medical journals nor have any therapeutic trials of oral antifungal agents been published. Chronic use of oral antifungal agents has the potential for hepatotoxicity and must be monitored closely.

Intravenous immunoglobulin. Three case series reported on the use of intravenous immunoglobulin (IVIG) in children with ASDs. Two studies cited marked clinical improvement (Gupta et al. 1996; Plioplys 1998), whereas one found no improvement in seven subjects over 6 months (DelGiudice-Asch et al. 1999). IVIG is an expensive therapy that requires intravenous infusion. Because of the limited supply of this medication, many hospitals are beginning to restrict use of IVIG to proven therapeutic uses. Adverse effects may include flushing and hypotension, chills and fever, headache, low back pain, nausea, and chest tightness. Acute renal failure, aseptic meningitis, neutropenia, and elevations of serum creatinine have been reported following administration. Anaphylactic reactions are rare but have been known to occur ("IVIG"

2006). IVIG is considered a blood product, and there is a small but real risk of blood-borne infection (Levy and Hyman 2005).

Dimethylglycine.   Dimethylglycine (DMG) is classified as a food compound that is similar in composition to the water-soluble B vitamins ("Dimethylglycine [DMG]" 2006). This substance has been touted to cure many ills, from cancer to hepatitis, but has little scientific investigation surrounding its use. The mechanism of action of DMG is unknown, but DMg is proposed to be an immunomodulatory agent. However, there is no proven immunologic effect of this agent. Two placebo-controlled trials of DMG have been conducted in children with autism and have produced negative results (Bolman and Richmond 1999; Kern et al. 2001). Despite this, DMG is still being promoted as a therapeutic agent for autism by many alternative medical practitioners. The usual starting total daily dose in autism is 60–125 mg, with the dose gradually increased to 200–400 mg. Normal pediatric dosing is not known. Fatty infiltration of the liver has been reported with long-term use of pangamic acid, a closely related compound (Ziemlanski et al. 1984).

Metabolic Therapies and Nutritional Supplements

Impaired Heavy Metal Detoxification in Autism Spectrum Disorders

Those who believe that autistic children have impaired ability to detoxify the body of heavy metals point to a basic science article showing a genetic susceptibility to effects of mercury in certain strains of mice (Hornig et al. 2004). These genetically susceptible mice demonstrated developmental delays and decreased socialization after exposure to mercury.

Metallothionein is a cellular protein that neutralizes harmful influences of exposure to toxic metals such as mercury. It also plays a role in the intracellular fixation of zinc and copper. Unpublished data from the Pfeiffer Institute labs in 500 individuals with ASDs showed that many individuals had abnormal serum zinc and copper levels. These data were presented at Defeat Autism Now! meetings across the country, with the conclusion that metallothionein dysfunction occurs in autism, causing poor detoxification of heavy metals and leading to impaired neuronal development and impaired immune function. Peer-reviewed data on metallothionein, copper, and zinc metabolism are lacking, although one group in the 1970s published data that this group of children has normal copper and zinc levels compared with control subjects (Jackson and Garrod 1978).

The well-known mercury/thimerosal vaccine controversy has stimulated much discussion in academic and nonacademic circles. This issue continues to be hotly debated despite fairly strong scientific evidence against the hypothesis of mercury or thimerosal in vaccines as a causative agent of autism (Andrews et al. 2004; Hviid et al. 2003; Madsen et al. 2003). The controversy is spurred on by articles such as the Geier and Geier (2005) analysis of the Vaccine Adverse Event Reporting System (VAERS), in which the authors cited increased reports to VAERS of speech delay, mental retardation, and autism after receiving thimerosal-containing vaccines. The clear reporting biases inherent to this type of database were not discussed in the article, yet this article is frequently cited as evidence of the vaccine/autism connection.

Heavy Metal Treatments/Detoxification

Treating metallothionein dysfunction. Proponents of metallothionein dysfunction theory often recommend treating patients with a cocktail of the 14–amino acid precursors to metallothionein as well as selenium and glutathione, which are hypothesized to become depleted in the face of a high body heavy-metal burden. No trials of this cocktail have been reported in peer-reviewed publications to date. The potential adverse effects are unknown.

Chelation therapy. DMSA (dimercaptosuccinic acid) and CaEDTA (edetate calcium disodium) are chelation agents that pull heavy metals from body tissues and excrete them from the urine. Chelating is intended to be used after an acute exposure to a heavy metal. Data from lead poisoning studies show that once neurological damage from heavy metal exposure has occurred, chelation treatment is of little value (Levy and Hyman 2005). Chelation therapy is untested in children with autism. Common adverse side effects of chelation agents are rash, diarrhea, nausea, vomiting, and increased liver function tests. Numerous potentially serious adverse effects have been reported and include hematological, renal, and liver toxicity ("Edetate Calcium" 2007; "Succimer" 2007; see also Levy and Hyman 2005). These serious side effects, plus the recent report of child deaths during intravenous injection of CaEDTA (Centers for Disease Control and Prevention 2006), make this a treatment with little evidence base and a real potential for harm.

Abnormalities in Fatty Acid Metabolism in Autism Spectrum Disorders

Polyunsaturated fatty acids are naturally occurring lipids that must be taken in through the diet and are essential for normal brain development and function

(Clandinin and Jumpsen 1997). Polyunsaturated fatty acids are incorporated into phospholipids, which make up a large portion of neuronal cell membranes. Phospholipids have many important neural functions, including cell signaling, neurotransmission, and second-messaging (Bennett and Horrobin 2000; Horrobin 1998; Horrobin and Bennett 1999; Horrobin et al. 1994). Two laboratories have reported that autistic individuals have depletion of polyunsaturated omega-3 fatty acids in their red blood cell membranes (Bell et al. 2004) and plasma (Vancassel et al. 2001), but a recent report found normal levels (Bu et al. 2006), except for an increase in a few of the minor fatty acids of children with autism and regression.

Omega-3 fatty acid supplementation.   Omega-3 supplements are available as health food supplements. Common names for these supplements include fish oil, evening primrose oil, and flax oil. All contain slightly different ratios or blends of omega-3 and omega-6 fatty acids. Clinical trials of supplementation with polyunsaturated fatty acids have shown some promise in treating patients with depression (Nemets et al. 2002; Peet and Horrobin 2002; Puri et al. 2002), and developmental coordination disorders (Richardson and Montgomery 2005). Mixed results have been found in trials of other conditions such as schizophrenia (Peet et al. 2001; Puri and Richardson 1998) and attention-deficit/hyperactivity disorder (L. E. Arnold et al. 1989; Stevens et al. 2003; Voigt et al. 2001). A recent pilot study (Amminger et al. 2007) using an EPA (eicosapentaenoic acid) + DHA (docosahexaenoic acid) supplement found improvements in hyperactivity and stereotypy as measured by the Aberrant Behavior Checklist. This study needs to replicated with a larger sample size and stronger statistical analysis. Commonly cited side effects are increased belching, fishy odor, skin rash, abdominal distention, diarrhea, increased risk of nosebleed, and easy bruising ("Docosahexaenoic Acid [DHA]" 2007).

Impaired Methylation Capacity in Autism Spectrum Disorders

Methionine is an amino acid whose metabolism is important in many cellular processes, including methylation of DNA, RNA, and membrane phospholipids, as well as protection of cells from oxidative stress. Theoretically, abnormalities in this metabolic pathway could lead to altered neurotransmission and cell signaling and maladaptive immune responses, although this has not been demonstrated clinically. Cofactors for methionine metabolic reactions include a number of enzymes, vitamins (B_6 and B_{12}), and DMG. Recently, James et al. (2004) reported abnormalities in the methionine cycle among autistic individuals, including decreased levels of a number of the breakdown products of this cycle.

Treatment of impaired methylation capacity/oxidative damage

Glutathione. Glutathione is an antioxidant produced as a result of the methionine breakdown pathway. Since James et al. (2004) demonstrated reduced levels of this antioxidant in serum of autistic patients, the popularity of glutathione treatments has increased. This supplement is given either in patch form or intravenously. Currently there are no published trials demonstrating the safety or efficacy of glutathione as a treatment for symptoms of autism. No serious adverse effects have been reported to date ("Glutathione" 2006).

Vitamin B_6 and magnesium. Vitamin B_6 and magnesium have been used as an alternative treatment for symptoms of autism since the 1960s, when reports of speech and language improvements were observed after administration of megadoses of vitamin B_6 (Bonisch 1968). Despite some initial promise of positive effects in open-label or single-blind studies (Barthelemy et al. 1980; Jonas et al. 1984; Martineau et al. 1985; Rimland et al. 1978), two randomized, double-blind clinical trials were negative (Findling et al. 1997; Tolbert et al. 1993). However, even these well-designed studies have their limitations. The Tolbert et al. (1993) study used smaller doses of vitamin B_6 than typically reported in previous studies, and the Findling et al. (1997) study used a very small sample size of 12 children, only 10 of whom completed the entire study protocol. Therefore, at this time there is not enough evidence to support or refute the use of megadoses of vitamin B_6 in combination with magnesium for the treatment of ASD symptoms (Nye and Brice 2005). Peripheral neuropathy has been reported after prolonged use of vitamin B_6 or use at dosages higher than 100 mg/day. Photosensitivity, nausea, vomiting, and abdominal pain have also been reported. Magnesium in high doses has been associated with cardiovascular effects. Sweating, flushing, nausea, vomiting, prolonged bleeding time, and central nervous system effects have been reported.

Vitamin B_{12}. Vitamin B_{12} is a water-soluble vitamin that is being explored as a possible alternative treatment for autism. It is a cofactor in the conversion of homocysteine back to methionine. One open trial (James et al. 2004) demonstrated a return to normal levels on several markers of methionine metabolism, but measures of change in autistic symptoms were not included in the study design. The laboratory findings are of interest, and further study into this area is needed. Currently there is not enough data to comment on the efficacy of this treatment in ASDs.

Treatments Targeting Neurotransmitters

Evidence of Impaired Neurotransmitter Function in Autism Spectrum Disorders

Evidence from brain imaging and clinical pharmacology studies suggests that multiple neurotransmitter systems are disrupted in autism (Polleux and Lauder 2004). Evidence is strongest for abnormalities in the γ-aminobutyric acid (GABA)–ergic, glutaminergic, and serotonergic systems (Mulder et al. 2004; Ritvo et al. 1970; Spivak et al. 2004). Drug studies featuring medications that act on these neurotransmitters (i.e., risperidone, fluoxetine, fluvoxamine) show some promise in treating symptoms of autism and lend further evidence to the potential role of these neurotransmitter systems in the pathophysiology of autism. Many herbal supplements claim effects on the neurotransmitter systems.

Supplements Aimed at Restoring Neurotransmitter Function

L-Carnosine.   The mechanism of action of carnosine on brain functioning is not well defined at this time, but hypotheses include actions as a general neuroprotective agent or modulator of GABA activity. In one randomized, placebo-controlled clinical trial of L-carnosine, treatment children showed improvements in the Gilliam Autism Rating Scale and the Peabody Picture Vocabulary Test compared with control subjects (Chez et al. 2002). This study has not been replicated.

Vitamin C.   Vitamin C is a cofactor in the conversion of tryptophan to serotonin and theoretically could be of benefit in treating symptoms of autism (Levy and Hyman 2005). One double-blind crossover trial of institutionalized children with autism showed a reduction of autistic symptoms in treatment children. This trial has not been replicated, and for unknown reasons vitamin C has not gained popularity as an alternative therapy for children with autism (Levy and Hyman 2005).

Tryptophan.   Tryptophan is an amino acid precursor to serotonin. G.L. Arnold et al. (2003) demonstrated a trend for children with autism to have lower plasma amino acid levels of tryptophan and tyrosine, both dietary precursors to serotonin. One study demonstrated that dietary tryptophan depletion exacerbates autistic symptoms, theoretically by reducing the available supply of serotonin in the brain (McDougle et al. 1993). Another study demonstrated that an oral dose of tryptophan increased excretion of urinary metabolites of serotonin production, but no clinical correlation to change in autistic symptoms was made (Hanley et al. 1977).

Melatonin. Melatonin (*N*-acetyl-5-methoxytryptamine) is a hormone derived from serotonin in the pineal gland. Secretion of melatonin is stimulated by darkness, and it is known to be involved in the regulation of the circadian rhythm (Brzezinski 1997). Melatonin is available as an over-the-counter dietary supplement. It has become popular among parents for treating sleep problems in their children with autism, and there is some evidence that it improves sleep latency in children with neurodevelopmental disabilities (Phillips and Appleton 2004).

St. John's wort. St. John's wort is an extract of the plant *Hypericum perforatum.* Although the exact mechanism of action is unknown, several substances in this plant are thought to have antidepressant activity. St. John's wort has been compared with selective serotonin reuptake inhibitors (SSRIs) and placebo in several trials of depression, and some of these studies suggest that it is effective in the treatment of mild to moderate depression (Charrois et al. 2007). There are no published trials regarding the use of St. John's wort in treating symptoms of autism.

S-adenosylmethionine. *S*-adenosylmethionine (SAM-e) is metabolically derived from the amino acid methionine. Acting primarily as a methyl donor, SAM-e is involved in many important biological reactions, including methylation of DNA, phospholipids, and synthesis of several neurotransmitters. SAM-e was shown to be as effective as tricyclic antidepressants in several controlled trials of depression, but a few studies showed equivocal results to placebo. No published studies of SAM-e in treatment of autistic disorder are available.

Naltrexone. Naltrexone is an opioid agonist that was hypothesized to work by lowering high β-endorphin levels as documented in several studies of subjects with autism (Bouvard et al. 1995; Cazzullo et al. 1999; Gillberg 1995; Weizman et al. 1984; Willemsen-Swinkels et al. 1996). Initial excitement about naltrexone was generated when several uncontrolled open-label studies found reduction in hyperactivity, self-injurious behavior, and stereotyped and compulsive behavior (Campbell et al. 1993; Herman et al. 1989; Panksepp and Lensing 1991), but subsequent randomized, double-blind, placebo-controlled trials found only marginal benefits over use of placebo (Cazzullo et al. 1999; Feldman et al. 1999; Kolmen et al. 1997; Willemsen-Swinkels et al. 1996).

Nonbiological Treatments

Auditory Integration Training

Auditory integration training is a therapy in which children are screened for sound sensitivities and then delivered a tailored program of auditory input that filters out the sound frequencies to which they are sensitive (American Academy of Pediatrics 1998). These sessions are delivered over several months and can be rather costly.

The American Academy of Pediatrics and the Cochrane Developmental, Psychosocial and Learning Problems Group have reviewed the literature on auditory integration training (American Academy of Pediatrics 1998; Sinha et al. 2004). None of the nine studies assessing this treatment are adequately blinded, and some studies did not assign treatment groups randomly. In three studies parents reported improvements on standardized checklists, but parents were aware of the therapy their child was receiving. Bettison's (1996) study assigned 80 children to receive either filtered or unfiltered music. Both groups showed significant improvements in IQ, suggesting that the act of listening to music itself may be a useful intervention in this population (Baranek 2002; Bettison 1996). The American Academy of Pediatrics and the Cochrane group both concluded that there is not enough evidence to recommend this therapy to families with autistic children at this time.

Sensory Integration Therapy

Classical sensory integration therapy and variations thereof involve exposing the child to a series of sensory-based experiences, such as swinging, joint compressions, brushing, holding, and squeezing. These experiences are designed to address the observed hypo- and hyperresponses to sensory stimuli seen in children with ASDs. These therapies are often used in conjunction with a holistic occupational therapy treatment plan.

Quite a few articles have been written about these therapies, but few well-designed clinical trials exist. Two small crossover studies have evaluated classical sensory integration therapy (Baranek 2002). Case-Smith and Bryan (1999) showed that young autistic boys in sensory integration therapy had improvements in play skills that were directly related to therapy but, only one had improvements in peer and adult social interactions. Linderman and Stewart (1999) showed that both children studied demonstrated gains in social interactions and improvements in other outcomes. Only one case report describes improvements in tantrums, activity level, and coordination in a young boy with autism, who was prescribed a "sensory diet" of joint compressions and brushing (Stagnitti et al. 1999). One controlled study comparing touch pressure with alternative treatment conditions suggested that this therapy may increase responsiveness to sound and social communication in children with ASDs (Edelson et al. 1999).

Massage Therapy

One randomized clinical trial assessed the effect of massage therapy on 3- to 6-year-old children with ASDs. The parents were trained by a massage therapist and were instructed to deliver massage for 15 minutes prior to bedtime. The control group children were read Dr. Seuss stories nightly. The intervention group had less stereotypic behaviors, improvement in on-task behaviors, improved social relatedness, and fewer sleep problems (Escalona et al. 2001). This is an area that warrants further scientific exploration.

Craniosacral Therapy

Craniosacral therapy is a form of therapeutic touch in which the therapist "senses waves of spinal fluid" and applies touch to manipulate these flows. There are no controlled studies evaluating this therapy. It may be that the massage or touch itself lends some benefits to child with autism, but this is yet to be explored in controlled studies.

Facilitated Communication

Facilitated communication is a method of providing assistance in communication to patients with severe deficits in motor skills or motor apraxia by a typewriter or other communication device. Given that motor skills deficits have been observed in autism, this method was proposed to be helpful in assisting with communication deficits in this population. A facilitator supports the autistic individual's hand to make it easier for him or her to choose the letters on the communication device. Several cleverly designed studies looked at the issue of facilitator influence on the subject's communication (Eberlin et al. 1993; Regal et al. 1994). These studies bring the whole concept of facilitated communication into question because it appears that autistic children were not able to answer questions presented to them correctly unless their facilitator knew the answer to the question.

Music Therapy

In music therapy, the therapist uses musical experiences to engage the child in a relationship-focused dyadic exchange (Gold et al. 2006). Listening to music is embedded in an interactive process and exchange with the therapist. Only case reports and preexperimental designs have evaluated this therapy in subjects with ASDs. Edgerton (1994) reported a case series of 11 children exposed to music therapy and found a continuous increase in communicative acts. Another qualitative article was written on how relationship patterns develop in autistic children exposed to music therapy (Schumacher and Calvet-Kruppa 1999). To date no studies with control groups or experimental designs have assessed the utility of this therapy.

Conclusions

The current state of the literature makes it premature to recommend use of most supplements in the treatment of autism. However, some of the clinical trial research has shown promising results and calls for well-designed, large-scale clinical trials to answer definitively questions about their therapeutic utility. It could be that some of these treatments are best used as an adjunct to standard therapies. Research in this field has significant methodological limitations. Future studies need to give careful attention to use of clear diagnostic criteria, adequate sample size, control groups, subject treatment status, and correlation with biochemical and physiologic measures.

References

AltMedDex. Thomson Micromedex. Available at: http://www.thomsonhc.com. Accessed April 22, 2007.

American Academy of Pediatrics: Auditory integration training and facilitated communication for autism. Committee on Children With Disabilities. Pediatrics 102 (part 1):431–433, 1998

American Academy of Pediatrics: Counseling families who choose complementary and alternative medicine for their child with chronic illness or disability. Committee on Children With Disabilities. Pediatrics 107:598–601, 2001

Amminger PG, Berger GE, Schafer MR, et al: Omega-3 fatty acids supplementation in children with autism: a double-blind, randomized, placebo-controlled pilot study. Biol Psychiatry 61:551–553, 2007

Andrews N, Miller E, Grant A, et al: Thimerosal exposure in infants and developmental disorders: a retrospective cohort study in the United Kingdom does not support a causal association. Pediatrics 114:584–591, 2004

Arnold GL, Hyman SL, Mooney RA, et al: Plasma amino acids profiles in children with autism: potential risk of nutritional deficiencies. J Autism Dev Disord 33:449–454, 2003

Arnold LE, Kleykamp D, Votolato NA, et al: Gamma-linolenic acid for attention-deficit hyperactivity disorder: placebo-controlled comparison to D-amphetamine. Biol Psychiatry 25:222–228, 1989

Baranek GT: Efficacy of sensory and motor interventions for children with autism. J Autism Dev Disord 32:397–422, 2002

Barthelemy C, Garreau B, Leddet I, et al: [Biological and clinical effects of oral magnesium and associated magnesium-vitamin B6 administration on certain disorders observed in infantile autism]. Therapie 35:627–632, 1980

Bell JG, MacKinlay EE, Dick JR, et al: Essential fatty acids and phospholipase A2 in autistic spectrum disorders. Prostaglandins Leukot Essent Fatty Acids 71:201–204, 2004

Bennett CN, Horrobin DF: Gene targets related to phospholipid and fatty acid metabolism in schizophrenia and other psychiatric disorders: an update. Prostaglandins Leukot Essent Fatty Acids 63:47–59, 2000

Bettison S: The long-term effects of auditory training on children with autism. J Autism Dev Disord 26:361–374, 1996

Black C, Kaye JA, Jick H: Relation of childhood gastrointestinal disorders to autism: nested case-control study using data from the UK General Practice Research Database. BMJ 325:419–421, 2002

Bolman WM, Richmond JA: A double-blind, placebo-controlled, crossover pilot trial of low dose dimethylglycine in patients with autistic disorder. J Autism Dev Disord 29:191–194, 1999

Bonisch E: [Experiences with pyrithioxin in brain-damaged children with autistic syndrome]. Prax Kinderpsychol Kinderpsychiatr 17:308–310, 1968

Bouvard MP, Leboyer M, Launay JM, et al: Low-dose naltrexone effects on plasma chemistries and clinical symptoms in autism: a double-blind, placebo-controlled study. Psychiatry Res 58:191–201, 1995

Brudnak MA, Rimland B, Kerry RE, et al: Enzyme-based therapy for autism spectrum disorders—is it worth another look? Med Hypotheses 58:422–428, 2002

Brzezinski A: Melatonin in humans. N Engl J Med 336:186–195, 1997

Bu B, Ashwood P, Harvey D, et al: Fatty acid composition of red blood cell phospholipids in children with autism. Prostaglandins Leukot Essent Fatty Acids 74:215–221, 2006

Cade R, Privette M, Fregley M: Autism and schizophrenia: intestinal disorders. Nutr Neurosci 3:57–72, 2000

Campbell M, Anderson LT, Small AM, et al: Naltrexone in autistic children: behavioral symptoms and attentional learning. J Am Acad Child Adolesc Psychiatry 32:1283–1291, 1993

Case-Smith J, Bryan T: The effects of occupational therapy with sensory integration emphasis on preschool-age children with autism. Am J Occup Ther 53:489–497, 1999

Cazzullo AG, Musetti MC, Musetti L: Beta-endorphin levels in peripheral blood mononuclear cells and long-term naltrexone treatment in autistic children. Eur Neuropsychopharmacol 9:361–366, 1999

Centers for Disease Control and Prevention: Deaths associated with hypocalcemia from chelation therapy—Texas, Pennsylvania, and Oregon, 2003–2005. MMWR Morb Mortal Wkly Rep 55(8):204–207, 2006

Charrois TL, Sadler C, Vohra S; American Academy of Pediatrics Provisional Section on Complementary, Holistic, and Integrative Medicine: Complementary, holistic, and integrative medicine: St John's wort. Pediatr Rev 28(2):69–72, 2007

Chez MG, Buchanan CP, Aimonovitch MC, et al: Double-blind, placebo-controlled study of L-carnosine supplementation in children with autistic spectrum disorders. J Child Neurol 17:833–837, 2002

Clandinin M, Jumpsen J: Fatty acids metabolism in relation to development, membrane structure and signaling, in Handbook of Essential Fatty Acid Biology: Biochemistry, Physiology, and Behavioral Neurobiology. Totowa, NJ, Human Press, 1997, pp 16–65

Comi AM, Zimmerman AW, Frye VH, et al: Familial clustering of autoimmune disorders and evaluation of medical risk factors in autism. J Child Neurol 14:388–394, 1999

Connolly AM, Chez MG, Pestronk A, et al: Serum autoantibodies to brain in Landau-Kleffner variant, autism, and other neurologic disorders. J Pediatr 134:607–613, 1999

Cremonini F, Di Caro S, Nista EC, et al: Meta-analysis: the effect of probiotic administration on antibiotic-associated diarrhoea. Aliment Pharmacol Ther 16:1461–1467, 2002

Croonenberghs J, Bosmans E, Deboutte D, et al: Activation of the inflammatory response system in autism. Neuropsychobiology 45:1–6, 2002

D'Eufemia P, Celli M, Finocchiaro R, et al: Abnormal intestinal permeability in children with autism. Acta Paediatr 85:1076–1079, 1996

De Groote MA, Frank DN, Dowell E, et al: Lactobacillus rhamnosus GG bacteremia associated with probiotic use in a child with short gut syndrome. Pediatr Infect Dis J 24:278–280, 2005

DelGiudice-Asch G, Simon L, Schmeidler J, et al: Brief report: a pilot open clinical trial of intravenous immunoglobulin in childhood autism. J Autism Dev Disord 29:157–160, 1999

Dimethylglycine (DMG), in AltMedDex System, Thomson Micromedex. Available at http://www.thomsonhc.com. Accessed September 10. 2006.

Docosahexaenoic acid (DHA), in AltMedDex System, Thomson Micromedex. Available at http://www.thomsonhc.com. Accessed June 6, 2007.

D'Souza AL, Rajkumar C, Cooke J, et al: Probiotics in prevention of antibiotic associated diarrhoea: meta-analysis. BMJ 324:1361, 2002

Eberlin M, McConnachie G, Ibel S: Facilitated communication: a failure to replicate the phenomenon. J Autism Dev Disord 23:507–530, 1993

Edelson S, Goldberg M, Edelson MG, et al: Behavioral and physiological effects of deep pressure on children with autism: a pilot study evaluating the efficacy of Grandin's hug machine. Am J Occup Ther 53:145–152, 1999

Edetate calcium disodium, in AltMedDex System, Thomson Micromedex. Available at http://www.thomsonhc.com. Accessed June 6, 2007.

Edgerton C: Effect of improvisational music therapy on the communicative behaviors of autistic children. J Music Ther 21:31–62, 1994

Elder J, Shankar M, Shuster J, et al: The glutein-free, casein-free diet in autism: results of a preliminary double-blind clinical trial. J Autism Devel Disord 36(3):413–420, 2006

Escalona A, Field T, Singer-Strunck R, et al: Brief report: improvements in the behavior of children with autism following massage therapy. J Autism Dev Disord 31:513–516, 2001

Feldman HM, Kolmen BK, Gonzaga AM: Naltrexone and communication skills in young children with autism. J Am Acad Child Adolesc Psychiatry 38:587–593, 1999

Findling RL, Maxwell K, Scotese-Wojtila L, et al: High-dose pyridoxine and magnesium administration in children with autistic disorder: an absence of salutary effects in a double-blind, placebo-controlled study. J Autism Dev Disord 27:467–478, 1997

Fiorica-Howells E, Maroteaux L, Gershon MD: Serotonin and the 5-HT(2B) receptor in the development of enteric neurons. J Neurosci 20:294–305, 2000

Geier MR, Geier DA: The potential importance of steroids in the treatment of autistic spectrum disorders and other disorders involving mercury toxicity. Med Hypotheses 64:946–954, 2005

Gillberg C: Endogenous opioids and opiate antagonists in autism: brief review of empirical findings and implications for clinicians. Dev Med Child Neurol 37:239–245, 1995

Glutathione, in AltMedDex System, Thomson Micromedex. Available at http://www.thomsonhc.com. Accessed September 12, 2006.

Gold C, Wigram T, Elefant C: Music therapy for autistic spectrum disorder. Cochrane Database of Systematic Reviews 2006, Issue 2. Art. No.: CD004381. DOI: 10.1002/14651858.CD004381.pub2

Gupta S, Aggarwal S, Heads C: Dysregulated immune system in children with autism: beneficial effects of intravenous immune globulin on autistic characteristics. J Autism Dev Disord 26:439–452, 1996

Gupta S, Aggarwal S, Rashanravan B, et al: Th1- and Th2-like cytokines in CD4+ and CD8+ T cells in autism. J Neuroimmunol 85:106–109, 1998

Hanley HG, Stahl SM, Freedman DX: Hyperserotonemia and amine metabolites in autistic and retarded children. Arch Gen Psychiatry 34:521–531, 1977

Hediger ML England L, Molloy CA, et al: Reduced cortical thickness in boys with autism or autistic spectrum disorders. Paper presented at the Pediatric Academic Societies Meeting, Washington, DC, 2005

Herman BH, Hammock MK, Arthur-Smith A, et al: Effects of acute administration of naltrexone on cardiovascular function, body temperature, body weight and serum concentrations of liver enzymes in autistic children. Dev Pharmacol Ther 12:118–127, 1989

Hollander E, Novotny S, Hanratty M, et al: Oxytocin infusion reduces repetitive behaviors in adults with autistic and Asperger's disorders. Neuropsychopharmacology 28:193–198, 2003

Hornig M, Chian D, Lipkin WI: Neurotoxic effects of postnatal thimerosal are mouse strain dependent. Mol Psychiatry 9:833–845, 2004

Horrobin DF: The membrane phospholipid hypothesis as a biochemical basis for the neurodevelopmental concept of schizophrenia. Schizophr Res 30:193–208, 1998

Horrobin DF, Bennett CN: Depression and bipolar disorder: relationships to impaired fatty acid and phospholipid metabolism and to diabetes, cardiovascular disease, immunological abnormalities, cancer, ageing and osteoporosis. Possible candidate genes. Prostaglandins Leukot Essent Fatty Acids 60:217–234, 1999

Horrobin DF, Glen AI, Vaddadi K: The membrane hypothesis of schizophrenia. Schizophr Res 13:195–207, 1994

Horvath K, Perman JA: Autism and gastrointestinal symptoms. Curr Gastroenterol Rep 4:251–258, 2002

Horvath K, Stefanatos G, Sokolski KN, et al: Improved social and language skills after secretin administration in patients with autistic spectrum disorders. J Assoc Acad Minor Phys 9:9–15, 1998

Horvath K, Papadimitriou JC, Rabsztyn A, et al: Gastrointestinal abnormalities in children with autistic disorder. J Pediatr 135:559–563, 1999

Hviid A, Stellfeld M, Wohlfahrt J, et al: Association between thimerosal-containing vaccine and autism. JAMA 290:1763–1766, 2003

IVIG, in AltMedDex System, Thomson Micromedex. Available at http://www.thomsonhc.com. Accessed September 10, 2006.

Jackson MJ, Garrod PJ: Plasma zinc, copper, and amino acid levels in the blood of autistic children. J Autism Child Schizophr 8:203–208, 1978

James SJ, Cutler P, Melnyk S, et al: Metabolic biomarkers of increased oxidative stress and impaired methylation capacity in children with autism. Am J Clin Nutr 80:1611–1617, 2004

Jonas C, Etienne T, Barthelemy C, J et al: [Clinical and biochemical value of magnesium + vitamin B6 combination in the treatment of residual autism in adults]. Therapie 39:661–669, 1984

Jyonouchi H, Sun S, Le H: Proinflammatory and regulatory cytokine production associated with innate and adaptive immune responses in children with autism spectrum disorders and developmental regression. J Neuroimmunol 120:170–179, 2001

Kalliomaki M, Salminen S, Arvilommi H, et al: Probiotics in primary prevention of atopic disease: a randomised placebo-controlled trial. Lancet 357:1076–1079, 2001

Kane V, Linn V: Boy dies during autism treatment. Post Gazette, 2005

Kern JK, Miller VS, Cauller PL, et al: Effectiveness of N,N-dimethylglycine in autism and pervasive developmental disorder. J Child Neurol 16:169–173, 2001

Knivsberg A-M, Reichelt KL, Høien T, et al: Randomised, controlled study of dietary intervention in autistic syndromes. Nutr Neurosci 5:251–261, 2002

Kolmen BK, Feldman HM, Handen BL, et al: Naltrexone in young autistic children: replication study and learning measures. J Am Acad Child Adolesc Psychiatry 36:1570–1578, 1997

Kunz AN, Noel JM, Fairchok MP: Two cases of Lactobacillus bacteremia during probiotic treatment of short gut syndrome. J Pediatr Gastroenterol Nutr 38:457–458, 2004

Levy SE, Hyman SL: Use of complementary and alternative treatments for children with autistic spectrum disorders is increasing. Pediatr Ann 32:685–691, 2003

Levy SE, Hyman SL: Novel treatments for autistic spectrum disorders. Ment Retard Dev Disabil Res Rev 11:131–142, 2005

Levy SE, Mandell DS, Merhar S, et al: Use of complementary and alternative medicine among children recently diagnosed with autistic spectrum disorder. J Dev Behav Pediatr 24:418–423, 2003

Linderman TM, Stewart KB: Sensory integrative-based occupational therapy and functional outcomes in young children with pervasive developmental disorders: a single-subject study. Am J Occup Ther 53:207–213, 1999

Lucarelli S, Frediani T, Zingoni AM, et al: Food allergy and infantile autism. Panminerva Med 37:137–141, 1995

Madsen KM, Lauritsen MB, Pedersen CB, et al: Thimerosal and the occurrence of autism: negative ecological evidence from Danish population-based data. Pediatrics 112 (part 1):604–606, 2003

Martineau J, Barthelemy C, Garreau B, et al: Vitamin B6, magnesium, and combined B6-Mg: therapeutic effects in childhood autism. Biol Psychiatry 20:467–478, 1985

McDougle CJ, Naylor ST, Goodman WK, et al: Acute tryptophan depletion in autistic disorder: a controlled case study. Biol Psychiatry 33:547–550, 1993

Molloy CA, Manning-Courtney P: Prevalence of chronic gastrointestinal symptoms in children with autism and autistic spectrum disorders. Autism 7:165–171, 2003

Mulder EJ, Anderson GM, Kema IP, et al: Platelet serotonin levels in pervasive developmental disorders and mental retardation: diagnostic group differences, within-group distribution, and behavioral correlates. J Am Acad Child Adolesc Psychiatry 43:491–499, 2004

Nemets B, Stahl Z, Belmaker RH: Addition of omega-3 fatty acid to maintenance medication treatment for recurrent unipolar depressive disorder. Am J Psychiatry 159:477–479, 2002

Nickel R: Controversial therapies for young children with developmental disabilities. Infants Young Child 8:29–40, 1996

Nye C, Brice A: Combined vitamin B6-magnesium treatment in autism spectrum disorder. Cochrane Database of Systematic Reviews 2005, Issue 4. Art. No.: CD003497. DOI: 10.1002/14651858.CD003497.pub2

Pangborn J: Biomedical assessment options for children with autism and related problems. A consensus report of the Defeat Autism Now! (DAN!) Scientific Effort. Paper presented at the Defeat Autism Now! Conference, San Diego, CA, 2002

Panksepp J, Lensing P: Brief report: a synopsis of an open-trial of naltrexone treatment of autism with four children. J Autism Dev Disord 21:243–249, 1991

Peet M, Horrobin DF: A dose-ranging study of the effects of ethyl-eicosapentaenoate in patients with ongoing depression despite apparently adequate treatment with standard drugs. Arch Gen Psychiatry 59:913–919, 2002

Peet M, Brind J, Ramchand CN, et al: Two double-blind placebo-controlled pilot studies of eicosapentaenoic acid in the treatment of schizophrenia. Schizophr Res 49:243–251, 2001

Phillips L, Appleton RE: Systematic review of melatonin treatment in children with neurodevelopmental disabilities and sleep impairment. Dev Med Child Neurol 46:771–775, 2004

Plioplys AV: Intravenous immunoglobulin treatment of children with autism. J Child Neurol 13:79–82, 1998

Polleux F, Lauder JM: Toward a developmental neurobiology of autism. Ment Retard Dev Disabil Res Rev 10:303–317, 2004

Posey DJ, Kem DL, Swiezy NB, et al: A pilot study of D-cycloserine in subjects with autistic disorder. Am J Psychiatry 161:2115–2117, 2004

Probiotics, in AltMedDex System, Thomson Micromedex. Available at http://www.thomsonhc.com. Accessed June 12, 2007.

Puri BK, Richardson AJ: Sustained remission of positive and negative symptoms of schizophrenia following treatment with eicosapentaenoic acid. Arch Gen Psychiatry 55:188–189, 1998

Puri BK, Counsell SJ, Richardson AJ, et al: Eicosapentaenoic acid in treatment-resistant depression. Arch Gen Psychiatry 59:91–92, 2002

Regal RA, Rooney JR, Wandas T: Facilitated communication: an experimental evaluation. J Autism Dev Disord 24:345–355, 1994

Reichelt K, Knivesberg AM, Lind G, et al: Probable etiology and possible treatment of childhood autism. Brain Dysfunction 4:308–319, 1991

Richardson AJ, Montgomery P: The Oxford-Durham study: a randomized, controlled trial of dietary supplementation with fatty acids in children with developmental coordination disorder. Pediatrics 115:1360–1366, 2005

Rimland B, Callaway E, Dreyfus P: The effect of high doses of vitamin B6 on autistic children: a double-blind crossover study. Am J Psychiatry 135:472–475, 1978

Ritvo ER, Yuwiler A, Geller E, et al: Increased blood serotonin and platelets in early infantile autism. Arch Gen Psychiatry 23:566–572, 1970

Sandler A: Placebo effects in developmental disabilities: implications for research and practice. Ment Retard Dev Disabil Res Rev 11:164–170, 2005

Sandler RH, Finegold SM, Bolte ER, et al: Short-term benefit from oral vancomycin treatment of regressive-onset autism. J Child Neurol 15:429–435, 2000

Schumacher K, Calvet-Kruppa C: The AQR-analysis system to evaluate the quality of relationship during music therapy. Nordic Journal of Music Therapy 8:1888–1191, 1999

Secretin, in AltMedDex System, Thomson Micromedex. Available at http://www.thomsonhc.com. Accessed September 5, 2006.

Shattock P, Kennedy A, Rowell F, et al: The role of neuropeptides in autism and their relationship to classical neurotransmitters. Brain Dysfunction 3:328–345, 1990

Sinha Y, Silove N, Wheeler D, et al: Auditory integration training and other sound therapies for autism spectrum disorders. Cochrane Database of Systematic Reviews 2004, Issue 1. Art. No.: CD003681. DOI: 10.1002/14651858.CD003681.pub2

Smith MD, Haas PJ, Belcher RG: Facilitated communication: the effects of facilitator knowledge and level of assistance on output. J Autism Dev Disord 24:357–367, 1994

Spivak B, Golubchik P, Mozes T, et al: Low platelet-poor plasma levels of serotonin in adult autistic patients. Neuropsychobiology 50:157–160, 2004

Stagnitti K, Raison P, Ryan P: Sensory defensiveness syndrome: a pediatrics perspective and case study. Australian Occupational Therapy Journal 46:175–187, 1999

Stevens L, Zhang W, Peck L, et al: EFA supplementation in children with inattention, hyperactivity, and other disruptive behaviors. Lipids 38:1007–1021, 2003

Succimer, in AltMedDex System, Thomson Micromedex. Available at http://www.thomsonhc.com. Accessed June 6, 2007.

Sweeten TL, Bowyer SL, Posey DJ, et al: Increased prevalence of familial autoimmunity in probands with pervasive developmental disorders. Pediatrics 112:e420, 2003

Szajewska H, Mrukowicz JZ: Probiotics in the treatment and prevention of acute infectious diarrhea in infants and children: a systematic review of published randomized, double-blind, placebo-controlled trials. J Pediatr Gastroenterol Nutr 33 (suppl 2):S17–S25, 2001

Tolbert L, Haigler T, Waits MM, et al: Brief report: lack of response in an autistic population to a low dose clinical trial of pyridoxine plus magnesium. J Autism Dev Disord 23:193–199, 1993

Vancassel S, Durand G, Barthelemy C, et al: Plasma fatty acid levels in autistic children. Prostaglandins Leukot Essent Fatty Acids 65:1–7, 2001

Van Niel CW, Feudtner C, Garrison MM, et al: Lactobacillus therapy for acute infectious diarrhea in children: a meta-analysis. Pediatrics 109:678–684, 2002

Voigt RG, Llorente AM, Jensen CL, et al: A randomized, double-blind, placebo-controlled trial of docosahexaenoic acid supplementation in children with attention-deficit/hyperactivity disorder. J Pediatr 139:189–196, 2001

Wakefield AJ, Murch SH, Anthony A, et al: Ileal-lymphoid-nodular hyperplasia, non-specific colitis, and pervasive developmental disorder in children. Lancet 351:637–641, 1998

Weizman R, Weizman A, Tyano S, et al: Humoral-endorphin blood levels in autistic, schizophrenic and healthy subjects. Psychopharmacology (Berl) 82:368–370, 1984

Willemsen-Swinkels SH, Buitelaar JK, Weijnen FG, et al: Plasma beta-endorphin concentrations in people with learning disability and self-injurious and/or autistic behaviour. Br J Psychiatry 168:105–109, 1996

Williams KW, Wray JJ, Wheeler DM: Intravenous secretin for autism spectrum disorder. Cochrane Database of Systematic Reviews 2005, Issue 3. Art. No.: CD003495. DOI: 10.1002/14651858.CD003495.pub2

Ziemlanski S, Wielgus-Serafinsak E, Panczenko-Kresowska B, et al: Effect of long-term diet enrichment with selenium, vitamin E and vitamin B15 on the degree of fatty infiltration of the liver. Acta Physiol Pol 35(4):382–397, 1984

Promising New Avenues of Treatment and Future Directions for Patients With Autism

Evdokia Anagnostou, M.D.

Geoffrey Collins, B.A.

Eric Hollander, M.D.

Although there is a plethora of treatment options available for individuals with autism, many of these options are lacking scientific data, and families find themselves overwhelmed with the responsibility of choosing the appropriate treatments for their child. The scientific community needs to provide controlled data for efficacy or nonefficacy of available treatments, as well as in identifying predictors of response to specific treatments. There is also an urgency to identify distinct endophenotypes (based on genetics, neurobiology, or response to treatment) that may be associated with characteristic and/or unique response to various interventions.

Preparation of this chapter supported with funding from STAART Autism Center of Excellence Grant 5 U54 MH06673–02 and the Seaver Foundation.

Pharmacological Treatments

Psychopharmacological agents such as mood-stabilizing antiepileptic drugs, antidepressants, atypical neuroleptics, stimulants, and anticholinergic agents have been used to treat specific symptoms of autism. Double-blind, placebo-controlled trials are emerging supporting the use of neuroleptics and antidepressants, but further work is needed to confirm safety and efficacy of these medications. Future research needs to explore new chemical systems to address issues related to cognition and social and language deficits in autism. Glutamate and oxytocin seem promising in this regard.

Glutamatergic Drugs in the Treatment of Autism

Several studies have demonstrated activation of the glutamatergic system in persons with autism, which could play a role in brain maturation alterations in autism. Patients with autism or Asperger's disorder have been found to have raised levels of glutamate in plasma compared with healthy control subjects in multiple studies (Aldred et al. 2003; Moreno-Fuenmayor et al. 1996; Rolf et al. 1993). Glutamic acid decarboxylase protein, the enzyme responsible for normal conversion of glutamate to γ-aminobutyric acid in the brain, has been noted to be reduced in the brain of autistic subjects in postmortem studies, suggesting increased levels of glutamate or transporter receptor density in autistic brains (Fatemi 2002). In addition, further postmortem studies have revealed decreased α-amino-3-hydroxy-5-methyl-4-isoxazolepropionic acid (AMPA)–type glutamate receptor density in the cerebellum of autistic individuals. In the same study, the messenger RNA levels of several genes involved in the glutamatergic pathways were significantly increased in autistic subjects, including the excitatory amino acid transporter 1 and the glutamate receptor $AMPA_1$ (Purcell et al. 2001). Genetic studies have so far revealed a mutation in the glutamate receptor gene *GRIK2* in 6q21 that is present in 8% of autistic subjects and 4% of control subjects and seems to be transmitted from mothers to autistic males (Phillipe et al. 1999). Furthermore, evidence for the presence of a susceptibility mutation in linkage disequilibrium with variants in the metabotropic glutamate receptor 8 gene was recently found on chromosome 7 (Serajee et al. 2003). In the one published study of magnetic resonance spectroscopy in autism (Friedman et al. 2003), no differences were found in the Glx (glutamate + glutamine) peak (used to estimate glutamate concentrations) among 3- to 4-

year-old children with autism, children with developmental delay, and healthy volunteers. However, recent work by Murphy and colleagues (D. Murphy, personal communication, 2006) in older autistic subjects (adolescents and young adults) did demonstrate increased brain glutamate concentrations estimated by the Glx peak. Lastly, in pediatric obsessive-compulsive disorder, there is evidence of increased glutamate in the caudate (Rosenberg et al. 2000). Decrease in glutamate concentration in this region was noted upon successful treatment.

Amantadine

Amantadine was shown to have N-methyl-D-aspartate (NMDA) noncompetitive inhibitor activity at doses routinely used for influenza and Parkinson's disease (Kornhuber et al. 1994) without having any psychomimetic side effects. On the basis of this finding, a double-blind, placebo-controlled trial of amantadine was carried out in autistic children. Although amantadine was tolerated, it was noted to have, at best, modest effect on irritability and hyperactivity. However, amantadine has very low affinity for the NMDA receptor, therefore 10- to 20-fold higher doses than that used for memantine may need to be used (Kornhuber et al. 1994).

D-Cycloserine

D-Cycloserine is a partial agonist of the NMDA receptor in lower doses and becomes an antagonist of the same receptor at higher doses (U response); it has different affinities for different NMDA receptor subtypes and therefore may exert some of its effects through NMDA antagonism. A double-blind, placebo-controlled trial of this medication in autistic children resulted in significant improvement on the Clinical Global Impression Scale (Guy 1976) and Social Withdrawal subscale of the Aberrant Behavior Checklist (Aman et al. 1985), and it was tolerated at most of the doses used (Posey et al. 2004).

Dextromethorphan

Dextromethorphan is an NMDA receptor antagonist. In a series of children with autism reported in case studies and single-subject design studies, it has been reported to improve problem behaviors such as tantrums and self-injurious behavior, as well as anxiety, motor planning, socialization, and language (Welch and Sovner 1992; Woodard et al. 2005).

Memantine

Memantine is a noncompetitive NMDA inhibitor. It has, however, moderate affinity for the receptor, with strong voltage dependency and rapid blocking/ unblocking properties (Mobius 2003). Memantine has recently been approved by the U.S. Food and Drug Administration for the treatment of memory loss in moderate to severe Alzheimer's disease based on three randomized, placebo-controlled trials that showed significant improvements in cognitive, functional, and global endpoints in this population (Farlow 2004; Reisberg et al. 2003; Winblad and Poritis 1999). Similar results were seen in two trials in vascular dementia (Wilcock et al. 2002; Orgogozo et al. 2002). Memantine has been used in Germany for a variety of neurological syndromes and cognitive deficits since 1982, with good tolerability. In animal models, memantine has been shown to prolong the duration of long-term potentiation in vivo and to improve learning and memory (Barnes et al. 1996; Zajaczkowski et al. 1996). Neuroprotection has been demonstrated in animals (Danysz et al. 2000), but the clinical data are still pending.

Chez et al. (2004) reported on 30 children and adolescents with autism spectrum disorders treated with memantine for 8–40 months at a mean dosage of 8.1 mg/day. Sixteen subjects showed significant improvements, and 10 showed mild improvements. These improvements were noted in the areas of language, attention, motor planning, and self-stimulation. No side effects were reported at the doses used. This cohort now includes approximately 400 children with ASD and the clinical observations remain the same (M.G. Chez, personal communication, 2005). Well-controlled randomized trials are needed to clarify further any potential improvements in cognition, core, and associated symptoms of autism.

Oxytocin and Autism

Oxytocin and the related peptide vasopressin are synthesized in the magnocellular neurons of the paraventricular and supraoptic nuclei of the hypothalamus and are released into the circulation via axon terminals in the neurohypophysis. They are structurally similar, comprising nine amino acids and differing only in two. Neurons from the paraventricular nucleus project to various sites within the brain and brainstem (Sofroniew and Weindl 1981) and receptors for both peptides are found throughout the limbic system and brainstem autonomic centers (Barberis and Tribollet 1996).

Accumulating evidence points to a possible association of the social deficits as well as the repetitive behaviors seen in autism with oxytocin. Oxytocin has been reported to facilitate social memory (Popik et al. 1992), and oxytocin knockout mice show deficits in social memory (Winslow and Insel 2002). Oxytocin also appears to be implicated in maternal and psychosexual behaviors in rats and sheep (Insel 1990; Witt et al. 1992) and in prairie voles (Insel and Hulihan 1995), suggesting it is important in social attachment. The related peptide vasopressin has also been implicated in facilitation of social memory, especially in male rats, and seems to be androgen dependent (Bluthe et al. 1990). Brattleboro rats with an inability to make vasopressin due to a point mutation leading to a frame shift in the vasopressin gene were found to have decreased social memory, in addition to diabetes insipidus and other cognitive deficits (de Wied et al. 1988). Vasopressin has also been implicated in paternal behavior (Wang et al. 1993) and appears to facilitate aggression consistent with nest defense (Ferris 1992; Winslow et al. 1993). Its effect on maternal behavior is weaker than oxytocin, and it may have an opposite effect than oxytocin in the case of female sociosexual behaviors (Pedersen et al. 1982; Sodersten et al. 1983). In the case of stereotypy, intracranioventricular administration of both peptides has been shown to increase repetitive behaviors, such as grooming, stretching, startle, and squeaking responses in mice (Meisenberg and Simmons 1983); repetitive grooming in rats (Drago et al. 1986; van Wimersma Greidanus et al. 1990); and wing flapping in chicks (Panksepp 1992). However, treatment of children with obsessive-compulsive disorder with clomipramine increased oxytocin levels and decreased stereotypies (Altemus et al. 1994). Intravenous administration of oxytocin was attempted; decrease of repetitive behaviors compared with placebo was observed in adults with autism (Hollander et al. 2003). Other studies in autistic children have revealed decreased blood levels of oxytocin and a failure to show the normal developmental increase in levels with age (Green et al. 2001; Modahl et al. 1998). There is some evidence that oxytocin peptide processing may partially explain this reduction. Although there is little relationship between blood and cerebrospinal fluid oxytocin levels, abnormalities in gene structure or expression are likely in both cases (Insel et al. 1999). Deficits in either peptide system may not so far explain adequately all deficits in autism; still, the available preclinical data suggest that these pathways are reasonable candidates of abnormalities in this population.

In summary, there is enough evidence suggesting possible glutamate and/or oxytocin abnormalities in subjects with autism. Further intervention studies targeting these systems may be of great value.

Other Approaches

Secretin, gluten-/casein-free diets, and chelation therapy are some of the many alternative treatments whose efficacy has not been established despite widespread use (see Chapter 12, "Complementary and Alternative Therapies for Autism," in this book). Given the potential for toxicity and the fact that they often replace efficacious treatments, such approaches need to be rigorously evaluated. Lastly, studies targeting associated symptoms such as sleep disturbance and possible dysfunction in other systems (i.e., immune and gastrointestinal systems) are also needed.

Educational and Psychosocial Interventions

Great progress has been made in generating several ideas and models of psychosocial and educational interventions. We already know that intensive early intervention is effective (Schreibman 2000), although there is a lot of heterogeneity in outcome. Future studies need to focus on

- Developing individualized programs to meet specific needs in specific children.
- Identifying the important variables in each program that are responsible for the treatment effect.
- Identifying appropriate intensity of treatment.
- Identifying prognostic factors specific to treatments.
- Developing interventions for older individuals.

Advocacy

Advocacy groups have been vital in increasing federal funding for research in autism. Some of these organizations have also developed their own funding mechanisms. However, a lot of work remains to be done.

There is a multitude of such groups, and there is a need either to combine them into larger, more efficient units or to develop networks with common visions and approaches to autism research. There is also a need to fund underserved areas of research, such as translational research, research in transitional care, vocational training, and independent living. The urgency is also there to fund only quality research, which often is not easy because the most interesting questions to parents may not be answered rigorously with the funding provided by such organizations. Lastly, parent/advocacy organizations can help to assure that the data collected in research studies do translate into improvement in services that children and adults with autism receive.

Continuous lobbying for increased funding will continue to be a primary responsibility of these advocacy organizations.

References

Aldred S, Moore KM, Fitzgerald M, et al: Plasma amino acid levels in children with autism and their families. J Autism Dev Disorder 33: 93–97, 2003

Altemus M, Pigott T, Kalogeras K, et al: Abnormalities in the regulation of vasopressin and corticotropin releasing factor secretion in obsessive compulsive disorder. Arch Gen Psychiatry 49:9–20, 1994

Aman MG, Singh NN, Stewart AW, et al: The Aberrant Behavior Checklist: a behavior rating scale for the assessment of treatment effects. Am J Ment Defic 89:485–491, 1985

Barberis C, Tribollet E: Vasopressin and oxytocin receptors in the central nervous system. Crit Rev Neurobiol 10:119–154, 1996

Barnes CA, Danysz W, Parsons CG: Effects of the uncompetitive NMDA receptor antagonist memantine on hippocampal long-term potentiation, short-term exploratory modulation and spatial memory in awake, freely moving rats. Eur J Neurosci 8:565–571, 1996

Bluthe RM, Schoenen J, Dantzer R: Androgen dependent vasopressinergic neurons are involved in social recognition in rats. Brain Res 519:150–157, 1990

Chez MG, Hung PC, Chin K: Memantine experience in children and adolescents with autism spectrum disorders (abstract). Ann Neurol 56(8, suppl):109, 2004

Danysz W, Parsons CG, Quack G: NMDA channel blockers: memantine and aminoalkylcyclohexanes—in vivo characterization. Amino Acids 19:167–172, 2000

de Wied D, Joels M, Burbach JPH: Vasopressin effects on the central nervous system, in Peptide Hormones: Effects of Mechanism of Action. Edited by Conn PM, Negro Villar A. Boca Raton, FL, CRC Press, 1988, pp 97–140

Drago F, Pedersen C, Caldwell J, et al: Oxytocin potently enhances novelty induced grooming behavior in the rat. Brain Res 368:287–295, 1986

Farlow MR: NMDA receptor antagonists: a new therapeutic approach for Alzheimer's disease. Geriatrics 59:22–27, 2004

Fatemi SH: The role of Reelin in pathology of autism. Mol Psychiatry 7:919–920, 2002

Ferris C: Role of vasopressin in aggressive and dominant/subordinate behaviors. Ann NY Acad Sci 652:212–226, 1992

Friedman SD, Shaw DW, Artru AA, et al: Regional brain chemical alterations in young children with autism spectrum disorder. Neurology 60:100–107, 2003

Green L, Fein D, Modahl C, et al: Oxytocin and autistic disorder: alterations in peptide forms. Biol Psychiatry 50:609–613, 2001

Guy W: ECDEU assessment manual for psychopharmacology (NIMH Publ No 76–338). Rockville, MD, National Institute of Mental Health, 1976

Hollander E, Novotny S, Hanratty M: Oxytocin infusion reduces repetitive behaviors in adults with autistic and Asperger's disorders. Neuropsychopharmacology 28:193–198, 2003

Insel TR: Oxytocin and maternal behavior, in Mammalian Parenting: Biochemical, Neurobiological and Behavioral Determinants. Edited by Krasnegor N, Bridges R. New York, Oxford University Press, 1990, pp 260–280

Insel TR, Hulihan TJ: A gender specific mechanism for pair bonding: oxytocin and partner preference formation in monogamous voles. Behav Neurosci 109:782–789, 1995

Insel TR, O'Brien D, Beckman J: Oxytocin, vasopressin and autism: is there a connection? Biol Psychiatry 45:145–157, 1999

Kornhuber J, Weller M, Schoppmeyer K, et al: Amantadine and memantine are NMDA receptor antagonists with neuroprotective properties. J Neural Transm Suppl 43:91–104, 1994

Meisenberg G, Simmons W: Centrally mediated effects of neurohypophyseal hormones. Neurosci Biobehav Rev 7:263–280, 1983

Mobius HJ: Memantine: update on the current evidence. Int J Geriatr Psychiatry 18 (suppl 1):S47–S54, 2003

Modahl C, Green L, Fein D, et al: Plasma oxytocin levels in autistic children. Biol Psychiatry 43:270–277, 1998

Moreno-Fuenmayor H, Borjas L, Arrieta A, et al: Plasma excitatory amino acids in autism. Invest Clín 37:113–128, 1996

Orgogozo JM, Rigaud AS, Stoffler A, et al: Efficacy and safety of memantine in patients with mild to moderate vascular dementia: a randomized, placebo-controlled trial (MMM 300). Stroke 33:1834–1839, 2002

Panksepp J: Oxytocin effects on emotional processes: separation distress, social bonding and relationships to psychiatric disorders, in Oxytocin in Maternal Sexual and Social Processes, Vol 652. Edited by Pedersen C, Caldwell J, Jirikowski G, et al. New York, New York Academy of Sciences, 1992, pp 243–252

Pedersen C, Ascher J, Monroe Y, et al: Oxytocin induces maternal behavior in virgin female rats. Science 216:648–649, 1982

Phillipe A, Martinez M, Guilloud-Bataille M, et al: Genome-wide scan for autism susceptibility genes. Paris Autism Research International Sibpair Study. Hum Mol Genet 8:805–812, 1999

Popik P, Vos P, van Ree J: Neurohypophyseal hormone receptors in the septum are implicated in social recognition in the rat. Behav Pharmacol 3:351–358, 1992

Posey DJ, Kem DL, Swiezy NB, et al: A pilot study of D-cycloserine in subjects with autistic disorder. Am J Psychiatry 161:2115–2117, 2004

Purcell AE, Jeon OH, Zimmerman AW, et al: Postmortem brain abnormalities of the glutamate neurotransmitter system in autism. Neurology 57:1618–1628, 2001

Reisberg B, Doody R, Stoffler A, et al: Memantine in moderate-to-severe Alzheimer's disease. N Engl J Med 348:1333–1341, 2003

Rolf LH, Haarmann FY, Grotemeyer KH, et al: Serotonin and amino acid content in platelets of autistic children. Acta Psychiatr Scand 87:312–316, 1982

Rolf LH, Haarmann FY, Grotemeyer KH, et al: Serotonin and amino acid content in platelets of autistic children. Acta Psychiatr Scand 87(5):312–316, 1993

Rosenberg DR, MacMaster FP, Keshavan MS, et al: Decrease in caudate glutamatergic concentrations in pediatric obsessive-compulsive disorder patients taking paroxetine. J Am Acad Child Adolesc Psychiatry 39:1096–1103, 2000

Schreibman L: Intensive behavioral/psychoeducational treatments for autism: research needs and future directions. J Autism Dev Disord 30:373–378, 2000

Serajee FJ, Zhong H, Nabi R, et al: The metabotropic glutamate receptor 8 gene at 7q31: partial duplication and possible association with autism. J Med Genet 40:e42, 2003

Sodersten P, Henning M, Melin P, et al: Vasopressin alters female sexual behavior by acting on the brain independently of alterations in blood pressure. Nature 301:608–610, 1983

Sofroniew M, Weindl A: Central nervous system distribution of vasopressin, oxytocin, and neurophysin, in Endogenous Peptides and Learning and Memory Processes. Edited by Martinez J, Jensen R, Mesing R, et al. New York, Academic Press, 1981, pp 327–369

van Wimersma Greidanus T, Kroodsma J, Pot M, et al: Neurohypophyseal hormones and excessive grooming behavior. Eur J Pharmacol 187:1–8, 1990

Wang Z, Ferris CF, De Vries G: The role of septal vasopressin innervation in paternal behavior in prairie voles (Microtus ochrogaster). Proc Natl Acad Sci U S A 91:400–404, 1993

Welch L, Sovner R: Treatment of a chronic organic mental disorder with dextromethorphan in a man with severe mental retardation. Br J Psychiatry 161:118–120, 1992

Wilcock G, Mobius HJ, Stoffler A: A double-blind, placebo-controlled multicenter study of memantine in mild to moderate vascular dementia. Int Clin Psychopharmacol 17:297–305, 2002

Winblad B, Poritis N: Memantine in severe dementia: results of the 9M-Best Study (Benefit and efficacy in severely demented patients during treatment with memantine). Int J Geriatr Psychiatry 14:135–146, 1999

Winslow J, Insel T: The social deficits of the oxytocin knockout mouse. Neuropeptides 36:221–229, 2002

Winslow J, Hastings N, Carter C, et al: A role for central vasopressin in pair bonding in monogamous prairie voles. Nature 365:545–548, 1993

Witt D, Winslow J, Insel T: Enhanced social interactions in rats following chronic centrally infused oxytocin. Pharmacol Biochem Behav 43:855–861, 1992

Woodard C, Groden J, Goodwin M, et al: The treatment of the behavioral sequelae of autism with dextromethorphan: a case report. J Autism Dev Disord 35:515–518, 2005

Zajaczkowski W, Quack G, Danysz W: Infusion of (+) -MK-801 and memantine—contrasting effects on radial maze learning in rats with endorhinal cortex lesion. Eur J Pharmacol 296:239–246, 1996

Index

*Page numbers printed in **boldface** type refer to tables or figures.*